T0195196

Robotic Urology: The Next Frontier

Editors

JIM C. HU

JONATHAN E. SHOAG

UROLOGIC CLINICS
OF NORTH AMERICA

www.urologic.theclinics.com

Editor-in-Chief
KEVIN R. LOUGHLIN

February 2021 • Volume 48 • Number 1

ELSEVIER

1600 John F. Kennedy Boulevard • Suite 1800 • Philadelphia, Pennsylvania, 19103-2899

http://www.theclinics.com

UROLOGIC CLINICS OF NORTH AMERICA Volume 48, Number 1
February 2021 ISSN 0094-0143, ISBN-13: 978-0-323-77783-4

Editor: Kerry Holland
Developmental Editor: Julia McKenzie

Urologic Clinics of North America (ISSN 0094-0143) is published quarterly by Elsevier Inc., 360 Park Avenue South, New York, NY 10010-1710. Months of issue are February, May, August, and November. Business and Editorial Offices: 1600 John F. Kennedy Blvd., Suite 1800, Philadelphia, PA 19103-2899. Periodicals postage paid at New York, NY and additional mailing offices. Subscription prices are $395.00 per year (US individuals), $1033.00 per year (US institutions), $100.00 per year (US students and residents), $450.00 per year (Canadian individuals), $1059.00 per year (Canadian institutions), $100.00 per year (Canadian students/residents), $520.00 per year (foreign individuals), $1059.00 per year (foreign institutions), and $240.00 per year (foreign students/residents). Foreign air speed delivery is included in all *Clinics* subscription prices. All prices are subject to change without notice. **POSTMASTER:** Send address changes to *Urologic Clinics of North America*, Elsevier Health Sciences Division, Subscription Customer Service, 3251 Riverport Lane, Maryland Heights, MO 63043. **Customer Service: 1-800-654-2452 (US). From outside the United States, call 1-314-447-8871. Fax: 1-314-447-8029. E-mail: JournalsCustomerService-usa@elsevier.com (for print support)** and **JournalsOnlineSupport-usa@elsevier.com (for online support).**

Reprints. For copies of 100 or more, of articles in this publication, please contact the Commercial Reprints Department, Elsevier Inc., 360 Park Avenue South, New York, New York 10010-1710. Tel.: 212-633-3874; Fax: 212-633-3820; E-mail: reprints@elsevier.com.

Urologic Clinics of North America is covered in MEDLINE/PubMed (*Index Medicus*), *Excerpta Medica, Current Contents/Clinical Medicine, Science Citation Index,* and *ISI/BIOMED.*

Printed in the United States of America.

Contributors

EDITOR-IN-CHIEF

KEVIN R. LOUGHLIN, MD, MBA
Emeritus Professor of Surgery (Urology),
Harvard Medical School, Visiting Scientist,
Vascular Biology Research Program at Boston
Children's Hospital, Boston, Massachusetts,
USA

EDITORS

JIM C. HU, MD, MPH
Professor, Department of Urology, NewYork-
Presbyterian Hospital/Weill Cornell Medicine,
New York, New York, USA

JONATHAN E. SHOAG, MD, MS
Assistant Professor of Urology, University
Hospitals Cleveland Medical Center, Case
Western Reserve University School of
Medicine, Cleveland, Ohio, USA; Adjunct
Clinical Assistant Professor of Urology, Weill
Cornell Medical College, New York, New York,
USA

AUTHORS

MATHEW J. ALLAWAY, DO
Urology Associates and UPMC Western
Maryland, Cumberland, Maryland, USA

SAPAN N. AMBANI, MD
Assistant Professor, Department of Urology,
Michigan Medicine, Ann Arbor, Michigan, USA

CAMILO ARENAS-GALLO, MD
Graduated, School of Medicine, Universidad
Industrial de Santander, Santander, Colombia

KETAN BADANI, MD
Director, Vice Chair of Robotic Operations,
Department of Urology, Mount Sinai Hospital,
Professor of Urology, Icahn School of Medicine
at Mount Sinai Hospital, New York, New York,
USA

YASIN BHANJI, MD
Department of Urology, The James Buchanan
Brady Urological Institute, Johns Hopkins
School of Medicine, Baltimore, Maryland, USA

ROBERT E. BRANNIGAN, MD
Professor, Department of Urology,
Northwestern University Feinberg School of
Medicine, Chicago, Illinois, USA

JILL C. BUCKLEY, MD
Department of Urology, University of California,
San Diego, San Diego, California, USA

LAURA BUKAVINA, MD, MPH
University Hospitals Cleveland Medical Center,
Urology Institute, Case Western Reserve
University School of Medicine, Cleveland,
Ohio, USA

PETER Y. CAI, MD
Department of Urology, NewYork-
Presbyterian, Weill Cornell Medicine, New
York, New York, USA

ADAM C. CALAWAY, MD, MPH
Assistant Professor, University Hospitals
Cleveland Medical Center, Urology Institute,

Case Western Reserve University School of Medicine, Cleveland, Ohio, USA

REBECCA A. CAMPBELL, MD
Department of Urology, Glickman Urological & Kidney Institute, Cleveland Clinic, Cleveland, Ohio, USA

TIMOTHY C. CHANG, MD
Clinical Assistant Professor, Department of Urology, Stanford University School of Medicine, Stanford, California, USA; Veterans Affairs Palo Alto Health Care System, Palo Alto, California, USA

ANNIE DARVES-BORNOZ, MD
Department of Urology, Northwestern University Feinberg School of Medicine, Chicago, Illinois, USA

MEGHAN DAVIS, MD, MPH
Department of Urology, MedStar Georgetown University Hospital, Washington, DC, USA

ALICE DRAIN, MD, MS
Resident, NYU Langone Health Department of Urology, New York, New York, USA

JILLIAN EGAN, MD
Department of Urology, MedStar Georgetown University Hospital, Washington, DC, USA

OKYAZ EMINAGA, MD, PhD
Researcher, Department of Urology, Stanford University School of Medicine, Stanford, California, USA

ANTONIO GALFANO, MD
Department of Urology, ASST Grande Ospedale Metropolitano Niguarda, Milano, Italy

MICHAEL A. GORIN, MD
Urology Associates and UPMC Western Maryland, Cumberland, Maryland, USA

KARISHMA GUPTA, MD
Urology Institute–University Hospitals Cleveland Medical Center, Case Western Reserve University School of Medicine, Cleveland, Ohio, USA

JOSHUA A. HALPERN, MD, MS
Assistant Professor, Department of Urology, Northwestern University Feinberg School of Medicine, Chicago, Illinois, USA

JIM C. HU, MD, MPH
Professor, Department of Urology, NewYork-Presbyterian Hospital/Weill Cornell Medicine, New York, New York, USA

MIN SUK JUN, DO, MS
Fellow, NYU Langone Health Department of Urology, New York, New York, USA

ALEEM I. KHAN, BS
Department of Urology, NewYork-Presbyterian - Weill Cornell Medicine, New York, New York, USA

HYUNG L. KIM, MD
Professor of Surgery, Academic Urology Program Director, Cedars-Sinai Medical Center, Los Angeles, California, USA

SUNCHIN KIM, MD
Department of Urology, University of California, San Diego, San Diego, California, USA

KEITH J. KOWALCZYK, MD
Director, Urologic Oncology, Associate Professor, Department of Urology, Georgetown University Medical Center, Lombardi Cancer Center, MedStar Georgetown University Hospital, Washington, DC, USA

BYRON H. LEE, MD, PhD
Department of Urology, Glickman Urological & Kidney Institute, Cleveland Clinic, Cleveland, Ohio, USA

JOSEPH C. LIAO, MD
Associate Professor, Department of Urology, Stanford University School of Medicine, Stanford, California, USA; Department of Urology, Veterans Affairs Palo Alto Health Care System, Palo Alto, California, USA

ERIC M. LO, BS
Baylor College of Medicine, Houston, Texas, USA

SHAWN MARHAMATI, MD
Department of Urology, Austin Hospital, Heidelberg, Victoria, Australia

KIRTISHRI MISHRA, MD
University Hospitals Cleveland Medical Center, Urology Institute, Case Western Reserve University School of Medicine, Cleveland, Ohio, USA

SAMEER MITTAL, MD, MS, FAAP
Assistant Professor of Urology in Surgery, Children's Hospital of Philadelphia, Perelman School of Medicine, University of Pennsylvania, Philadelphia, Pennsylvania, USA

PRITHVI B. MURTHY, MD
Department of Urology, Glickman Urological & Kidney Institute, Cleveland Clinic, Cleveland, Ohio, USA

DANLY O. OMIL-LIMA, MD
Urology Institute, University Hospitals– Cleveland Medical Center, Cleveland, Ohio, USA

EVAN PANKEN, BS
Department of Urology, Northwestern University Feinberg School of Medicine, Chicago, Illinois, USA

LEE PONSKY, MD
Professor and Chairman, Urology Institute, Leo and Charlotte Goldberg Chair of Advanced Surgical Therapies, Master Clinician in Urologic Oncology, University Hospitals Cleveland Medical Center, Case Western Reserve University School of Medicine, Cleveland, Ohio, USA

DOUGLAS S. SCHERR, MD
Professor of Urology, Clinical Director of Urologic Oncology, Weill Cornell Medical College, New York, New York, USA

CALEB SEUFERT, MD
Resident, Department of Urology, Stanford University School of Medicine, Stanford, California, USA

EUGENE SHKOLYAR, MD
Resident, Department of Urology, Stanford University School of Medicine, Stanford, California, USA

JONATHAN E. SHOAG, MD, MS
Assistant Professor of Urology, University Hospitals Cleveland Medical Center, Case Western Reserve University School of Medicine, Cleveland, Ohio, USA; Adjunct Clinical Assistant Professor of Urology, Weill Cornell Medical College, New York, New York, USA

ARUN SRINIVASAN, MD
Assistant Professor of Urology in Surgery, Children's Hospital of Philadelphia, Perelman School of Medicine, University of Pennsylvania, Philadelphia, Pennsylvania, USA

ROBERT S. WANG, MD
Department of Urology, Michigan Medicine, Ann Arbor, Michigan, USA

MICHAEL WILSON, DO
Department of Urology, Icahn School of Medicine at Mount Sinai, New York City, New York, USA

MICHAEL A. ZELL, MD
Urology Institute–University Hospitals Cleveland Medical Center, Case Western Reserve University School of Medicine, Cleveland, Ohio, USA

LEE C. ZHAO, MD, MS
Assistant Professor, NYU Langone Health Department of Urology, New York, New York, USA

Contents

technique, and robotic platforms, but integration of a variety of imaging techniques. We believe with developing robotic expertise, practicing urologists will continue to push the envelope in nephron preservation and complication-free recovery.

Robotically assisted laparoscopic techniques may be used for proximal and distal ureteral strictures. Distal strictures may be approached with ureteroneocystotomy, psoas hitch, and Boari flap. Ureteroureterostomy, buccal mucosa graft ureteroplasty, and appendiceal flap ureteroplasty are viable techniques for strictures anywhere along the ureter. Ileal ureteral substitution is reserved for more extensive disease, and autotransplantation is reserved for salvage situations.

Lower urinary tract reconstruction has traditionally been approached in an open fashion but select complications or disease processes may be suitable for robotic reconstruction, including bladder neck contractures, proximal urethral strictures, and genitourinary fistulas. Here, the authors discuss the novel techniques used and the feasibility of robotic reconstruction for these conditions. The robotic approach is relatively novel, and more data and studies will be required to make definitive statements regarding success rate and complications from the procedure. Preliminary data suggest that the robotic approach may offer comparable success compared with open techniques.

 Video content accompanies this article at http://www.urologic.theclinics.com.

Almost 30 years have passed since the inception of minimally invasive surgery in urology and specifically in pediatric urology. Laparoscopy has now become an essential tool in the pediatric urologic armamentarium. The application of robot-assisted surgery in pediatrics has allowed for widespread utilization for common reconstructive procedures such as pyeloplasty and ureteral reimplantation. Understanding the implementation, technical considerations, and outcomes are critical for continued success and adoption. This has allowed for increased use in more complex urologic procedures such as redo pyeloplasty, dismembered ureteral reimplantation, catheterizable channel creation, and bladder augmentation.

The robotic platform offers theoretical and practical advantages to microsurgical male infertility surgery. These include reduction or elimination of tremor, 3-dimensional visualization, and decreased need for skilled surgical assistance. This article reviews the application of robotic surgery to each of the 4 primary male infertility procedures: vasectomy reversal, varicocelectomy, testicular sperm extraction, and spermatic cord denervation. Historical perspective is presented alongside the available outcomes data, which are limited in most cases. Before the robotic approach can be widely adopted, further clinical trials are needed to compare outcomes and costs with those of other validated surgical techniques.

UROLOGIC CLINICS OF NORTH AMERICA

SERIES OF RELATED INTEREST
Surgical Clinics of North America
https://www.surgical.theclinics.com/

Foreword
Robotic Urology: Remember the Future

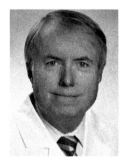

Kevin R. Loughlin, MD, MBA
Consulting Editor

My favorite line from my favorite play, *Camelot*, is when King Arthur says of his friend, Merlin, the magician, "He remembers the future." Doctors Jim Hu and Jonathan Shoag have assembled an array of urologic Merlins in this issue of *Urologic Clinics* devoted to Robotic Urology: The Next Frontier. It is wise to recognize that urologic robotic surgery is not a finished product; it is kinetic, a work in progress, if you will. Recently I wrote, "Relentlessly Make Yourself Obsolete."[1] I think that phrase captures the quiddity of urology in general and robotic urology in particular.

Urologic laparoscopy has only been part of urologic practice for 3 decades and urologic robotics for less than two. To put the rapidity of change into perspective, Tyson and colleagues[2] reviewed the trends in radical prostatectomy from 1998 to 2011 and found that during that period, the number of open prostatectomies decreased by 70%, and 18% of hospitals stopped performing open radical prostatectomies altogether.[2,3] They further reported that from 2008 to 2011, the number of laparoscopic radical prostatectomies declined by 90%.[2,3] The inexorable rise of robotics in urology has continued over the past decade.

One can divide the evolution of robotic urology into 3 phases: diagnostic, extirpative, and reconstructive, and each phase leads to the next. This issue of *Urologic Clinics* serves as an ecphoneme of where robotic urology is at presently.

Not only has every urologic malignancy been approached robotically, but also, we are firmly entrenched in the reconstructive robotic urology era. As evidenced in this issue, robotic reconstruction extends from the collecting system to the urethra. Complex reconstruction like Boari flaps and bladder neck contracture repairs are now routine. Not only are robotic radical cystectomies being increasingly performed, but also intracorporeal construction of ileal conduits is becoming widely embraced. The article on pediatric urologic reconstruction in this issue provides many insights specific to pediatric urologic reconstruction.

One of the joys of being a pediatric surgeon is exchanging technical nuances with your peers. Again, in this issue, guest editors, Drs Hu and Shoag, have gathered urologic Merlins to review the technical advances that have accrued over the past decade. The reader of this issue will find rich surgical tips regarding many aspects of robotic surgery.

The history of urologic surgery is replete with the advances provided by urologic devices, and this continues to be true of robotics. For the past 20 years, the Intuitive DaVinci system has dominated the market. Intuitive has continued to innovate with

Urol Clin N Am 48 (2021) xiii–xiv
https://doi.org/10.1016/j.ucl.2020.10.001
0094-0143/21/© 2020 Published by Elsevier Inc.

the development of the Si, X, Xi, and SP systems. However, what we see in this issue and what makes the future so exciting is that the robotic revolution has truly gone global. As reviewed within, advances in robotic research and development are occurring worldwide in Korea, Germany, Japan, and Canada, in addition to continuing in the United States. Work has already commenced to make robots smaller and less expensive.

The next major challenge in robotic surgery will be the further development of teleoperation, telementoring, telesurgery, and telepresence. There is not only a urologist shortage in the United States but also a urologist maldistribution.[4] Seventy percent of the counties in the United States have only one or no urologist. Maganty and colleagues[5] have correctly cautioned about the undertreatment of prostate cancer in rural areas. This maldistribution will likely be further exacerbated as the country becomes more urbanized.[6] Telerobotics and telementoring are 2 strategies to provide modern robotic technology and expertise to underserved areas, and this will likely accelerate in the future.

NASA has plans for manned missions to Mars and beyond by 2030. It is estimated that a manned mission to Mars and return to Earth will take 21 months.[7] Even with young, healthy astronauts, a trip of that duration mandates that the capability for remote surgical intervention will be critical. This need will undoubtedly drive the need for telerobotics even more. The logical extension of this need has already been envisioned: autonomous robots in the operating room.[8] Autonomous robots are no more fanciful now than urologic robotic surgery was in 1990.

We would do well to remember the words of Ralph Waldo Emerson: "Man is a shrewd inventor, and is ever taking the hint of a new machine from our own structure." We are faced with an exciting future. However, unlike Merlin, we cannot remember the future, but we can remember the past and learn from it.

Kevin R. Loughlin, MD, MBA
Vascular Biology Research Program at
Boston Children's Hospital
300 Longwood Avenue
Boston, MA 02115, USA

E-mail address:
kloughlin@partners.org

REFERENCES

1. Loughlin KR. Relentlessly make yourself obsolete: robot-assisted radical cystectomy, the emerging standard of care. Urol Oncol 2020. available online September 5, 2020.
2. Tyson MD, Andrew PE, Ferrigni RF, et al. Contemporary trends in radical prostatectomy in the United States, 1998-2011. Mayo Clin Proc 2016;91(1):10–6.
3. Dalela D, Menon M. Re: contemporary trends in radical prostatectomy in the United States: open versus minimally invasive surgery 1998-2011. Mayo Clin Proc 2016;91(1):1–2.
4. Loughlin KR. The confluence of the aging of the American population and the urological workforce: the Parmenides Fallacy. Urology Practice 2019;6(3): 198–203.
5. Maganty A, Sabik LM, Sun Z, et al. Undertreatment of prostate cancer in rural locations. J Urol 2020;203: 108–14.
6. Loughlin KR. Re: undertreatment of prostate cancer in rural locations. J Urol 2020;203(6):1211.
7. How long would a trip to Mars take? Extracted from course notes for Physics 6, Professor Craig Patten, UC San Diego. Available at: https://image.gsfc.nasa/poetry/venus/q2811.html. Accessed October 2, 2020.
8. Castellanos S. Autonomous robots in the OR. The future of everything/health. Wall Street Journal 2020; 11:R6.

Preface

Two Decades of Robotics in Urology: Origins, Current Practice, and Directions

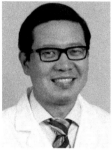　　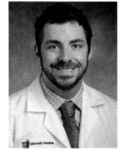

Jim C. Hu, MD, MPH　　　Jonathan E. Shoag, MD, MS

Editors

Robotics and new technologies have changed urologic surgery profoundly. This issue of *Urologic Clinics* explores some of these changes. The operation that led to the widespread adoption of robotics by urologists, radical prostatectomy, has likely been irreversibly transformed by this technology. We describe how the conversion to robotics has been accompanied by efforts to improve training, quality, diagnostics, and oncologic control, while limiting morbidity. Despite early concerns about cost, and oncologic control, it is increasingly clear that the changes to this operation are, to a certain extent, irreversible; most urologic trainees currently have minimal training and exposure to many major open operations.

In this issue, we focus on recent robotic innovations in urothelial cancer treatment, including wider adoption of intracorporeal diversion. We also discuss how routine urinary reconstruction and partial nephrectomy have been changed in many practices. We highlight clinical areas with less robotic adoption and adoption of robotics has been more controversial, such as pediatric urology, male infertility, and endourology. Throughout, we attempted to highlight many of the limitations of robotics as well as promising future directions, such as utilization of artificial intelligence. In summary, for better or worse, over the past 20 years, robotic surgery has profoundly changed urologic practice. Who knows what the next 20 years will bring?

Jim C. Hu, MD, MPH
Weill Cornell Medical College
525 East 68th Street
Starr 900
New York, NY 10065, USA

Jonathan E. Shoag, MD, MS
University Hospitals Cleveland Medical Center
Case Western Reserve University
School of Medicine
Wolstein Research Building
4th Floor 4541
2103 Cornell Road
Cleveland, OH 44106, USA

E-mail addresses:
Jch9011@med.cornell.edu (J.C. Hu)
Jxs218@case.edu (J.E. Shoag)

Urol Clin N Am 48 (2021) xv
https://doi.org/10.1016/j.ucl.2020.10.002
0094-0143/21/© 2020 Published by Elsevier Inc.

urologic.theclinics.com

Optimizing Surgical Techniques in Robot-Assisted Radical Prostatectomy

Camilo Arenas-Gallo, MD[a], Jonathan E. Shoag, MD, MS[b,c],*,
Jim C. Hu, MD, MPH[d]

KEYWORDS

- Prostatectomy • Prostate cancer • Robotic surgical procedures • Prostate

KEY POINTS

- Robot-assisted radical prostatectomy (RARP) is the most common surgical treatment of localized prostate cancer, which has almost completely replaced standard laparoscopic and open radical prostatectomy in the United States.
- Surgeon experience and surgical technique are associated with better RARP outcomes.
- The benefit of new techniques and maneuvers are best assessed by randomized trials. To date, there are few such trials to guide technique.

INTRODUCTION

The initial description of radical prostatectomy to treat prostate cancer is generally attributed to Hugh Hampton Young, who published the procedure in 1905.[1] The most important subsequent technical modification was the description of the neurophysiology and anatomy of the prostate in the 1980s, by Patrick Walsh, who developed the nerve-sparing technique.[2] The rapid adoption of robot-assisted radical prostatectomy (RARP) over the past 20 years constitutes the most recent major change technical modification to this procedure.[3]

RARP has rapidly become the preferred modality for radical prostatectomy. Although the benefits of RARP versus open retropubic radical prostatectomy in experienced hands may be minimal, the robotic technique is associated with less blood loss and shorter hospital stays than open surgery.[4,5] RARP has almost completely replaced

standard laparoscopic radical prostatectomy, and in 2010, it was estimated that 80% of radical prostatectomies in the United States were performed robotically.[3] More recent data estimate that RARP comprises more than 90% of all radical prostatectomies performed. This modality has now been adopted in both community and academic centers.[6]

Several anatomic descriptions and technical modifications have been proposed to improve functional outcomes after RARP. Here, the authors review critical maneuvers to preserve urinary and sexual function following RARP.[3]

Overview of the Nerve-Sparing Technique

The first nerve-sparing prostatectomy was performed in 1982 by Patrick Walsh.[2] The discovery and description of the anatomy of the neurovascular bundle (NVB) that surrounds the prostate

Funding: J. Shoag and J.C. Hu are supported by the Wallace Fund of the New York Community Trust. J. Shoag is supported by the Damon Runyon Cancer Research Foundation Physician Scientist Training Award.
[a] School of Medicine, Universidad Industrial de Santander, Cra 21 No 158-80 Casa 83, Floridablanca, Santander 681004, Colombia; [b] Department of Urology, University Hospitals Cleveland Medical Center, Case Western Reserve University School of Medicine, Case Comprehensive Cancer Center, 11100 Euclid Ave, Cleveland, OH 44106, USA; [c] Department of Urology, New York Presbyterian Hospital, Weill Cornell Medicine, 24610 Sittingbourne Drive, Bechwood, NY 44122, USA; [d] Department of Urology, New York Presbyterian Hospital, Weill Cornell Medicine, 413 East 69th Street, Starr 946, New York, NY 10021, USA
* Corresponding author.
E-mail address: Jonathan.shoag@uhhospitals.org

defined a new era in prostatectomy, allowing the preservation of erectile function in a greater number of patients.[7] Before this, it was universally accepted that radical prostatectomy led to the absence of any erectile function. It is now recognized that even in the presence of high tumor volume or extracapsular disease, nerve sparing can often be performed to some degree.

It is now widely recognized that preoperative erectile function is the main predictor of recovery from postprostatectomy erectile function.[8] In addition, cardiovascular risk factors such as dyslipidemia, diabetes mellitus, hypertension, coronary artery disease, and smoking have also been found to be independent predictors of erectile dysfunction.[9] In addition to these factors, it is widely accepted that optimal nerve-sparing technique plays a critical role in maintaining erectile function following surgery.[10]

The nerve-sparing technique can be broadly classified as antegrade or retrograde depending on the direction of dissection. The antegrade approach advances from the prostatic base to the apex and includes ascending traction of the vessels and seminal vesicles, athermal control of the prostatic pedicle, and exposure of the lateral pelvic fascia. The NVB is exposed when entering the space between Denonvilliers fascia, lateral pelvic fascia, and the prostate. Reflection of the lateral pelvic fascia outside the prostate exposes the interfascial or intrafascial planes for dissection[11] (**Figs. 1** and **2**).

The retrograde approach begins from the prostatic apex and continues toward the base. It includes dissection of the seminal vesicles and development of the posterior plane. The prostate is then retracted away from the side of interest,

and the levator fascia is opened to expose the NVB. Subsequently, the dissection between the prostate and the NVB is performed in an inter- or intrafascial approach, depending on disease burden, until the previously developed posterior plane is reached and the NVB is completely separated from the prostate.[11]

Apical dissection is a critical step in radical prostatectomy because the nerves responsible for erection and continence come in close proximity to the prostatic apex. The pudendal nerve perforates the levator ani at the apex of the prostate and sends branches to the sphincter in this position.[3] Damage to the nerves responsible for erection may be more likely to occur at this location because of its proximity to the prostatic apex.

Sometimes, in locally advanced prostate cancer more extensive excision must be performed and preservation of the NVB may be challenging. However, studies have shown that extracapsular extension of prostate cancer rarely extends histologically beyond 3 mm,[12] whereas anatomic studies have shown that the distance between the prostate capsule and the cavernous nerves (found in a bundle of the posterolateral fascial compartment) is around 5 mm.[13] Therefore, even if preoperative MRI of the prostate suggests extracapsular extension, the nerves may not have to be completely resected. If the extracapsular disease is unilateral, then preservation of the contralateral side can preserve functional outcomes.[3]

Based on the plane of dissection, a nerve-sparing technique can be classified as intrafascial or interfascial[14] (**Fig. 3**). Dissection in the intrafascial plane, located between the capsule and the

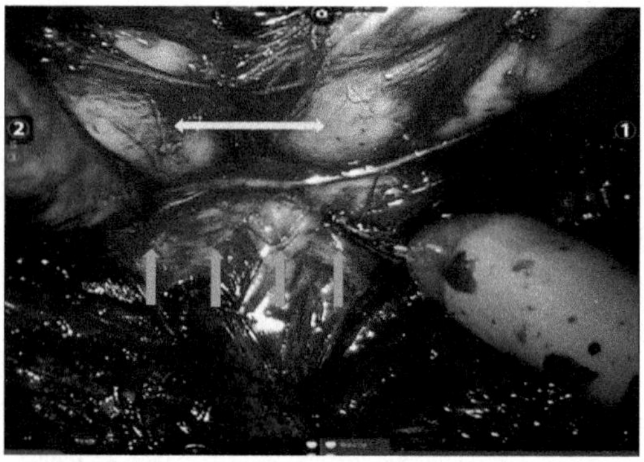

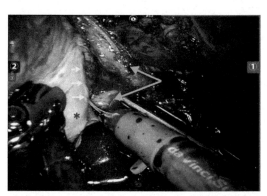

Fig. 1. Posterior prostatic dissection plane. Yellow arrow means vas deferens; blue arrows mean Denonvillier fascia; asterisk means seminal vesicles tissue. (*From* Tavukçu HH, Aytac O, Atug F. Nerve-sparing techniques and results in robot assisted radical prostatectomy. Investig Clin Urol. 2016;57(166):S172–84.)

Fig. 2. Right intrafascial dissection; prostate and right neurovascular bundle (NVB). Yellow arrows mean dissection plane; blue arrow means NVB; asterisk means prostate capsule. (*From* Tavukçu HH, Aytac O, Atug F. Nerve-sparing techniques and results in robot assisted radical prostatectomy. Investig Clin Urol. 2016;57(166):S172–84.)

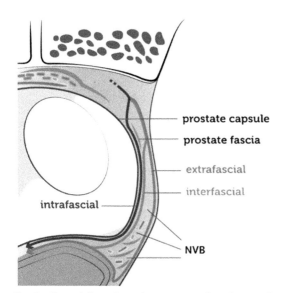

Fig. 3. The axial section of prostate and periprostatic fasciae at midprostate with 3 different dissection planes (intrafascial [*red line*], interfascial [*green line*], and extrafascial [*blue line*]). NVB, neurovascular bundle. (*From* Salonia A, Burnett AL, Graefen M, Hatzimouratidis K, Montorsi F, Mulhall JP, et al. Prevention and management of postprostatectomy sexual dysfunctions part 1: Choosing the right patient at the right time for the right surgery. Eur Urol. 2012;62(2):261–72.)

prostatic fascia, allows total preservation of the NVB. In contrast, dissection in the interfascial plane, located between the prostatic fascia and the lateral pelvic fascia, allows a greater probability of negative surgical margins at the expense of partial preservation of the NVB. The surgeon selects the appropriate plane for each patient based on the anatomy and extent of the cancer.[15] Kowalczyk and colleagues[16] described splitting the capsular vein along the NVB as a landmark for interfascial nerve sparing, as the vein is often the most medial component of the anterior medial aspect of the NVB.

Potdevin and colleagues[17] retrospectively compared 147 patients undergoing interfascial versus intrafascial athermic nerve sparing to assess the benefit of the latter's conservation of more anterolateral nerve fibers. They found potency rates at 9 months in the intrafascial group of 90.9% versus 66.7% in the interfascial group (P<.01). However, the improvement in functional outcome came at the tradeoff of increased rates of positive surgical margins in pT3 disease, 41.18% in intrafascial versus 22.2% in interfascial (P<.05). No differences were found in complication rates, continence rates at 6 months, and positive margin rates in patients with pT2 disease.

A systematic review and meta-analysis published in 2017 by Weng and colleagues[18] compared intrafascial versus interfascial nerve-sparing prostatectomy for localized prostate cancer. They included 6 trials of open, laparoscopic, and robotic prostatectomy and demonstrated that the intrafascial approach was associated with better continence rates at 6 months (risk ratio [RR] = 1.18, 95% confidence interval [CI] 1.08–1.30, $P = .0002$) and 36 months (RR = 1.13, 95% CI 1.02–1.25, $P = .02$). In addition, the intrafascial approach was associated with better potency recovery at 6 months (RR = 1.49, 95% CI 1.01–2.18, $P = .04$) and 12 months (RR = 1.40, 95% CI 1.24–1.57, $P<.00001$). However, the quality of evidence was very low for oncologic outcomes.

Neuropraxia or tension on the NVB is also thought to affect recovery of erectile function: minimizing lateral displacement of the NVB is associated with earlier and better recovery of erectile function. Kowalczyk and colleagues[16] made a retrospective study comparing sexual function outcomes for nerve sparing without countertraction versus with assistant and/or surgeon NVB countertraction. They measured the sexual function using the Expanded Prostate Cancer Index Composite (EPIC), scored from 0 to 100, with higher scores representing better outcomes, and found that nerve sparing without assistant countertraction was associated with higher 5-month sexual function (20 vs 10; $P<.001$). However, no difference in sexual function or potency was observed at 12 months dependent on this approach. There were no significant differences in positive surgical margins between techniques.

Surgeon experience has also been shown to play a role in outcomes. Alemozaffar and colleagues[19] in a retrospective study of 400 consecutive RARPs demonstrated greater surgeon experience was associated with better 5-month sexual function (parameter estimate [PE]: 5.21; 95% CI, 1.4 to 9.02) and with a trend for better 12-month sexual function (PE: 0.06; 95% CI, 0–0.12). In addition, trainee robotic console involvement during nerve sparing was associated with worse 12-month sexual function (PE: −12.58; 95% CI, −23.23 to −1.92), demonstrating a learning curve effect.

Several studies have suggested that meticulous preservation of the NVB in radical prostatectomy improves the results of postoperative continence. Possible reasons for this include the preservation of intrapelvic somatic supply to the external striated rhabdosphincter.[20] A 2015 meta-analysis of 27 cohort studies with a total of 13,749 patients demonstrated that postoperative continence was achieved faster with the nerve-sparing technique compared with non–nerve-sparing technique in the first 6 months after surgery (RR 1.20, CI 1.04–1.39; P = .02). However, there was no difference in incontinence outcomes beyond 6 months (RR 1.09, CI 0.97–1.22), regardless of whether or not a nerve-sparing procedure was performed.[21] Additional studies are needed to improve the understanding of male urinary continence and the pathophysiology of postradical prostatectomy incontinence and its relationship to nerve sparing.[20]

The Veil of Aphrodite Technique or "High Anterior Release"

The technique known as high anterior release or "the veil of Aphrodite" to preserve the NVB was described in 2006 by Menon and colleagues.[22] In this approach, the surgeon develops a plane between the prostatic capsule and the prostatic fascia at the base of the seminal vesicles. The next step is a meticulous bilateral interfascial dissection between 1 and 5 o'clock on the right side, as well as 6 and 11 o'clock on the left side. At the end of the dissection, the curtains of periprostatic tissue are suspended from the pubourethral ligament, which is also known as the "veil of Aphrodite." This approach involves resection of the periprostatic fascia on the lateral sides of the prostate to drop the fascia and prevent damage to the NVB below.[3] It is suggested that this technique may improve potency compared with conventional nerve-sparing while not compromising oncologic outcomes. The original technique was later modified by extending the anterior interfascial dissection and preserving the pubovesical ligaments and the dorsal vein plexus ("superveil technique").[23] The rationale for this technique has been questioned in a subsequent cadaveric analysis of the distribution of the periprostatic nerves, where the level of the cavernous nerves in the neurovascular bundle was examined.[24,25] This study found that most of the nerves of the NVB were located inferolateral to the prostate above the rectum; therefore, the high release of the fascia above the midline of the prostate may have little effect in preserving these important nerves.[3]

Preservation of the Urethral Smooth Muscle Preservation

The urethral sphincter is made up of 2 muscle types: the outer, horseshoe-shaped striated muscle fibers and inner elastic tissue and smooth muscle fibers that are completely circular in men and are present mainly at the proximal urethra.[26] *Schlomm and colleagues* described a full-length preservation of the urethral sphincter by identifying and dissecting the distinct striated and smooth muscle part of the sphincter inside the prostate apex until the colliculus seminalis is encountered. This technique allows preservation of the full functional-length urethra and of the anatomic fixation of the urethral sphincter complex. This approach resulted in early continence results in 406 consecutive patients compared with standard RARP: 50.1% versus 30.9% 1 week after catheter removal ($P<.0001$) and 96.9% versus 94.7% (P = .59) at 12 months after surgery.[27] However, others contend that the urethral sphincter smooth muscle supplies only passive continence and true active continence is mediated by the striated muscle, which is innervated by the pudendal nerve,[28] therefore, preservation of urethral smooth muscle does not have an anatomic basis for improving postoperative continence after radical prostatectomy. Nevertheless, as a general anatomic principle, most of the urethra and the surrounding muscle should be preserved.

The Suburethral Plication Stitch

Some studies have suggested that a plication stitch, also known as a Rocco stitch, which extends suburethrally at the apex of the prostate to the Denonvilliers layer below the bladder, aids in the restoration of postoperative continence. In addition to making the anastomosis technically easier, theorized benefits of the stitch include restoration of the length of the urethrosphincteric complex, avoiding its retraction, withdrawal of excessive tension in the posterior vesicourethral anastomosis, and provision of a posterior pillar to the urethral sphincter complex to facilitate its effective contraction.[29]

A meta-analysis published in 2012 concluded that factors that affect the risk for urinary incontinence after RARP include patient preoperative characteristics (age and preoperative potency), surgeon experience, surgical technique, and the methods used to collect the report data and that the reconstruction posterior muscle fascial with the Rocco stitch seems to offer a slight advantage at 1 month after surgery but not afterward.[30] A prospective, randomized trial of this approach found no benefit with rhabdosphincter reconstruction versus standard vesicourethral anastomosis in terms of early return of urinary continence after RARP.[31] Similarly, Woo and colleagues[32] in a retrospective analysis found no statistically significant difference in outcomes depending on whether the stitch was used.

Urethral suspension techniques have also been studied for improving urinary function. Canvasser and colleagues[33] explored a posterior urethral suspension technique at the time of anastomosis in a case control study of 83 patients. This suspension is made with the intention of lightly and minimally elevating the anastomosis to avoid urethral compression while limiting membranous urethra/sphincter complex descent with increases in intra-abdominal pressure. Patients with the urethral suspension required less protective incontinence products at 1 and 2 weeks after catheter removal ($P<.03$) and had pad-free rates of 60% compared with 36% among controls at 12 weeks after catheter removal ($P = .07$).[33]

Others have studied the effect of vas suspension on urinary continence. *van der Poel and colleagues*[34] conducted a randomized trial of 112 patients evaluating a vas deferens urethral support technique. They hypothesized that ventral rather than cranial support of the dorsal urethral plate is required for proper sphincter function. Accordingly, the investigators used a ventral support technique using the vas deferens and compared with standard anastomosis during RARP. Vas suspension improved early continence at 1 month (59% vs 35%, $P = .02$); however, men also reported loss of urine significantly more often due to urgency (ICIQ-SF question 4b) at the 1-month interval (26% vs 11%, $P = .03$). No significant differences in full urine continence or pad use was observed at later time points.[34]

Seminal Vesicle-Sparing Prostatectomy

Thermal injury and traction may also contribute to poor functional outcomes after prostatectomy. Anatomic studies demonstrate the proximity of neurovascular tissue to the seminal vesicles and the posterior neck of the bladder,[35] leading to the proposition that seminal vesicle preservation may be beneficial.[36] A 2017 randomized controlled trial of 140 patients assessing this hypothesis compared functional outcomes after standard nerve-sparing RARP versus enhanced nerve-sparing technique with the preservation of the seminal vesicles.[37] The study found no differences in sexual and continence functional scores, surgical margin status, or PSA biochemical recurrence between the groups and concluded that preservation of the seminal vesicles was not an effective intervention.

This conclusion was supported by anatomic studies by a group at the Royal Melbourne Hospital, which showed that the autonomic neural components of the NVB were within a reasonable distance from the ends of the seminal vesicles.[38] The parasympathetic autonomic nerves S2 to S4

join a ganglion 1 to 2 cm from the ends of the seminal vesicles, near the base of the prostate. Therefore, dissection of the seminal vesicles is unlikely to alter the autonomic function or improve functional outcomes.

Prostatic Vasculature as a Landmark

Patel and colleagues[39] described the use of vascular landmarks to aid in identification of the proper plane for nerve sparing during prostatectomy. This technique relies on identification of an artery that runs along the lateral edge of the prostate, which could correspond to a prostate or capsular artery, that can be recognized after opening the levator fascia at the base of the prostate. The prostate artery is a larger tortuous vessel seen on the medial aspect of the NVB. In contrast, the capsular arteries are smaller without tortuosity, which makes them more difficult to visualize, and are located more distally in relation to the prostatic artery. The dissection plane is identified between one of these landmark arteries and the prostate at the midprostate. Dissection then continues retrograde to the posterior plane and the base of the prostate. After controlling the prostatic pedicles at the base, the dissection is performed antegrade to the apex.[15]

Retrograde Release of the Neurovascular Bundle with Preservation of the Dorsal Venous Complex

In 2018, de Carvalho and colleagues[40] introduced a technical modification of the RARP with nerve preservation, in which the retrograde release of NVB allows the preservation of nervous and vascular structures. In this study, the functional and oncological results were described in 128 patients operated by a single surgeon. This technique involves incision of the anterior peritoneum to access the space of Retzius, dissection of the overlying fatty tissue, and dissection of the anterior neck of the bladder without entering the endopelvic fascia or ligating the dorsal venous complex (DVC). Next, an incision is made in the posterior neck of the bladder, and dissection of the vas deferens and seminal vesicles is performed. The NVB is released starting at the level of the bladder neck, developing an avascular plane below the DVC, and thereafter the dissection continues laterally. Prostatectomy with complete nerve preservation is performed when the NVB is dissected medially to the prostate artery, fusing this plane with the previously developed posterior plane. So far there have been no randomized trials comparing this approach with the standard one.

Retzius-Sparing Radical Prostatectomy

Galfano and colleagues[41] in 2010 described a surgical technique for RARP known as a posterior or "Retzius-sparing." It has been suggested that this could enable earlier continence recovery compared with the traditional technique.[42] This approach is based on the idea of performing an RARP exclusively through the pouch of Douglas space, thus avoiding any interruption of the anterior anatomic structures that surround the prostate gland such as the pubovesical ligaments, puboprostatic fascia, NVBs, and the dorsal venous complex. It is thought that preserving these structures may result in better functional results.[43]

In 2014, Lim and colleagues[44] reported a similar RARP technique with the preservation of the space of Retzius. In this approach, surgery begins with an incision through the peritoneum posterior to the bladder, and the seminal vesicles are dissected as a first step. Initial reports on this technique described a high T2-positive margin rate of 12% compared with 5.3% in another robot-assisted laparoscopic prostatectomy (RALP) cohort. This high positivity rate of the T2 margin was suggested to be the resultant from a steep learning curve associated with performing this technique.

Another study published in 2018 investigated functional recovery, cancer outcomes, and postoperative complications in 120 patients after S-RARP versus RS-RARP.[45] The investigators concluded that in patients with low-risk or intermediate-risk prostate cancer, the results at a 12-month follow-up point were not significantly different on any of the measurable parameters and that the return to continence after RS-RARP was not different from conventional RARP ($P = .001$).[46] However, the RS-RARP approach is technically difficult, associated with a high learning curve (plateau after 200–300 cases)[47,48] and must be performed by surgeons skilled in the standard RARP technique.

A systematic review and comparative analysis of standard RARP (S-RARP) and RARP with preservation of Retzius (RS-RARP) was recently published.[49] The investigators included 8 clinical studies. The results showed a shorter operating time with the RS-RARP; however, this was only a 14.7-minute time difference (weighted mean difference 14.7 min, $P = .03$). No significant differences were found in terms of estimated blood loss or postoperative complications; however, the positive surgical margin rate was lower for the S-RARP group (rate 15.2% vs 24%; odds ratio 1.71, $P = .01$), which may be influenced by the RS-RARP learning curve. This is an important issue

because the investigators suggest that higher rates of positive margins could translate into greater need for adjuvant or salvage radiation therapy, with the potential for associated morbidity. The cumulative analysis did show a statistically significant advantage for RS-RARP compared with S-RARP in terms of continence recovery at 3, 6, and 12 months ($P = .004$). A recently published comparative analysis of a single surgeon series of 70 RS-RARP versus 70 S-RARP showed no differences in sexual function but improved overall continence rates at total follow-up (95.7% vs 85.7%, $P = .042$).[50]

DISCUSSION

Radical prostatectomy remains the most common treatment of localized prostate cancer.[51] More than 90% of radical prostatectomies in the United States are performed robotically.[52] Patient, surgeon, and technical modifications affect functional outcomes after RARP.[53] Surgeon experience and technique matters. Among 2000 prostatectomies performed by 11 high surgeons at a cancer center, the adjusted probability of erectile function 12 months after prostatectomy ranged from 10% to 50% after adjustment for patient age and baseline erectile function.[54]

Despite the widespread use of robotic surgery, the results for RARP compared with open prostatectomy do not seem to have improved in recent years. In fact, in centers where only a few robotic procedures are performed annually, the results may be worse as compared with open prostatectomy.[4,5] It is well known that even in the best hands, sexual function will be affected to some degree by prostatectomy. To effectively preserve the cavernous nerves during prostatectomy, it is crucial to minimize the mechanisms that can injure them, including transection, traction, and thermal injury. Traction and transection injuries can occur when there is excessive bleeding that obscures the surgeon's visualization or as a result of poorly positioned surgical instruments. Common examples of the latter include misplaced retractors during open prostatectomy and traction created by assistant suction during laparoscopic and robotic cases. The risk of thermal injury can be eliminated with the use of cautery-free techniques.[55] Furthermore, neuropraxia results from crush injuries of the NVB grasped with instruments or with excessive lateral retraction. It can be minimized with delicate surgical techniques that prevent stretching of the nerves.[16]

The absence of a standardized method for reporting results, as well as the paucity of randomized controlled trials, has posed a significant challenge for the systematic comparison of nerve-sparing techniques. The Sexual Health Inventory for Men, the EPIC 26-item as well as the International Index of Erectile Function are tools that have been used in the evaluation of pre- and post-operative sexual function. The use of different assessment tools and also the use of variable cut-off points could potentially introduce variability in the results of sexual potency. As new techniques and maneuvers are explored, attention to rigorous, randomized trials will be critical.

CLINICS CARE POINTS

- The goal of a RARP is to achieve cancer cure and minimize its impact on the quality of life and functional outcomes. The surgeon's experience, surgical technique, and presurgical characteristics of the patient are critical factors associated with a successful outcome after RARP.
- With current evidence, patients should be informed that robotic-assisted prostatectomy offers comparable outcomes in urinary and sexual function compared to the open or laparoscopic approach. These outcomes are more surgeon vs. approach dependent.
- Most patients with prostate cancer are candidates for a nerve-sparing technique which can generally be performed to some degree, even in men with extracapsular disease.
- The decision to perform a nerve-sparing RARP and the appropriate nerve-sparing plane is guided by preoperative sexual function, biopsy and MRI characteristics and tailored to goals of treatment through shared decision making.

REFERENCES

1. Young HH. Conservative Perineal Prostatectomy: The Results of Two Years' Experience and Report of Seventy-Five Cases. Ann Surg 1905;41(4):549–54957.
2. Walsh PC, Donker PJ. Impotence Following Radical Prostatectomy: Insight into Etiology and Prevention. J Urol 1982;128:492–7.
3. Costello AJ. Considering the role of radical prostatectomy in 21st century prostate cancer care. Nat Rev Urol 2020;17(3):177–88.
4. Yaxley JW, Coughlin GD, Chambers SK, et al. Robot-assisted laparoscopic prostatectomy versus open radical retropubic prostatectomy: early outcomes from a randomised controlled phase 3 study. Lancet 2016;388(10049):1057–66.
5. Carlsson S, Jäderling F, Wallerstedt A, et al. Oncological and functional outcomes 1 year after radical prostatectomy for very-low-risk prostate cancer: results from the prospective LAPPRO trial. BJU Int 2016;118(2):205–12.
6. Meng MV. Smith & Tanagho's General Urology. In: McAninch JW, Lue TF, editors. 18a ed. New York: McGraw-Hill Medical; 2013. p. 151–3.
7. Haglind E, Carlsson S, Stranne J, et al. Urinary Incontinence and Erectile Dysfunction after Robotic Versus Open Radical Prostatectomy: A Prospective, Controlled, Nonrandomised Trial. Eur Urol 2015;68(2):216–25.
8. Salonia A, Burnett AL, Graefen M, et al. Prevention and management of postprostatectomy sexual dysfunctions part 1: Choosing the right patient at the right time for the right surgery. Eur Urol 2012;62(2):261–72.
9. Teloken PE, Nelson CJ, Karellas M, et al. Defining the impact of vascular risk factors on erectile function recovery after radical prostatectomy. BJU Int 2013;111(4):653–7.
10. Sanda MG, Dunn RL, Michalski J, et al. Quality of Life and Satisfaction with Outcome among Prostate-Cancer Survivors. N Engl J Med 2008;358(12):1250–61.
11. Ko YH, Coelho RF, Sivaraman A, et al. Retrograde versus antegrade nerve sparing during robot-assisted radical prostatectomy: Which is better for achieving early functional recovery? Eur Urol 2013;63(1):169–77.
12. Sohayda C, Kupelian PA, Levin HS, et al. Extent of extracapsular extension in localized prostate cancer. Urology 2000;55(3):382–6.
13. Costello AJ, Brooks M, Cole OJ. Anatomical studies of the neurovascular bundle and cavernosal nerves. BJU Int 2004;94(7):1071–6.
14. Berry A, Korkes F, Hu JC. Landmarks for consistent nerve sparing during robotic-assisted laparoscopic radical prostatectomy. J Endourol 2008;22(8):1565–7.
15. Tavukçu HH, Aytac O, Atug F. Nerve-sparing techniques and results in robot-assisted radical prostatectomy. Investig Clin Urol 2016;57(166):S172–84.
16. Kowalczyk KJ, Huang AC, Hevelone ND, et al. Stepwise approach for nerve sparing without countertraction during robot-assisted radical prostatectomy: Technique and outcomes. Eur Urol 2011;60(3):536–47.
17. Potdevin L, Ercolani M, Jeong J, et al. Functional and oncologic outcomes comparing interfascial and intrafascial nerve sparing in robot-assisted laparoscopic radical prostatectomies. J Endourol 2009;23(9):1479–84.
18. Weng H, Zeng XT, Li S, et al. Intrafascial versus interfascial nerve sparing in radical prostatectomy for localized prostate cancer: A systematic review and meta-analysis. Sci Rep 2017;7(1):1–11.
19. Alemozaffar M, Duclos A, Hevelone ND, et al. Technical refinement and learning curve for attenuating

neurapraxia during robotic-assisted radical prostatectomy to improve sexual function. Eur Urol 2012; 61(6):1222–8.

20. Murphy DG, Costello AJ. How can the autonomic nervous system contribute to urinary continence following radical prostatectomy? A "boson-like" conundrum. Eur Urol 2013;63(3):445–7.

21. Reeves F, Preece P, Kapoor J, et al. Preservation of the neurovascular bundles is associated with improved time to continence after radical prostatectomy but not long-term continence rates: Results of a systematic review and meta-analysis. Eur Urol 2015;68(4):692–704.

22. Menon M, Shrivastava A, Kaul S, et al. Vattikuti Institute Prostatectomy: Contemporary Technique and Analysis of Results. Eur Urol 2007;51(3): 648–58.

23. Menon M, Shrivastava A, Bhandari M, et al. Vattikuti Institute Prostatectomy: Technical Modifications in 2009. Eur Urol 2009;56(1):89–96.

24. Clarebrough EE, Challacombe BJ, Briggs C, et al. Cadaveric analysis of periprostatic nerve distribution: An anatomical basis for high anterior release during radical prostatectomy? J Urol 2011;185(4): 1519–25.

25. Savera AT, Kaul S, Badani K, et al. Robotic Radical Prostatectomy with the "Veil of Aphrodite" Technique: Histologic Evidence of Enhanced Nerve Sparing. Eur Urol 2006;49(6):1065–74.

26. Wallner C, Dabhoiwala NF, DeRuiter MC, et al. The Anatomical Components of Urinary Continence. Eur Urol 2009;55(4):932–44.

27. Schlomm T, Heinzer H, Steuber T, et al. Full functional-length urethral sphincter preservation during radical prostatectomy. Eur Urol 2011;60(2):320–9.

28. Koraitim MM. The Male Urethral Sphincter Complex Revisited: An Anatomical Concept and its Physiological Correlate. J Urol 2008;179(5):1683–9.

29. Grasso AAC, Mistretta FA, Sandri M, et al. Posterior musculofascial reconstruction after radical prostatectomy: an updated systematic review and a meta-analysis. BJU Int 2016;118(1):20–34.

30. Ficarra V, Novara G, Ahlering TE, et al. Systematic review and meta-analysis of studies reporting potency rates after robot-assisted radical prostatectomy. Eur Urol 2012;62(3):418–30. http://ovidsp. ovid.com/ovidweb.cgi?T=JS&PAGE=reference& D=emed10&NEWS=N&AN=2012451567.

31. Menon M, Muhletaler F, Campos M, et al. Assessment of Early Continence After Reconstruction of the Periprostatic Tissues in Patients Undergoing Computer Assisted (Robotic) Prostatectomy: Results of a 2 Group Parallel Randomized Controlled Trial. J Urol 2008;180(3):1018–23.

32. Woo JR, Shikanov S, Zorn KC, et al. Impact of posterior rhabdosphincter reconstruction during robot-assisted radical prostatectomy: Retrospective analysis of time to continence. J Endourol 2009;23(12):1995–9.

33. Canvasser NE, Lay AH, Koseoglu E, et al. Posterior Urethral Suspension during Robot-Assisted Radical Prostatectomy Improves Early Urinary Control: A Prospective Cohort Study. J Endourol 2016;30(10): 1089–94.

34. van der Poel HG, de Blok W, van Muilekom HAM. Vas deferens urethral support improves early post-prostatectomy urine continence. J Robot Surg 2012;6(4):289–94.

35. Ganzer R, Stolzenburg JU, Neuhaus J, et al. Anatomical study of pelvic nerves in relation to seminal vesicles, prostate and urethral sphincter: Immunohistochemical staining, computerized planimetry and 3-dimensional reconstruction. J Urol 2015; 193(4):1205–12.

36. John H, Hauri D. Seminal vesicle-sparing radical prostatectomy: A novel concept to restore early urinary continence. Urology 2000;55(6):820–4.

37. Gilbert SM, Dunn RL, Miller DC, et al. Functional Outcomes Following Nerve Sparing Prostatectomy Augmented with Seminal Vesicle Sparing Compared to Standard Nerve Sparing Prostatectomy: Results from a Randomized Controlled Trial. J Urol 2017; 198(3):600–7.

38. Costello AJ. Editorial Comment. J Urol 2017;198(3): 606.

39. Patel VR, Schatloff O, Chauhan S, et al. The role of the prostatic vasculature as a landmark for nerve sparing during robot-assisted radical prostatectomy. Eur Urol 2012;61(3):571–6.

40. de Carvalho PA, Barbosa JABA, Guglielmetti GB, et al. Retrograde Release of the Neurovascular Bundle with Preservation of Dorsal Venous Complex During Robot-assisted Radical Prostatectomy: Optimizing Functional Outcomes. Eur Urol 2018. https:// doi.org/10.1016/j.eururo.2018.07.003.

41. Galfano A, Ascione A, Grimaldi S, et al. A new anatomic approach for robot-assisted laparoscopic prostatectomy: A feasibility study for completely intrafascial surgery. Eur Urol 2010; 58(3):457–61.

42. Galfano A, Di Trapani D, Sozzi F, et al. Beyond the learning curve of the Retzius-sparing approach for robot-assisted laparoscopic radical prostatectomy: Oncologic and functional results of the first 200 patients with ≥1 year of follow-up. Eur Urol 2013;64(6): 974–80.

43. Galfano A, Secco S, Di Trapani D, et al. Robotics in Genitourinary Surgery. In: Hemal AK, Menon M, editors. 2a ed. London, UK: Springer; 2018. p. 299–316. https://doi.org/10.1007/978-3-319-20645-5.

44. Lim SK, Kim KH, Shin TY, et al. Retzius-sparing robot-assisted laparoscopic radical prostatectomy: Combining the best of retropubic and perineal approaches. BJU Int 2014;114(2):236–44.

45. Menon M, Dalela D, Jamil M, et al. Functional Recovery, Oncologic Outcomes and Postoperative Complications after Robot-Assisted Radical Prostatectomy: An Evidence-Based Analysis Comparing the Retzius Sparing and Standard Approaches. J Urol 2018;199(5):1210–7.

46. Dalela D, Jeong W, Prasad MA, et al. A Pragmatic Randomized Controlled Trial Examining the Impact of the Retzius-sparing Approach on Early Urinary Continence Recovery After Robot-assisted Radical Prostatectomy. Eur Urol 2017;72(5):677–85.

47. Abboudi H, Khan MS, Guru KA, et al. Learning curves for urological procedures: A systematic review. BJU Int 2014;114(4):617–29.

48. Thompson JE, Egger S, Böhm M, et al. Superior quality of life and improved surgical margins are achievable with robotic radical prostatectomy after a long learning curve: A prospective single-surgeon study of 1552 consecutive cases. Eur Urol 2014;65(3):521–31.

49. Checcucci E, Veccia A, Fiori C, et al. Retzius-sparing robot-assisted radical prostatectomy vs the standard approach: systematic review and analysis of comparative outcomes. BJU Int 2020;125(1):8–16.

50. Qiu X, Li Y, Chen M, et al. Retzius-sparing robot-assisted radical prostatectomy improves early recovery of urinary continence: a randomized, controlled, single-blind trial with a 1-year follow-up. BJU Int 2020. https://doi.org/10.1111/bju.15195.

51. Cooperberg MR, Broering JM, Carroll PR. Time trends and local variation in primary treatment of localized prostate cancer. J Clin Oncol 2010;28(7):1117–23.

52. Guru AK, Hussain A, Chandrasekhar R, et al. Current status of robot-assisted surgery in urology: a multi-national survey of 297 urologic surgeons. Can J Urol 2009;16(4):4736–41.

53. Alemozaffar M, Regan MM, Cooperberg MR, et al. Prediction of Erectile Function Following Treatment for Prostate Cancer. JAMA 2011;306(11):1205–14.

54. Vickers A, Savage C, Bianco F, et al. Cancer control and functional outcomes after radical prostatectomy as markers of surgical quality: Analysis of heterogeneity between surgeons at a single cancer center. Eur Urol 2011;59(3):317–22.

55. Ahlering TE, Skarecky D, Borin J. Impact of cautery versus cautery-free preservation of neurovascular bundles on early return of potency. J Endourol 2006;20(8):586–9.

Retzius-Sparing Robot-Assisted Robotic Prostatectomy
Past, Present, and Future

Meghan Davis, MD, MPH[a], Jillian Egan, MD[a], Shawn Marhamati, MD[b], Antonio Galfano, MD[c], Keith J. Kowalczyk, MD[a],*

KEYWORDS

- Robotic-assisted surgery • Retzius sparing prostatectomy • Urinary function • Incontinence
- Outcomes • Prostate cancer

KEY POINTS

- Radical prostatectomy has undergone many modifications since its inception, including the Retzius-sparing robotic-assisted radical prostatectomy developed by Galfano and his team in 2010.
- Compared with standard anterior robotic-assisted radical prostatectomy, the Retzius-sparing robotic-assisted radical prostatectomy preserves many structures thought to play a role in urinary continence.
- Comparative studies have demonstrated improved early continence outcomes and equivalent oncologic efficacy with a Retzius sparing approach.
- Further research is needed to evaluate sexual function outcomes as well as long-term oncologic outcomes.

INTRODUCTION

Prostate cancer (PCa) is the most common non-dermatologic malignancy affecting men with an estimated 191,930 new cases diagnosed in the United States in 2020.[1] One-third of patients with localized PCa receive treatment with radical prostatectomy (RP), which is considered the gold standard for treatment.[2] However, urinary incontinence after RP is a significant and under-reported long-term consequence that substantially decreases quality of life. For instance, the US Preventive Services Task Force cites urinary incontinence among the harms of prostate-specific antigen screening, and a US Preventive Services Task Force infographic quotes a 19% incontinence rate after RP.[3] Additionally, 3.7% of men undergoing RP have been reported to go on to have surgery to correct severe incontinence.[4]

Multiple technical modifications have been proposed to improve urinary continence, including the periurethral suspension stitch,[5] bladder neck (BN) preservation,[6] preservation of the puboprostatic ligaments, nerve-sparing, pubovesical complex preservation, and urethral length preservation, as well as anterior and posterior reconstructive strategies, all in an attempt to maintain or restore as much normal pelvic anatomy as possible.[7,8] In

[a] Department of Urology, MedStar Georgetown University Hospital, 3800 Reservoir Road Northwest, Washington, DC 20007, USA; [b] Austin Hospital, Department of Urology, 145 Studley Rd, Heidelberg VIC 3084, Australia; [c] Department of Urology, ASST Grande Ospedale Metropolitano Niguarda, Piazza Ospedale Maggiore, 3, Milano 20162, Italy

* Corresponding author. Department of Urology, MedStar Georgetown University Hospital, 3800 Reservoir Road Northwest, Washington, DC 20007, USA.
E-mail address: keith.kowalczyk@medstar.net
Twitter: @MeghanDavisMD (M.D.); @JillianEganMD (J.E.); @KeithKow (K.J.K.)

Urol Clin N Am 48 (2021) 11–23
https://doi.org/10.1016/j.ucl.2020.09.012
0094-0143/21/© 2020 Elsevier Inc. All rights reserved.

2010, Galfano and colleagues[9] described the Retzius-sparing robot-assisted RP (RS-RARP), a technique that incorporates natural preservation of the pelvic fascial anatomy without a need for reconstruction, which has demonstrated improved short-term urinary continence.[10] However, urologists have been slow to adopt RS-RARP, with a recent poll of 250 respondents demonstrating that only 10.8% of RP are performed with this approach.[11] Therefore, further study is needed to demonstrate reproducibility of RS-RARP short-term outcomes, exhibit improved long-term outcomes, and confirm oncologic efficacy.

In this article, we trace the origins of RP leading to current techniques, review the theoretical anatomic basis of why RS-RARP preserves urinary continence, outline the key steps of the procedure, and summarize outcomes in published series. In our opinion, RS-RARP is not only feasible with equivalent oncologic outcomes compared with standard anterior RARP (S-RARP), but with more study and experience we believe this procedure should become the gold standard for the surgical management of PCa.

RADICAL PROSTATECTOMY: HISTORIC EVOLUTION

The notion of preserving pelvic anatomy during RP dates to 1905 with its conception as perineal RP (PRP) performed by Hugh Hampton Young.[12] At that time, most men with PCa presented at late stages of the disease, with survival estimated at 24 to 30 months after diagnosis. Therefore, surgical management was usually reserved for relief of urinary obstruction rather than for oncologic cure.[13] However, surgical management with PRP evolved and this approach was used for treatment in young and healthy men with palpable disease. In 1947, Millin[14] described the retropubic RP (RRP), which was widely adopted because the anatomy was more familiar and allowed for simultaneous pelvic lymph node dissection through the same incision. However, severe blood loss incurred during transection of the dorsal venous complex (DVC) deterred many from using this approach. Impotence and incontinence were nearly universal. Therefore, RRP failed to gain popularity owing to excessive morbidity, and with the introduction of external beam radiation, surgical management was not considered the gold standard of treatment.[15]

Thirty years later, significant anatomic discoveries by Walsh and colleagues led to RRP modifications that increased the feasibility of the operation and significantly decreased surgical morbidity. In 1979, Reiner and Walsh established

a technique for early DVC control to improve visualization and decrease blood loss, and open retropubic RRP soon became the most common surgical approach to PCa.[16] Further anatomic study of the autonomic nerves originating from the pelvic plexus, located on the lateral surface of the rectum and continuing to innervate the corpora cavernosa, eventually led to nerve-sparing procedures that improved sexual function following nerve-sparing RRP.[17]

Although RRP quickly gained popularity, PRP remained a surgical option, because continence and potency outcomes in contemporary PRP were comparatively favorable, with some reporting continence and potency rates of 95% and 70%, respectively.[18] There was also significantly less blood loss compared with RRP in some series, with no difference in positive surgical margins.[19] However, despite studies showing relatively equivalent outcomes, PRP decreased in popularity, perhaps owing to less familiar anatomy, difficulty in performing concomitant lymph node dissection, and questions regarding oncologic efficacy.

In 1993, Rigatti and colleagues[20] proposed a novel transcoccygeal approach that involved developing the plane between the prostate and rectum to reach the prostatovesical junction posteriorly. With this technique, the bladder remained in its normal anatomic position, although the DVC and puboprostatic ligaments still required transection and ligation.[20] The transcoccygeal approach did not gain traction, likely owing to the need for a separate pelvic lymph node dissection via laparotomy or laparoscopy, and also unfamiliar anatomic approach.[20]

In 2000, the first robotic-assisted RP (RARP) was performed and now makes up greater than 90% of RP performed worldwide,[21,22] with S-RARP the preferred approach for 82% of urologists in a recent online poll.[11] The benefits of RARP are mostly in the perioperative setting with reduced blood loss, pain, length of hospital stay, and earlier return to work. However, RARP functional outcomes reporting is inconsistent and dubious. Recent evidence suggests that the incidence of incontinence (defined as no pad) is between 4% and 31% and the incidence of erectile dysfunction is between 10% and 46% at 1 year after RARP.[23,24] Therefore, it is evident that although S-RARP is currently the most widely used RP approach, improvements in outcomes are still needed.

Traditional S-RARP involves an anterior approach to the prostate by releasing the bladder from its anterior abdominal wall attachments, including the bilateral medial umbilical ligaments and urachus, thus entering the retropubic space of Retzius. Like RRP, this anterior approach necessitates transection of the anterior detrusor apron, puboprostatic ligaments, and both arteries and veins contained within the DVC (**Fig. 1**). Subsequent techniques have evolved to preserve or reconstruct normal anatomy to achieve better sexual and urinary function.[22] The periurethral suspension stitch was introduced to mimic the support provided by the puboprostatic ligaments and some reports showed earlier return to continence as well as improved 3-month post–S-RARP continence rates.[5] Bladder Neck (BN) preservation has been shown to shorten time to continence, as well as possibly improve long-term continence outcomes at 1 year.[6] Other techniques reported include preservation of the puboprostatic ligaments, nerve sparing, preservation of the pubovesical complex or detrusor apron, and preservation of urethral length.[7] However, despite these modifications, urinary continence continues to have a negative impact on health-related quality of life after RARP.[25]

ANATOMIC BASIS OF RETZIUS-SPARING ROBOTIC-ASSISTED RADICAL PROSTATECTOMY

In 2010, Galfano and colleagues[9] described Retzius-sparing robot assisted prostatectomy (RS-RARP), a posterior approach to the prostate that spares all structures anterior to the prostate and bladder and showed earlier return of continence (**Fig. 2**). This result is thought to be due to the preservation of anatomic structures within the anterior pelvic compartment, including the DVC, pubovesical and puboprostatic ligaments, detrusor apron, and endopelvic fascia.[9] However, despite other studies confirming improved continence with RS-RARP, there has not yet been universal acceptance, with only 11% of respondents to a recent online poll stating that this was their preferred RP approach.[11] Concerns regarding this approach, justified or not, include unfamiliarity with the anatomic approach, a possible steep learning curve (although a recent study suggested this is not the case[26]), and an increased risk of positive surgical margins (although most studies show equivalence), as well as uncertainty regarding improvements in long-term continence rates.

One must have an intimate understanding of the fascial and vascular anatomy of the pelvis to understand the theoretic advantages of RS-RARP. Whereas S-RARP requires division and ligation of the DVC, RS-RARP spares the DVC as well as surrounding structures.[22] Anatomic studies revealed that the DVC leaves the penis under Buck's fascia between the corpora cavernosa and penetrates the urogenital diaphragm, dividing into the superficial branch, and the right and left lateral venous plexuses.[15] Up to 40% of the cross-sectional surface area of the urethral sphincter tissue is laterally overlapped by the DVC and might be injured during en bloc ligation.[27]

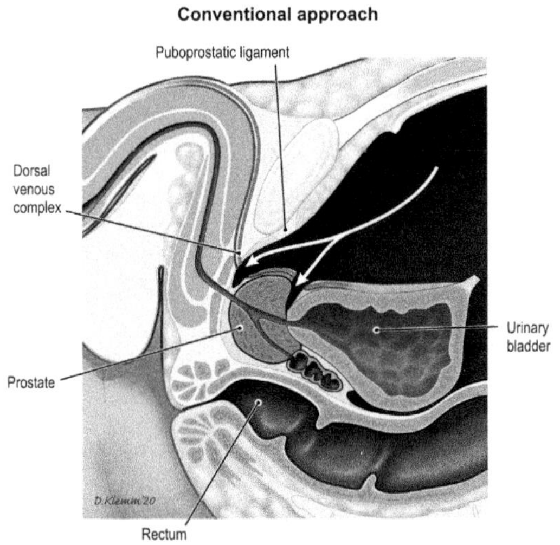

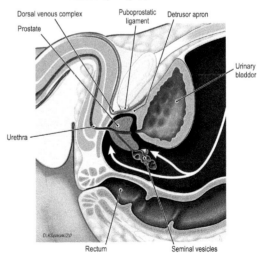

Fig. 1. Sagittal view of dissection planes for conventional anterior robot-assisted RP, which necessitates releasing the bladder from the anterior abdominal wall, division of the detrusor apron, as well as through the arterial and venous structures of the DVC.

Fig. 2. Sagittal view of surgical approach for Retzius sparing, or pelvic fascia sparing, robot-assisted RP. This approach preserves anterior bladder attachments as well as the detrusor apron, prostatic and endopelvic fascia, puboprostatic ligaments, as well as the arteries and veins within the DVC.

Denonvilliers' fascia covers the posterior surface of the prostate, while the lateral endopelvic fascia covers the pelvic musculature. Both of these fascial layers are intimately associated with the DVC, the neurovascular bundle (NVB), and the striated sphincter. The external striated urethral sphincter is thought to be the primary anatomic source of urinary continence. Anatomic studies by Myers and colleagues[28] found that at the apex of the prostate the muscular fibers of the urethral sphincter complex form a tubular striated sphincter surrounding the membranous urethra, with broad attachments over the fascia of the prostate near the apex. Given this, transection of the DVC by definition will injure a portion of the sphincteric complex, and this is a necessary step during the anterior approach of S-RARP that may result in injury to the sphincter and compromised continence.[27] Furthermore, during ligation of the DVC, small accessory arterioles from the pudenal artery are encountered that provide additional blood supply to the sphincter as well as the corpora cavernosum. Preserving these branches may potentially result in improved continence and erectile function postoperatively.[9,29] Last, incision of the endopelvic fascia, given its proximity to the urethral sphincter and the puboperinealis muscle, which functions to pull the perineal body ventrally to the pubic bone, may also compromise continence mechanisms in S-RARP.[7,27] Alternatively, RS-RARP completely spares the endopelvic fascia.

RS-RARP also preserves the pubovesical and puboprostatic ligaments in the anterior pelvis, which help to stabilize and support the bladder and urethra via suspension from the pubic bone.[29] Previous research has shown that a low BN to pubic symphysis ratio is associated with better continence outcomes after S-RARP.[30] Leaving these support structures untouched helps to maintain the normal position of the BN relative to the pubic symphysis. Chang and colleagues[31] evaluated the low BN to pubic symphysis ratio in men undergoing RS-RARP versus S-RARP, and found significantly less bladder descent among the RS-RARP (0.25 vs 0.46; $P = .000$),[30] and low BN to pubic symphysis ratio remained associated with continence recovery in a multivariate analysis.[31]

There are also theoretical anatomic advantages of RS-RARP that may lead to improved sexual function. Prior studies have suggested that preservation of pudendal arteries, DVC, and the endopelvic fascia may improve sexual function, and all of these structures are preserved during RS-RARP.[32] Although sparing the posterolateral NVBs is considered essential in promoting post-

RARP sexual function, a cadaveric study demonstrated that up to one-third of the periprostatic nerves course anteriorly and anterolaterally.[33] Preservation of these nerves as they continue to the cavernous nerves in RS-RARP may lead to improved sexual function outcomes. However, more study is needed to see if there are long-term sexual function advantages of RS-RARP.

SURGICAL TECHNIQUE
Port Placement and Robotic Set-Up

Our RS-RARP technique replicates that of Galfano and colleagues[9] with minor modifications. In contrast to S-RARP, the left second robotic arm is medial and more caudal, at the level of the camera, to decrease arm collisions. Prograsp forceps are placed in this arm. Bipolar Maryland forceps are placed in the left lateral third robotic arm (**Fig. 3**). If using the DaVinci Xi platform, there are no major changes other than changing the camera port to a robotic 8 mm port, side docking of the patient cart, and the ability to easily change from the 30° down lens to the 30° up lens after completion of the seminal vesicles (SV) dissection. Cautery is set at 35 W for monopolar and bipolar on the Si platform, and the ERBE VIO dVÒ 2.0 generator cautery setting is set to 3 for monopolar and bipolar on the Xi platform.

Incision of Peritoneum, Vas Deferens and Seminal Vesicles Dissection, Posterior Dissection

The 0° or 30° lens can be used to start based on surgeon preference and patient anatomy. A horizontal semicircular incision is made at the level of the vas deferens (VD) and SV, identified as an arch anterior to the rectum. Denovillier's fascia is

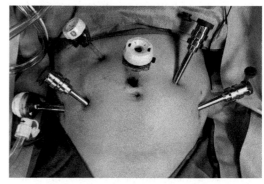

Fig. 3. Schematic of port placement for both RS-RARP and S-RARP. For RS-RARP, the Prograsp forceps placed in the left medial robotic port and a more caudal position, as this minimizes instrument clashing in the small operative space.

exposed posteriorly, and bilateral VD and SV are noted anteriorly. Each VD is dissected laterally and transected, with the SV commonly located inferior to the VD. The SV is bluntly dissected off Denovillier's fascia until lateral arterioles are encountered and dissected with bipolar cautery and sharp dissection. Dissection is continued to the base of the prostate. Continual adjustment of gentle traction with the Prograsp is critical for exposure.

The 30° up lens is used after the SV and VD dissection. Two 3-0 Prolene sutures on a Keith needle are placed through the anterior abdominal wall, through the anterior cut edge of peritoneum, and back through the abdomen for anterior peritoneal retraction. The sutures are clamped extracorporeally, with the SV and VD tucked under the sutures to provide exposure and free the Prograsp for the remainder of the procedure (**Fig. 4**).

The posterior plane is developed by incising Denovillier's fascia and continuing dissection toward the apex and bilateral NVB. During intrafascial nerve sparing, this plane is continued as lateral as possible, directly on the surface of the prostate. We develop this plane more extensively during RS-RARP compared with S-RARP, because it allows for identification of the prostatic arterial pedicles as dissection continues laterally.

Lateral Pedicles and Nerve Sparing

The fourth arm is positioned at the base of the ipsilateral SV for retraction and the medial edge of the pedicle is encountered. With the posterior prostate as a guide, each arteriole is skeletonized and clipped as dissection is carried out anterolaterally using 5-mm clips (Aesculap, Tuttlingen, Germany) and gentle bipolar cautery (**Fig. 5**). After pedicle dissection, the posterolateral intrafascial plane is encountered and the prostate is dissected from the remaining NVB, avoiding traction. With

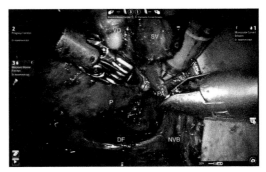

Fig. 5. The right lateral prostatic pedicle is skeletonized and taken athermally with either small clips or bipolar cautery. The posterior prostate is used as a guide during this step.

interfascial or extrafascial approaches, a wider margin is taken compared with an intrafascial approach. The Prograsp is continually repositioned as dissection is advanced toward the apex. Once the prostate is free posteriorly and laterally, the ipsilateral SV and VD are removed from the retraction sutures and the prostate is approached anteriorly, where more arterioles may be found. The anterior detrusor apron is gently teased from the anterolateral prostate and apex. This procedure is repeated on the contralateral side.

Apical and Anterior, Bladder Neck, and Urethral Dissection

The prostate is now retracted posteriorly with the Prograsp, allowing easy identification of detrusor fibers from the detrusor apron inserting into the anterolateral prostate bilaterally (**Fig. 6**). The bladder is retracted anteriorly to create a tension line, and detrusor fibers are gently dissected

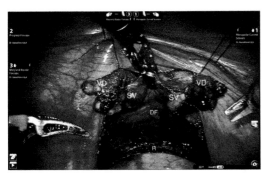

Fig. 4. Exposure of posterior plane after VD and SV dissection and placement of anterior suspension sutures.

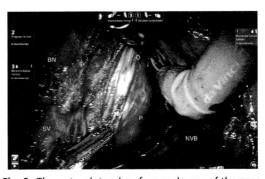

Fig. 6. The anterolateral surface and apex of the prostate are further developed before dissecting the bladder neck. Continuous upward traction on the bladder with the left hand along with posterior retraction with the Prograsp will often reveal the interface between the detrusor fibers and prostate.

away from the anterior and apical prostate bilaterally with light monopolar cautery, taking care to avoid excessive tissue char or desiccation. After dissection of the detrusor apron from the anterior and apical prostate bilaterally, the prostate is gently retracted posteriorly, further exposing the BN. The BN is dissected circumferentially, again with anterior retraction on the bladder and light monopolar cautery. Once skeletonized, the BN is transected exposing the Foley catheter, which is withdrawn, and the anterior BN mucosa is scored with monopolar cautery.

Beyond the BN, the anterior detrusor fibers are dissected with bipolar cautery and sharp dissection to avoid dissecting into the incorrect surgical plane (**Fig. 7**). The fourth arm is continually repositioned to provide posterior traction on the prostate, and the previously dissected anterolateral apex is used as a guide to maintain the correct surgical plane underneath the detrusor apron and DVC. The posterior DVC is entered if there is an anterior lesion. In our experience, DVC bleeding is minimal and rarely requires suturing, because this space is closed with the vesicourethral anastomosis. The anterior urethra is encountered, and anatomy resembles S-RARP. The prostate is gently rotated bilaterally to dissect any remaining apical attachments. The urethra is developed into a large stump and sharply divided just distal to the apex.

Anastomosis

Needle drivers are placed in the first and second arms, leaving the Maryland bipolar forceps in the third arm for hemostasis. A 15 cm 3-0 V-loc (Ethicon Inc., Somerville, NJ) with a CV-23 needle is placed through the anterior BN at the 1:00 position, outside to inside, and the needle is looped and secured to the BN. The suture is then placed

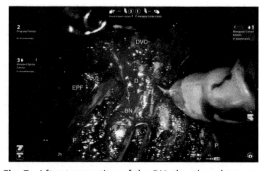

Fig. 7. After transection of the BN, the plane between the anterior prostate and DVC is developed. The prostatic apex is used as a visual guide during dissection. If necessary, the posterior portion of the DVC can be entered if the plane is difficult to establish or in men with anterior lesions.

through the anterior urethra from inside to outside and the BN and urethra are brought together. A second 3-0 V-Loc suture is placed outside to inside on the anterior BN at 11:00. Both sutures are then run to 6:00. Before closing the posterior BN, the catheter is inserted across the anastomosis, which remains at a 90° "coude" angle to the urethra. The right-sided suture is passed inside to outside through the posterior BN and the sutures are tied together. The anastomosis is tested with 120 mL of saline irrigation and drain is omitted if there is no leak.

EARLY RESULTS WITH RETZIUS-SPARING ROBOTIC-ASSISTED RADICAL PROSTATECTOMY
Urinary Outcomes

Nine studies have compared outcomes of RS-RARP and S-RARP (**Table 1**). Following initial description of RS-RARP in 2010, Galfano and colleagues[34] published outcomes from their first 200 patients. After their initial learning curve of 100 patients, 90% of men were using 0 to 1 safety pad within 7 days after catheter removal, and this increased to 96% at 1 year. Early continence rates have been consistently superior for RS-RARP versus S-RARP in other studies (**Table 2**).[10,31,35–39] A 2017 randomized, controlled trial demonstrated RS-RARP versus S-RARP continence rates of 71% versus 48%, respectively, 1 week after catheter removal.[35] Similarly, Chang and colleagues[31] demonstrated immediate continence rates of 73% versus 26% for RS-RARP versus S-RARP in a propensity score–matched analysis, however, 1-year continence rates were similar (RS-RARP 100% vs S-RARP 93.3%; $P = .150$). Sayyid and colleagues[36] also reported on continence at 1 year and found persistently improved continence at 12 months for RS-RARP versus S-RARP when measuring mean pad use (0.6 pads per day vs 1.5 pads per day; $P = .01$). In our own retrospective study of 140 patients undergoing S-RARP and RS-RARP, we saw continual improvements in EPIC-CP urinary incontinence scores out to 12 months that surpassed those seen the S-RARP group, and continence was also significantly improved at 12 months (95.7% vs 85.7%; $P = .042$). Finally, a Cox regression analysis showed a very strong reduction in incontinence risk at 12 months for RS-RARP (hazard ratio, 0.18; 95% confidence interval, 0.05–0.67; $P = .010$).[39]

Oncologic Outcomes

RS-RARP is first and foremost an oncologic operation and therefore ensuring equivalent oncologic

Table 1
Studies comparing RS-RARP versus S-RARP

Author, Year	Country	Study Design	N		Surgical Team	Follow-Up for RS-RARP
			RS-RARP	S-RARP		
Lim et al,[37] 2014	South Korea	Propensity score matched cohort	50	50	Single surgeon	4 wk
Delala et al,[35] 2017	USA	RCT	60	60	Single surgical team	3 mo
Sayyid et al,[36] 2017	USA	Retrospective cohort	100	100	Single surgeon	12 mo
Chang et al,[31] 2018	Taiwan	Propensity score matched cohort	30	30	Single surgeon	12 mo
Eden et al,[10] 2018	UK	Retrospective cohort	40	40	Single surgeon	4 wk
Menon et al,[40] 2018[a]	USA	RCT	60	60	Single surgical team	12 mo
Asimakopoulos et al,[38] 2019	Italy	RCT	45	57	Single surgeon	6 mo
Lee et al,[41] 2020	South Korea	Propensity score matched cohort	609	609	Two surgeons	6 mo
Egan et al,[39] 2020	USA	Retrospective cohort	70	70	Single surgeon	12 mo

Abbreviation: RCT, randomized controlled trial.
[a] One-year update on outcomes from Delala et al.[35]

Table 2
Continence outcomes in studies comparing RS-RARP versus S-RARP

Study	Notes	RS-RARP	S-RARP	P-Value
Lim et al,[37] 2014	At 1 mo postoperatively	Completely dry: 70% Drops ± safety liner: 22% >1 PPD: 8%	Completely dry: 50% Drops ± safety liner: 24% >1 PPD: 26%	.097
Delala et al,[35] 2017	0 PPD or 1 security PPD	Postoperatively[b]: 71% 1 mo: 83% 2 mo: 88%	Postoperatively: 48% 1 mo: 67% 2 mo: 72%	.02[c]
Sayyid et al,[36] 2017	Mean number of PPD	3 mo: 1.5 6 mo: 0.9 9 mo: 1.0 12 mo: 0.6	3 mo: 3.2 6 mo: 2.3 9 mo: 1.9 12 mo: 1.5	<.001 <.001 .03 .01
Chang et al,[31] 2018	<1 safety pad/d	Postoperatively: 73.3% 1 mo: 91.0% 3 mo: 94.2% 6 mo: 97.7% 12 mo: 100%	Postoperatively: 26.7% 1 mo: 30.0% 3 mo: 56.7% 6 mo: 76.7% 12 mo: 93.3%	<.001[c]
Eden et al,[10] 2018	At 4 wk postoperatively	0PPD: 90% 1 PPD 7.5% 2 PPD 2.5%	0PPD: 37.5% 1 PPD 32.5% 2 PPD 30%	<.001 .01 .002
Menon et al,[40] 2018[a]	0 PPD or 1 security PPD	3 mo: 93.3% 6 mo: 98.3% 12 mo: 98.3%	3 mo: 85.0% 6 mo: 93.3% 12 mo: 93.3%	.09[c]
Asimakopoulos et al,[38] 2019	0 PPD or no leakage	Postoperatively: 51%. 1 mo: 81.0% 3 mo: 90.5% 6 mo: 90.5%	Postoperatively: 21%. 1 mo: 47.4% 3 mo: 60.0% 6 mo: 64.1%	.02[c]
Lee et al,[41] 2020	<1 safety liner per day	1 mo: 45% 6 mo: 98%	1 mo: 9% 6 mo: 77%	<.001[c]
Egan et al,[39] 2020	EPIC-CP Urinary incontinence scores	Baseline 1.0 6 wk: 3.2 3 mo: 2.1 6 mo: 1.7 9 mo: 1.3 12 mo: 1.0	Baseline 0.7 6 wk: 4.4 3 mo: 3.4 6 mo: 2.4 9 mo: 2.4 12 mo: 2.3	.240 .014 .008 .076 .010 .033
	0–1 safety pad (12 mo)	97.6%	81.4%	.002

Abbreviations: EPIC-CP, expanded prostate cancer index composite for clinical practice; PPD, pads per day.
[a] One-year update on outcomes from the Delala et al[35] RCT.
[b] Postoperatively refers to outcomes less than 4 weeks postoperatively.
[c] P value based on Kaplan–Meier curves with log-rank tests for comparison.

outcomes is critical (**Table 3**). Multiple studies demonstrate similar rates of positive surgical margins (PSMs) as well as similar 1-year biochemical recurrence-free survival.[10,31,35–37,39–41] When examining their own learning curve over their first 200 RS-RARP, Galfano and colleagues[34] found that that PSM decreased from 22% in the first 100 patients versus 9% second 100 patients, with the majority of the PSMs at the apex. This result has been similarly seen in past laparoscopic and robotic RP series early in the learning curve.[42–44] Menon and colleagues[40] found no difference in the rates of focal or nonfocal PSM, despite a significantly greater proportion of pT3 disease in the RS-RARP cohort. There were also no significant differences in the location of the positive margins or biochemical recurrence-free survival at 18 months. Asimakopoulos and colleagues[38] did find a significant difference in the PSM (28.2% PSM in RS-RARP vs 10% PSM S-RARP; P = .05); however, when evaluated by pathologic stage, there were no significant

Table 3
Oncologic outcomes in studies comparing RS-RARP versus S-RARP

Study	Positive Surgical Margin (%)[a]			BCRFS (%)		Time since Surgery (mo)	P Value
	RS-RARP	S-RARP	P Value	RS-RARP	S-RARP		
Lim et al,[37] 2014.	14%	14%	.42	NR	NR		NR
Delala et al,[35] 2017	Nonfocal: 11.7%	Nonfocal: 8.3%	.2	91	91	3	.5
Sayyid et al,[36] 2017	≤T2: 16.7% ≥T3: 47.1%	≤T2: 13% ≥T3: 47.8%	.54 .95	NR	NR	-	-
Chang et al,[31] 2018	23.3%	26.7%	.62	86.7	83.3	12	.718
Eden et al,[10] 2018	T2: 16.7% T3: 31.8%	T2: 7.7% T3: 14.3%	.65 .44	NR	NR	-	-
Menon et al,[40] 2018[b]	Focal: 13.3% Nonfocal: 11.7%	Focal: 5.0% Nonfocal: 8.3%	.2 .2	83.8	92.7	18	.3
Asimako-poulos et al,[38] 2019	T2: 19.0% T3: 41.2%	T2: 6.7% T3: 22.2%	.21 .33	91.4	92.7	12	NS
Lee et al,[41] 2020	T2: 11% T3: 36%	T2: 15% T3: 32%	.13 .45	NR	NR	-	-
Egan et al,[39] 2020	Focal: 27.1% Nonfocal: 7.1%	Focal: 21.4% Nonfocal: 8.6%	.43 .02	87.1	81.4	12	.357

Abbreviations: BCRFS, biochemical recurrence free survival; NR, not reported; NS, not significant.
[a] Overall positive surgical margin rate unless otherwise noted.
[b] One year update on outcomes from Delala et al[35] RCT.

differences. Lim and colleagues[37] did not note an overall difference in PSM; however, they did note that most PSM were anterior, which was thought to be due the absence of a definite plane between the prostate and the urinary sphincter at the apex. The surgeons modified their technique to direct their dissection more anteriorly at the expense of partial DVC resection.[37] All of these studies are limited by the relatively short follow-up for RS-RARP, and longer term data are needed to fully evaluate oncologic outcomes of this technique. However, the majority of series show no significant difference in PSM rates or biochemical recurrence-free survival, demonstrating that RS-RARP is likely oncologically equivalent to S-RARP.

Sexual Outcomes

Although RS-RARP is associated with early return of continence, there has been less comparative research on erectile and overall sexual function after RS-RARP (**Table 4**). Although theoretically the preservation of the DVC and pudendal arteries combined with complete intrafascial nerve sparing

may result in better sexual function outcomes, this result has yet to be demonstrated, although longer follow-up may be needed to actualize this benefit.[27,29]

Among the cohort from the Galfano and colleagues[34] series, the median 1-year International Index for Erectile Function score was 18, although baseline values were not reported, and this outcome was not compared with S-RARP outcomes. Menon and colleagues[40] found no significant differences in the potency rates or percentage of men regaining a Sexual Health Inventory for Men score of greater than 17 at 1 year. In our series, we also found no significant differences in EPIC-CP sexual function scores or potency at 12 months postoperatively.[39]

AREAS OF FUTURE STUDY

The preservation of the natural arterial and venous supply to the penis could result in less penile shortening, which is a known but sometimes neglected or forgotten side effect of RP.[45–48] Gontero and colleagues[49] studied penile shortening

Table 4
Sexual function outcomes

Study	Notes	RS-RARP	S-RARP	P Value
Galfano et al,[34] 2013	IIEF Score at 12 mo	18	NR	–
Menon et al,[40] 2018.	Potency (sufficient for penetrative at 1 y Postoperatively), %	86.5	69.2	.500
	SHIM >17, %	44.1	44.6	.9
Egan et al,[39] 2020	EPIC-CP Sexual Function scores	Baseline 2.9	Baseline 3.1	.701
		6 wk: 8.1	6 wk: 8.8	.218
		3 mo: 7.3	3 mo: 7.6	.653
		6 mo: 6.6	6 mo: 6.8	.764
		9 mo: 5.3	9 mo: 6.9	.091
		12 mo: 4.6	12 mo: 5.3	.417
	Potency (sufficient for sexual activity), %	65.7	62.9	.727

Abbreviations: EPIC-CP, expanded prostate cancer index; IIEF, international index of erectile function. Composite for Clinical Practice, NR, not reported; SHIM, Sexual Health Inventory for Men.

after RP, noting that maximal penile shortening measured by stretched length occurred at the time of catheter removal, with a lesser but still significant degree of shortening over 1 year postoperatively. Significant predictors of preserved penile length were a nerve-sparing procedure and recovery of erectile function. However, these patients underwent RRP and, although not noted specifically, likely also with division of the DVC. Therefore, the effect of DVC preservation on penile length and sexual function remains unknown, and there have yet to be any studies assessing penile length preservation following RS-RARP.

Another less reported complication of RP is the development of Peyronie's disease (PD), which is an inflammatory process leading to penile deformity and, in extreme cases, an inability to have penetrative intercourse. Tal and colleagues[50] reported a much higher incidence of PD in men undergoing RRP than the general population at 15.9%, with younger age and Caucasian race as independent predictive factors. However, the pathophysiology of this phenomenon after RP remains difficult to discern. Trauma remains a well-known cause in developing PD in the general population. It has been suggested that PD subsequently results from repetitive microvascular injury, resulting in fibrin deposition and trapping within the tunica albuginea that surrounds the corpora. This process results in fibroblast activation and proliferation, enhanced vessel permeability, and leukocyte proliferation, as in normal healing. However, in PD, the fibroblastic lesion fails to resolve, collagen also becomes trapped, and pathologic fibrosis ensues.[51] One potential source of microvascular injury during conventional RP and RARP is ligation of the DVC, which contains arterioles to the corpora, as mentioned elsewhere in this article. The ability to spare these structures during RS-RARP may lead to reduced incidence of PD; however, large collaborative studies are needed to test this theory.

Finally, inguinal hernia development is a known complication of both RRP and S-RARP. This entity was described in an RRP series by Regan and colleagues[52] at Georgetown University Hospital, with an incidence of up to 12% 6 months following surgery. Yamada and colleagues[53] found a 15.4% incidence of inguinal hernia development at 3 years after RARP, which was associated with poorer urinary outcomes. Therefore, inguinal hernia remains a significant but largely ignored complication after both RRP and RARP. With RS-RARP, there is no separation of the bladder from the anterior abdominal wall, and therefore one could reason that there should be fewer inguinal hernias with this approach. However, this notion also has yet to be studied.

SUMMARY

Although RP has undergone many changes since its first conception, RS-RARP has the potential to become the new gold standard for PCa treatment with improved early continence and equivalent oncologic efficacy as S-RARP. Future research and longer follow-up is needed to determine if there is improved sexual function outcomes given preservation of multiple structures in the anterior pelvis, and also to see if other less studied outcomes such as penile shortening and inguinal hernia rates improve with RS-RARP. Collaborative and randomized studies among urologists performing RS-RARP are needed to solidify RS-RARP as an accepted and gold standard treatment for PCa.

CLINICS CARE POINTS (KEY POINTS)

- Several comparative studies have demonstrated improved early continence outcomes with RS-RARP compared to S-RARP.
- Current data suggests equivalent oncologic outcomes, but this comparison is limited by short duration of follow-up. Study of sexual outcomes following RS-RARP has been limited.

ACKNOWLEDGMENTS

Medical illustrations by David Klemm, Georgetown University Medical Center, Washington DC USA

DISCLOSURES

None.

REFERENCES

1. Siegel R, Naishadham D, Jemal A. Cancer statistics, 2013. CA Cancer J Clin 2013;63(1):11–30.
2. Chen J, Oromendia C, Halpern JA, et al. National trends in management of localized prostate cancer: a population based analysis 2004-2013. Prostate 2018;78(7):512–20.
3. Holt JD, Gerayli F. Prostate cancer screening. Prim Care 2019;46(2):257–63.
4. Nelson M, Dornbier R, Kirshenbaum E, et al. Use of surgery for post-prostatectomy incontinence. J Urol 2020;203(4):786–91.
5. Patel VR, Coelho RF, Palmer KJ, et al. Periurethral suspension stitch during robot-assisted laparoscopic radical prostatectomy· description of the technique and continence outcomes. Eur Urol 2009;56(3):472–8.
6. Ma X, Tang K, Yang C, et al. Bladder neck preservation improves time to continence after radical prostatectomy: a systematic review and meta-analysis. Oncotarget 2016;7(41):67463–75.
7. Kojima Y, Takahashi N, Haga N, et al. Urinary incontinence after robot-assisted radical prostatectomy: pathophysiology and intraoperative techniques to improve surgical outcome. Int J Urol 2013;20(11):1052–63.
8. Vora AA, Dajani D, Lynch JH, et al. Anatomic and technical considerations for optimizing recovery of urinary function during robotic-assisted radical prostatectomy. Curr Opin Urol 2013;23(1):78–87.
9. Galfano A, Ascione A, Grimaldi S, et al. A new anatomic approach for robot-assisted laparoscopic prostatectomy: a feasibility study for completely intrafascial surgery. Eur Urol 2010;58(3):457–61.
10. Eden CG, Moschonas D, Soares R. Urinary continence four weeks following Retzius-sparing robotic radical prostatectomy: the UK experience. J Clin Urol 2018;11(1):15–20.
11. Kowalczyk KJ. Available at: https://twitter.com/KeithKow/status/1237406461686435842?s=20. Twitter. Accessed April 14, 2020.
12. Young HH. The early diagnosis and radical cure of carcinoma of the prostate. Being a study of 40 cases and presentation of a radical operation which was carried out in four cases. 1905. J Urol 2002;168(3):914–21.
13. Rolnick HC. Radical perineal prostatectomy for carcinoma. J Urol 1935;34(2):116–21.
14. Retropubic urinary surgery: by Terence Millin, M.D., Surgeon, all saints hospital for genito-urinary diseases, London. Pp. 208, with 163 illustrations. Baltimore, 1947, Williams & Wilkins Company. Surgery 1949;25(4):654.
15. Walsh PC. Anatomic radical prostatectomy. J Urol 1998;160(6 Pt 2):2418–24.
16. Reiner WG, Walsh PC. An anatomical approach to the surgical management of the dorsal vein and Santorini's plexus during radical retropubic surgery. J Urol 1979;121(2):198–200.
17. Walsh PC, Lepor H, Eggleston JC. Radical prostatectomy with preservation of sexual function: anatomical and pathological considerations. Prostate 1983;4(5):473–85.
18. Weldon VE, Tavel FR, Neuwirth H. Continence, potency and morbidity after radical perineal prostatectomy. J Urol 1997;158(4):1470–5.
19. Frazier HA, Robertson JE, Paulson DF. Radical prostatectomy: the pros and cons of the perineal versus retropubic approach. J Urol 1992;147(3 II):888–90.
20. Rigatti P, Da Pozzo L, Francesca F, et al. Transcoccygeal radical prostatectomy for localized prostate cancer: early clinical results. In: European Urology. Eur Urol 1993;24:29–33.
21. Pasticier G, Rietbergen JBW, Guillonneau B, et al. Robotically assisted laparoscopic radical prostatectomy: feasibility study in men. Eur Urol 2001;40(1):70–4.
22. Lepor H. A review of surgical techniques for radical prostatectomy. Rev Urol 2005;7(Suppl 2):S11–7. Available at: http://www.ncbi.nlm.nih.gov/pubmed/16985892. Accessed March 14, 2020.
23. Ficarra V, Novara G, Rosen RC, et al. Systematic review and meta-analysis of studies reporting urinary continence recovery after robot-assisted radical prostatectomy. Eur Urol 2012;62(3):405–17.
24. Ficarra V, Novara G, Ahlering TE, et al. Systematic review and meta-analysis of studies reporting potency rates after robot-assisted radical prostatectomy. Eur Urol 2012;62(3):418–30.

25. Hoffman KE, Penson DF, Zhao Z, et al. Patient-reported outcomes through 5 years for active surveillance, surgery, brachytherapy, or external beam radiation with or without androgen deprivation therapy for localized prostate cancer. JAMA 2020;323(2):149–63.

26. Olivero A, Galfano A, Piccinelli M, et al. Retzius-sparing robotic radical prostatectomy for surgeons in the learning curve: a propensity score–matching analysis. Eur Urol Focus 2020. https://doi.org/10.1016/j.euf.2020.03.002.

27. Walz J, Epstein JI, Ganzer R, et al. A critical analysis of the current knowledge of surgical anatomy of the prostate related to optimisation of cancer control and preservation of continence and erection in candidates for radical prostatectomy: an update. Eur Urol 2016;70(2):301–11.

28. Myers RP, Goellner JR, Cahill DR. Prostate shape, external striated urethral sphincter and radical prostatectomy: the apical dissection. J Urol 1987;138(3):543–50.

29. Walz J, Burnett AL, Costello AJ, et al. A critical analysis of the current knowledge of surgical anatomy of the prostate related to optimisation of cancer control and preservation of continence and erection in candidates for radical prostatectomy: an update. Eur Urol 2010;57(2):179–92.

30. Olgin G, Alsyouf M, Han D, et al. Postoperative cystogram findings predict incontinence following robot-assisted radical prostatectomy. J Endourol 2014;28(12):1460–3.

31. Chang LW, Hung SC, Hu JC, et al. Retzius-sparing robotic-assisted radical prostatectomy associated with less bladder neck descent and better early continence outcome. Anticancer Res 2018;38(1):345–51.

32. Secin FP, Touijer K, Mulhall J, et al. Anatomy and preservation of accessory pudendal arteries in laparoscopic radical prostatectomy. Eur Urol 2007;51(5):1229–35.

33. Alsaid B, Bessede T, Diallo D, et al. Division of autonomic nerves within the neurovascular bundles distally into corpora cavernosa and corpus spongiosum components: immunohistochemical confirmation with three-dimensional reconstruction. Eur Urol 2011;59(6):902–9.

34. Galfano A, Di Trapani D, Sozzi F, et al. Beyond the learning curve of the Retzius-sparing approach for robot-assisted laparoscopic radical prostatectomy: oncologic and functional results of the first 200 patients with ≥1 year of follow-up. Eur Urol 2013;64(6):974–80.

35. Dalela D, Jeong W, Prasad MA, et al. A pragmatic randomized controlled trial examining the impact of the Retzius-sparing approach on early urinary continence recovery after robot-assisted radical prostatectomy. Eur Urol 2017;72(5):677–85.

36. Sayyid RK, Simpson WG, Lu C, et al. Retzius-sparing robotic-assisted laparoscopic radical prostatectomy: a safe surgical technique with superior continence outcomes. J Endourol 2017;31(12):1244–50.

37. Lim SK, Kim KH, Shin TY, et al. Retzius-sparing robot-assisted laparoscopic radical prostatectomy: combining the best of retropubic and perineal approaches. BJU Int 2014;114(2):236–44.

38. Asimakopoulos AD, Topazio L, De Angelis M, et al. Retzius-sparing versus standard robot-assisted radical prostatectomy: a prospective randomized comparison on immediate continence rates. Surg Endosc 2019;33(7):2187–96.

39. Egan J, Marhamati S, Carvalho F, et al. Retzius-sparing robot-assisted radical prostatectomy leads to durable improvement in urinary function and quality of life versus standard robot-assisted radical prostatectomy without compromise of oncologic efficacy: single surgeon series and step-by-step. Eur Urol 2020. https://doi.org/10.1016/j.eururo.2020.05.010.

40. Menon M, Dalela D, Jamil M, et al. Functional recovery, oncologic outcomes and postoperative complications after robot-assisted radical prostatectomy: an evidence-based analysis comparing the Retzius sparing and standard approaches. J Urol 2018;199(5):1210–7.

41. Lee J, Kim HY, Goh HJ, et al. Retzius sparing robot-assisted radical prostatectomy conveys early regain of continence over conventional robot-assisted radical prostatectomy: a propensity score matched analysis of 1,863 patients. J Urol 2020;203(1):137–44.

42. Katz R, Salomon L, Hoznek A, et al. Positive surgical margins in laparoscopic radical prostatectomy: the impact of apical dissection, bladder neck remodeling and nerve preservation. J Urol 2003. https://doi.org/10.1097/01.ju.0000065822.15012.b7.

43. Williams SB, Chen MH, D'Amico AV, et al. Radical retropubic prostatectomy and robotic-assisted laparoscopic prostatectomy: likelihood of positive surgical margin(s). Urology 2010. https://doi.org/10.1016/j.urology.2009.11.079.

44. Checcucci E, Veccia A, Fiori C, et al. Retzius-sparing robot-assisted radical prostatectomy vs the standard approach: a systematic review and analysis of comparative outcomes. BJU Int 2020;125(1):8–16.

45. Mulhall JP. Penile length changes after radical prostatectomy. BJU Int 2005;96(4):472–4.

46. Frey AU, Sønksen J, Fode M. Neglected side effects after radical prostatectomy: a systematic review. J Sex Med 2014;11(2):374–85.

47. Carlsson S, Nilsson AE, Johansson E, et al. Self-perceived penile shortening after radical

prostatectomy. Int J Impot Res 2012;24(5): 179–84.

48. Munding MD, Wessells HB, Dalkin BL. Pilot study of changes in stretched penile length 3 months after radical retropubic prostatectomy. Urology 2001; 58(4):567–9.

49. Gontero P, Galzerano M, Bartoletti R, et al. New insights into the pathogenesis of penile shortening after radical prostatectomy and the role of postoperative sexual function. J Urol 2007;178(2): 602–7.

50. Tal R, Heck M, Teloken P, et al. Peyronie's disease following radical prostatectomy:

incidence and predictors. J Sex Med 2010; 7(3):1254–61.

51. Devine CJ, Somers KD, Jordan GH, et al. Proposal: trauma as the cause of the Peyronie's lesion. Elsevier Inc. J Urol 1997;157:285–90

52. Regan TC, Mordkin RM, Constantinople NL, et al. Incidence of inguinal hernias following radical retropubic prostatectomy. Urology 1996;47(4):536–7.

53. Yamada Y, Fujimura T, Fukuhara H, et al. Incidence and risk factors of inguinal hernia after robot-assisted radical prostatectomy. World J Surg Oncol 2017; 15(1). https://doi.org/10.1186/s12957-017-1126-3.

Recent Advances and Current Role of Transperineal Prostate Biopsy

Yasin Bhanji, MD[a], Mathew J. Allaway, DO[b], Michael A. Gorin, MD[b],*

KEYWORDS

- Transperineal prostate biopsy • Infection • Sepsis • Transrectal prostate biopsy • Prostate cancer
- MRI • Robot-assisted • Transrectal ultrasound

KEY POINTS

- Transrectal prostate biopsy remains the most commonly performed type of prostate biopsy, but is limited by a high false-negative rate and is associated with the risk of life-threatening infections.
- Transperineal prostate biopsy is associated with a decreased risk of infectious complications, whereas transrectal prostate biopsy has been shown to have a lower risk of post-biopsy acute urinary retention but a higher risk of hematochezia.
- Freehand transperineal prostate biopsy can be performed safely in an outpatient setting using local anesthesia.
- Targeted prostate biopsy using MRI and ultrasound-fusion in combination with the transperineal approach results in high detection rates of clinically significant cancer and more accurate sampling of the anterior prostate gland.
- Robot-assisted image-guided transperineal biopsy offers the potential of more accurate targeted biopsies that can be pre-planned and reduce interoperator variability; however, the benefits of this approach must be studied further, particularly with respect to issues of cost-effectiveness.

INTRODUCTION

In recent decades, the routine use of prostate-specific antigen (PSA) testing has led to an increase in the number of men undergoing a prostate biopsy.[1,2] By one estimate, up to 1 million prostate biopsies are performed annually in the United States alone.[3] Given the large number of prostate biopsies performed throughout the world, there has been significant effort to determine the most accurate method for performing this procedure with the lowest the risk of complications.

At the present time, prostate biopsy is most commonly performed via a transrectal (TR) approach using ultrasound guidance. In recent years, multiparametric MRI has been shown to greatly improve the detection of clinically significant prostate cancer.[4–7] As a result, multiple biopsy platforms have been developed that allow for the fusion of MRI and live transrectal ultrasound images to augment the user's ability to detect prostate cancer.[8,9] Although these advancements have improved accuracy, use of TR prostate biopsy is associated with a high risk of infectious

Conflicts of Interest: M.J. Allaway is the founder and CEO of Perineologic, a subsidiary of Corbin Clinical Resources, LLC. M.A. Gorin is a paid consultant for BK Medical ApS, KOELIS Inc., and Corbin Clinical Resources, LLC.
[a] The James Buchanan Brady Urological Institute and Department of Urology, Johns Hopkins University School of Medicine, 600 N. Wolfe Street, Marburg 134, Baltimore, MD 21287, USA; [b] Urology Associates and UPMC Western Maryland, 12234 Williams Road, Cumberland, MD 21502, USA
* Corresponding author.
E-mail address: mgorin@urologyassociatesmd.com

complications.[10] Thus, in recent years there has been growing interest in performing prostate biopsies percutaneously via a transperineal approach (TP), thereby avoiding rectal bacteria.

In this review, we offer a comparison of the TR and TP approaches to prostate biopsy with regard to rates of complications, cancer detection, and patient comfort. In addition, we provide a procedural overview of the most common approaches for performing TP prostate biopsy. Finally, we discuss recent innovations in this procedure including the incorporation of MRI guidance and the robotic approach.

COMPARISON OF TRANSRECTAL AND TRANSPERINEAL PROSTATE BIOPSY
Infectious Complications

TR prostate biopsy has a relatively short learning curve and can be performed quickly in the office setting under local anesthesia. These factors have led to its widespread adoption and popularity since it was first described in the 1980s.[11,12] However, prostate biopsy via the TR approach places men at risk of infectious complications due to the passage of needles through the rectal mucosa on their course to the prostate. As a result, fecal flora may enter into the prostate, a highly vascular organ, leading to a number of infectious complications including cystitis, prostatitis, epididymitis, and bacteremia. According to one report, the rates of infectious complications related to prostate biopsy range from 0.1% to 7.0%, and sepsis rates range from 0.3% to 3.1%.[10]

The risk of post-biopsy sepsis after TR prostate biopsy has long been recognized, and prophylactic antibiotics are routinely given in anticipation of this procedure. Despite the use of prophylactic antibiotics, the rates of post-TR biopsy infection continue to rise.[13] This is likely due to the emergence of multidrug-resistant bacteria, with recent reports suggesting rates as high as 20% to 30%.[14,15] One of the main drivers for severe infection is the presence of fluoroquinolone-resistant fecal bacteria, likely due to widespread use of this class of antibiotics in human and veterinary medicine as well as animal husbandry. To combat this, some clinicians who perform TR prostate biopsy now routinely use targeted prophylaxis after culturing the patient's rectal flora.[16,17] Although this practice is effective in reducing infectious complications from prostate biopsy, it risks contributing to the rise of multidrug-resistant bacteria[18] and continues to place patients at risk of complications of antibiotic administration

including gastrointestinal side effects and allergic reactions.[19,20]

TP prostate biopsy, which avoids violation of the rectal mucosa, reduces the chance of inoculating the prostate and bloodstream with rectal flora and has been shown to vastly reduce the rates of infectious complications, even in the absence of any periprocedural antibiotics. The case for TP prostate biopsy to reduce the risk of infectious complications is not entirely novel. In the early 1980s, Thompson and colleagues[21] found lower rates of bacteremia and plasma endotoxin levels in the bloodstream of patients who underwent a TP versus a TR prostate biopsy. Furthermore, of the patients studied, none of those who underwent a TP biopsy had a symptomatic infection and the organisms causing the bacteremia in these patients were predominantly skin contaminants. This is in contrast to the patients who underwent a TR prostate biopsy, of which 27% suffered symptomatic bacteremia.

At present, there have been no adequately powered randomized controlled trials comparing TR and TP prostate biopsy with respect to infectious complications. However, the available data from mostly single-arm studies does show lower rates of infectious complications when using a TP approach. In one prospective study of 577 patients who underwent a TP biopsy after receiving a single dose of intravenous cephalsporin antibiotics, no patients were readmitted to hospital with a post-biopsy infection.[22] Consistent with this, a recent systematic review of the literature that identified 16 mutually exclusive series of TP biopsies in a total of 6609 patients found that only 5 were readmitted to the hospital for sepsis for a rate of 0.076%.[23] This is further corroborated by a recent systematic review and meta-analysis of 11 studies comparing the complication rates and outcomes of more than 1600 patients who underwent either a TR or TP prostate biopsy.[24] Given the difficulty of obtaining positive blood cultures during a septic episode after prostate biopsy, this study examined the rate of fever as a surrogate for infection. The investigators found a nearly fivefold reduction in the rate of post-biopsy fever in those who underwent a TP prostate biopsy for a relative risk of 0.26 (95% confidence interval [CI] 0.14–0.48). Based on these data, some in the field have now even embraced performing TP prostate biopsy without any antibiotic prophylaxis.[25,26]

Noninfectious Complications

A number of noninfectious complications are possible after prostate biopsy, regardless of approach. These complications include hematuria, hematochezia, hematospermia, pain, and urinary retention. In the meta-analysis of 11 studies cited earlier, the investigators compared the relative risk for a number of noninfectious complications and found that the TP approach was associated with a lower risk of rectal bleeding, with a relative risk of 0.02 (95% CI 0.01–0.06).[24] Notably, there was no significant difference in the rates of acute urinary retention or hematuria in this particular study.

Some have noted that the risk of acute urinary retention after TP prostate biopsy as a reason not to pursue this approach. In one of the largest series of freehand TP prostate biopsy ever performed, urologists at North York General Hospital in Toronto, Canada, reported acute urinary retention in only 1.6% of 1237 patients studied.[27] On the other hand, in the PICTURE study, in which 249 men underwent multiparametric MRI followed by a TP template prostate mapping biopsy, 24% of men experienced post-biopsy acute urinary retention requiring a temporary catheter.[28] However, within this cohort, a median of 49 cores at 5-mm intervals were taken at the time of biopsy, possibly leading to significant periurethral swelling and therefore the higher rate of post-biopsy retention. There is no formal guideline on the recommended number of cores to be taken during TP prostate biopsy, and this number can vary greatly depending on the exact method used and size of the prostate gland. Some have considered as few as 12 to 14 cores to be adequate,[25] whereas others consider an average of more than 50 cores acceptable for a mapping biopsy.[29] As such, it is difficult to know if the increased risk of acute urinary retention after TP prostate biopsy is due to the approach used or simply related to the number of cores obtained.

Cancer Detection

In addition to significantly decreased rates of infectious complications, the possibility of improved cancer detection rates has also been considered an advantage of TP prostate biopsy. In one of the earliest systematic reviews and meta-analyses comparing TR with TP prostate biopsy, Shen and colleagues[30] found no significant difference in prostate cancer detection rates between the 2 procedures, even when the analysis was subdivided by extent of biopsy. However, it has previously been reported that TR prostate biopsy has a false-negative rate of 20% to 30%.[31] As early as 2000, Vis and colleagues[32] compared the diagnostic yield of the 2 approaches to prostate biopsy. Radical prostatectomy specimens

with TR prostate biopsy–detected cancer were used to perform simulated TP biopsies and repeat TR biopsies. The differences in simulated diagnostic yield were significant, with 82.5% of the known tumors detected with the TP approach versus 72.5% of cancers detection during repeat TR biopsy.

More recently, Hossack and colleagues[33] retrospectively reviewed 1132 radical prostatectomy specimens and found that although the TR and TP approaches identified cancers of similar size, stage, and significance, TP biopsy detected proportionally more anterior tumors and identified them at a smaller size and stage when compared with TR biopsy. Still others have found that men who underwent a TR biopsy were more likely to be upgraded to a higher clinical risk category at radical prostatectomy when compared with those who underwent a TP procedure.[34] This finding was echoed in a prospective, randomized comparison of the diagnostic accuracy of TP and TR prostate biopsies conducted by Takenaka and colleagues,[35] which found that in men with a PSA between 4.1 and 10 ng/mL, TP prostate biopsy was more likely to reveal positive biopsy cores, especially among transition zone cores.

The reason for the previously mentioned data suggesting the superiority of TP biopsy for diagnosing prostate cancer undoubtedly lies in the procedure's inherent ability to better sample the anterior prostate (**Fig. 1**). By one estimate, up to 40% of prostate tumors are found in the anterior portion of the gland.[36] In this same study, the investigators reported that approximately 80% of all tumors missed on temple-based TR prostate biopsy were found in the anterior prostate. Furthermore, anterior tumors appear to be more prominent in African American men, a population in which prostate cancer diagnosis is often delayed,[37] and these tumors tend to be more aggressive than tumors arising elsewhere in the gland.[38,39]

Patient Comfort

Another common hesitation among clinicians in considering the TP approach to prostate biopsy is the thought that this procedure requires general or spinal anesthesia, adding substantial time and risk. Although historically this had been the case, this is no longer true, and TP biopsy can now be safely and comfortably performed in the ambulatory setting under local anesthesia. In recent years, a variety of techniques have been described for achieving adequate local anesthesia during TP biopsy, including but not limited to subcutaneous perineal nerve block, periprostatic nerve block,

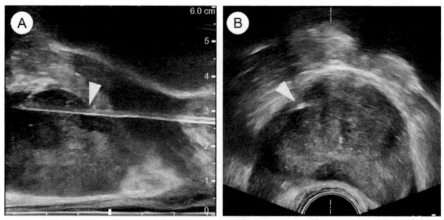

Fig. 1. Sampling of the anterolateral prostate using the transperineal approach. (*A*) Axial and (*B*) sagittal transrectal ultrasound images acquired during a freehand transperineal prostate biopsy. Yellow arrows point to the location of the biopsy needle.

pudendal nerve block, or prostatic apex nerve block.[40] Using the periprostatic nerve block, Kum and colleagues[41] found acceptable pain scores among patients undergoing TP prostate biopsy, as prospectively assessed using a visual analog scale. Patients reported a median pain score of 10.5 out of 100 with probe insertion, 37.5 with local anesthetic administration, and 28 with biopsy performance. These values are within acceptable limits for procedures performed under local anesthesia and these finding have been echoed in other reports such as a study by Marra and colleagues.[42]

PROCEDURAL ASPECTS OF TRANSPERINEAL PROSTATE BIOPSY
Mechanical Stepper-Based Approach

The most common method for performing transperineal prostate biopsy involves the use of a mechanical stepper unit equipped with a grid needle guide (**Fig. 2**). The ultrasound probe is mounted to the stepper unit and needles are passed through the grid, which is pressed against the perineal skin. This technique allows the urologist to sample the prostate in a systematic fashion following one of several previously described template patterns.[43] Although effective

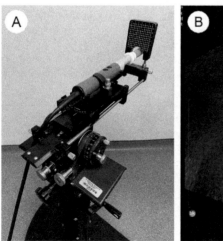

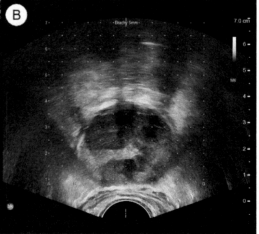

Fig. 2. Mechanical stepper-based transperineal prostate biopsy. (*A*) Image of a stepper unit equipped with a grid plate. The needle holes of the grid are spaced 5 mm apart. (*B*) Axial transrectal ultrasound image of the prostate with the overlaid grid template.

for sampling the prostate, this technique suffers from the shortcoming of requiring either general or spinal anesthesia in order for patients to tolerate the large number of perineal skin punctures. This is because of the nature of the grid plate, which is 7 to 8 cm in length and width. As a result, biopsy needles must puncture the perineal skin over a large area, which is difficult to adequately numb with local anesthetic. In addition, with the grid-stepper approach there is a not insignificant risk of post-biopsy complications. For example, in the previously mentioned PICTURE study, 24% of men experienced acute urinary retention, 26% experienced rectal pain, and 41% experienced perineal pain.[28] Furthermore, these men experienced poor urinary flow and a worsening in their erectile function and sexual desire as assessed with validated questionnaires.

Freehand Transperineal Prostate Biopsy

To overcome the disadvantages of the grid-stepper approach, some urologists have adopted a "freehand" technique that enables outpatient TP prostate biopsy to be performed using local anesthesia. In this technique, a common access cannula is introduced into the perineal skin and the biopsy needle is passed through the cannula multiple times during sampling of the prostate, thereby reducing the total area of tissue that must be anesthetized. The needle is steered freely by the urologist who can then select which areas of the gland to sample. In many instances, a simple angiocatheter serves as the cannula for the biopsy needle. In a 2016 retrospective review of freehand transperineal biopsies performed using an angiocatheter access cannula, 274 such procedures were performed in 244 patients under

local anesthesia, with each procedure taking an average of 7.9 minutes to complete.[44] There were no major complications reported, including systemic infection, urinary retention, hematuria, or pain requiring physician or hospital intervention. Others have also described their experience with a freehand technique with similar results.[27,42]

To facilitate the freehand approach to transperineal prostate biopsy, several purpose-built devices have been introduced. On example is the Cambridge Prostate Biopsy (CamPROBE) needle guide developed in the United Kingdom. This device includes an integrated needle to which a syringe can be attached for local anesthesia administration and is long enough to penetrate from the perineal skin to the prostate capsule. In a 2018 cohort study performed at a single institution using the CamPROBE device, 30 men were biopsied who had previously underwent a TR prostate biopsy while on active surveillance.[45] In this small cohort of men, there were no reported infections, episodes of sepsis, or acute urinary retention after freehand TP prostate biopsy with local anesthesia. Hematuria and hematospermia occurred in 67% and 62% of patients, respectively.

Although effective, one notable shortcoming of the originally described freehand technique is the fact that the access cannula is not coupled to the ultrasound probe. Thus, the urologist must constantly rotate the probe to keep the biopsy needle in view. This adds considerable time to the procedure and potentially sacrifices adequate sampling of prostate tissue. To improve on this, the PrecisionPoint Transperineal Access System (Perineologic, Cumberland, MD) was introduced, which uses a purpose-built access canula that is coupled to the ultrasound probe, ensuring

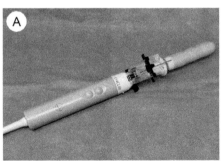 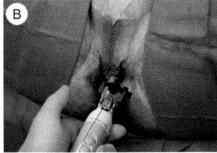

Fig. 3. Freehand transperineal prostate biopsy using the PrecisionPoint Transperineal Access System. (*A*) E14CL4b (9048) ultrasound probe from BK Medical equipped with the PrecisionPoint needle guide, which is designed to ensure alignment of the biopsy needle with the biplanar ultrasound arrays. (*B*) Biopsy being performed with the PrecisionPoint device. The access needle is engaged in the perineal skin allowing for multiple passes of the biopsy needle through a single puncture site.

alignment of the biopsy needle with the ultrasound probe (**Fig. 3**). This device was originally designed to be used in combination with any of the contemporary ultrasound units produced by BK Medical (Peabody, MA), allowing for the unique ability to view the biopsy needle simultaneously in the axial and sagittal views. This feature greatly improves the user's ability to steer the needle to areas of interest with a high degree of precision.

In a series of 43 patients undergoing transperineal prostate biopsy using the PrecisionPoint device without MRI targeting, the investigators reported a cancer detection rate of 48.8%.[25] In terms of complications, 4.7% experienced acute urinary retention and 2.3% experienced gross hematuria requiring catheterization. There were no infectious complications despite omission of periprocedural antibiotics in all cases. In a follow-up paper by this same group describing a technique to incorporate MRI targeting with use of the PrecisionPoint device, an overall cancer detection rate of 87.1% was achieved (36.4% for PI-RADS 3, 61.8% for PI-RADS 4, and 92.0% for PI-RADS 5).[46] In another series from Guy's Hospital in London,176 men underwent freehand TP prostate biopsies using the PrecisionPoint device.[41] Of the 75 patients who underwent a primary biopsy without MRI targeting, 61.3% were positive for cancer. When combined with MRI targeting, the cancer detection rate in this series rose to 88.6%.

MRI-Guided Transperineal Prostate Biopsy

In the modern era of prostate cancer diagnosis, the use of prebiopsy MRI plays a central role. Results from prospective, multicenter studies have shown that the detection of clinically significant prostate cancer is greater in men undergoing MRI-targeted biopsy compared with standard systematic biopsy (average improvement 10%–20%).[4–7] This leads to improved risk stratification of men with clinically localized prostate cancer and in turn optimizes treatment selection. More specifically, the most accurate knowledge of a patient's cancer grade is critical when deciding to enroll in active surveillance versus recommending radical therapy, as well as in administering the correct dose of radiotherapy and duration of androgen deprivation therapy if indicated.

A number of MRI-fusion biopsy systems are now commercially available, with the UroNav platform (Philips, Amsterdam, Netherlands)[47] having the largest user base. Other fusion platforms include the KOELIS Trinity (Princeton, NJ), Artemis (innoMedicus, Cham, Switzerland) and bkFusion (BK Medical). Although all of these systems now include the option of performing TP prostate biopsy with MRI fusion, as of only a few years ago most were strictly designed for TR procedures. Thus, early on those wishing to performing TP prostate biopsy with MRI-guidance had to do so using cognitive fusion (also known as visual estimation).[26,41,46,48] Many urologists, however, prefer to use a formal fusion platform driven by sophisticated hardware and software (**Fig. 4**). The advantages here are that one can record the biopsy core locations, which is important during active surveillance, when regular interval biopsies are planned to track changes in single or multiple lesions.[49] In addition, being able to record biopsy core locations allows one to reexamine biopsy accuracy in the event of an inconclusive or negative targeted biopsy result. In the United States, UroNav was

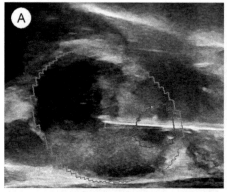 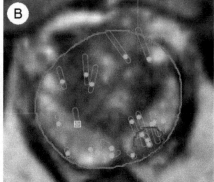

Fig. 4. MRI-guided freehand transperineal prostate biopsy using the bkFusion platform. (*A*) Sagittal transrectal ultrasound image of the contoured prostate and region of interest. The contours derived from the MRI are overlaid onto the real-time ultrasound images. A hypoechoic area on the ultrasound image corresponds to the region of interest on MRI. Using the transperineal approach, the biopsy needle has been precisely navigated to the target area. (*B*) Axial MRI image with overlaid biopsy needle locations. These data can be used at the time of a subsequent biopsy and/or a focal therapy procedure.

the first platform to offer the functionality of performing TP prostate biopsy with MRI fusion.[50] In the first version of this system biopsies were performed with a mechanical stepper unit. A new version now allows for the alternative option of a freehand approach.

Robot-Assisted Transperineal Prostate Biopsy

As prostate biopsy technology evolves to better and more accurately detect and risk-stratify prostate cancer, one potential downside to traditionally performed prostate biopsies, whether TR or TP, is the lack of ability to precisely pre-plan needle positions. As a result, adjustments in biopsy technique and needle trajectory must be made during the biopsy procedure, requiring additional time and room for error. In addition, there is a lack of consistency between users and it is well known that user experience impacts biopsy outcomes and cancer detection rates.[51–53] Automation, in the form of robotic prostate biopsy aims to overcome these limitations, albeit at a high cost. An automated system allows pre-planning of each biopsy so that it can be tailored to a patient's clinical needs, for instance in the case of planning for focal therapy or in a patient on active surveillance. Specific regions of the prostate or prior biopsy sites can be revisited and re-biopsied quickly when necessary, and the automatic, rapid positioning and targeting of the biopsy apparatus nearly eliminates the learning curve and interoperator variability inherent to the traditional prostate biopsy.

The robotic prostate device furthest along in development is the Bio-Xbot system (Biobot Surgical, Singapore). The Bio-Xbot uses a TP, dual-cone concept.[54,55] As in the freehand technique, the biopsy needles enter the perineal skin at a single point, one for each side of the prostate gland. This is then the "pivot point" and ensures that any part of the prostate, including the apex and anterior prostate, can be accessed with only 2 perineal skin punctures in total. Use of the Bio-Xbot follows a standardized workflow that entails image acquisition, 3D surface modeling, target planning, pivot point preparation, and execution. Included in the system are a mobile cart and a robot positioning system that houses the controls for the biopsy gun that operates in 3 axes ($x, y,$ and z). An ultrasound machine performs image acquisition. A touch screen monitor and computer are also part of the mobile unit, which the urologist uses for inputs. In an initial pilot study, 20 men who had undergone prior prostate biopsies underwent robot-assisted TP biopsies.[55] The mean number of biopsy cores taken was 28.5 with a mean total procedure time of 32.5 minutes,

performed under general anesthesia. Of the 20 patients, 2 had post-biopsy urinary retention requiring brief catheterization. There were no infectious complications, bleeding per rectum, or perineal hematoma. Further studies must be performed to better assess needle targeting accuracy, especially at the point where the biopsy needle interacts with perineal skin and within the tissue as it approaches the prostate, both instances in which the needle can bend, causing targeting error. In addition, further work is also needed to determine if any benefit to robotic systems truly exist compared with traditional biopsy methods, especially when considering issues of cost.

SUMMARY

TR prostate biopsy remains the most common technique for sampling the prostate, despite its limited sensitivity for the detection of clinically significant prostate cancer and increased risk of life-threatening sepsis. Although TP biopsy possibly poses a higher risk of post-biopsy urinary retention, it carries a much lower risk of infection and hematochezia. There are also data to suggest that this procedure is better at detecting clinically significant and anterior cancers. Multiple platforms are now commercially available that enable the performance of transperineal prostate biopsy with MRI-guidance. Robotic, image-guided biopsy platforms are also being developed to improve the ability to tailor each patient's biopsy and reduce interoperator variability between biopsy procedures.

REFERENCES

1. Farwell WR, Linder JA, Jha AK. Trends in prostate-specific antigen testing from 1995 through 2004. Arch Intern Med 2007;167(22):2497–502.
2. Neppl-Huber C, Zappa M, Coebergh JW, et al. Changes in incidence, survival and mortality of prostate cancer in Europe and the United States in the PSA era: Additional diagnoses and avoided deaths. Ann Oncol 2012;23(5):1325–34.
3. Loeb S, Carter HB, Berndt SI, et al. Complications after prostate biopsy: Data from SEER-Medicare. J Urol 2011;186(5):1830–4.
4. Ahmed HU, El-Shater Bosaily A, Brown LC, et al. Diagnostic accuracy of multi-parametric MRI and TRUS biopsy in prostate cancer (PROMIS): a paired validating confirmatory study. Lancet 2017; 389(10071):815–22.
5. Kasivisvanathan V, Rannikko AS, Borghi M, et al. MRI-targeted or standard biopsy for prostate-

cancer diagnosis. N Engl J Med 2018;378(19): 1767–77.

6. Rouvière O, Puech P, Renard-Penna R, et al. Use of prostate systematic and targeted biopsy on the basis of multiparametric MRI in biopsy-naive patients (MRI-FIRST): a prospective, multicentre, paired diagnostic study. Lancet Oncol 2019;20(1):100–9.

7. Ahdoot M, Wilbur AR, Reese SE, et al. MRI-targeted, systematic, and combined biopsy for prostate cancer diagnosis. N Engl J Med 2020; 382(10):917–28.

8. Sarkar D. The role of multi-parametric MRI and fusion biopsy for the diagnosis of prostate cancer – A systematic review of current literature. Adv Exp Med Biol 2018;1095:111–23.

9. O'Connor LP, Lebastchi AH, Horuz R, et al. Role of multiparametric prostate MRI in the management of prostate cancer. World J Urol 2020. https://doi.org/10.1007/s00345-020-03310-z.

10. Liss MA, Ehdaie B, Loeb S, et al. An update of the American Urological Association white paper on the prevention and treatment of the more common complications related to prostate biopsy. J Urol 2017;198(2):329–34.

11. Hodge KK, McNeal JE, Stamey TA. Ultrasound guided transrectal core biopsies of the palpably abnormal prostate. J Urol 1989;142(1):66–70.

12. Hodge KK, McNeal JE, Terris MK, et al. Random systematic versus directed ultrasound guided transrectal core biopsies of the prostate. J Urol 1989; 142(1):71–4.

13. Borghesi M, Ahmed H, Nam R, et al. Complications after systematic, random, and image-guided prostate biopsy. Eur Urol 2017;71(3):353–65.

14. Fasugba O, Gardner A, Mitchell BG, et al. Ciprofloxacin resistance in community- and hospital-acquired Escherichia coli urinary tract infections: A systematic review and meta-analysis of observational studies. BMC Infect Dis 2015;15(1):545.

15. Mortazavi-Tabatabaei SAR, Ghaderkhani J, Nazari A, et al. Pattern of antibacterial resistance in urinary tract infections: a systematic review and meta-analysis. Int J Prev Med 2019;10:169.

16. Taylor AK, Murphy AB. Preprostate biopsy rectal culture and postbiopsy sepsis. Urol Clin North Am 2015;42(4):449–58.

17. Cussans A, Somani BK, Basarab A, et al. The role of targeted prophylactic antimicrobial therapy before transrectal ultrasonography-guided prostate biopsy in reducing infection rates: A systematic review. BJU Int 2016;117(5):725–31.

18. Leahy OR, O'Reilly M, Dyer DR, et al. Transrectal ultrasound-guided biopsy sepsis and the rise in carbapenem antibiotic use. ANZ J Surg 2015;85(12): 931–5.

19. Wright J, Paauw DS. Complications of antibiotic therapy. Med Clin North Am 2013;97(4):667–79.

20. Ahmad N, Althemery A, Haseeb A, et al. Inclining trend of the researchers interest in antimicrobial stewardship: A systematic review. J Pharm Bioallied Sci 2020;12(1):11–5.

21. Thompson PM, Pryor JP, Williams JP, et al. The problem of infection after prostatic biopsy: the case for the transperineal approach. Br J Urol 1982;54(6): 736–40.

22. Pepdjonovic L, Tan GH, Huang S, et al. Zero hospital admissions for infection after 577 transperineal prostate biopsies using single-dose cephazolin prophylaxis. World J Urol 2017;35(8):1199–203.

23. Grummet JP, Weerakoon M, Huang S, et al. Sepsis and "superbugs": Should we favour the transperineal over the transrectal approach for prostate biopsy? BJU Int 2014;114(3):384–8.

24. Xiang J, Yan H, Li J, et al. Transperineal versus transrectal prostate biopsy in the diagnosis of prostate cancer: a systematic review and meta-analysis. World J Surg Oncol 2019;17(1):31.

25. Meyer AR, Joice GA, Schwen ZR, et al. Initial experience performing in-office ultrasound-guided transperineal prostate biopsy under local anesthesia using the precisionpoint transperineal access system. Urology 2018;115:8–13.

26. Ristau BT, Allaway M, Cendo D, et al. Free-hand transperineal prostate biopsy provides acceptable cancer detection and minimizes risk of infection: evolving experience with a 10-sector template. Urol Oncol Semin Orig Investig 2018;36(12):528. e15-20.

27. Stefanova V, Buckley R, Flax S, et al. Transperineal prostate biopsies using local anesthesia: experience with 1,287 patients. prostate cancer detection rate, complications and patient tolerability. J Urol 2019;201(6):1121–5.

28. Miah S, Eldred-Evans D, Simmons LAM, et al. Patient Reported Outcome Measures for transperineal template prostate mapping biopsies in the PICTURE etudy. J Urol 2018;200(6):1235–40.

29. Bittner N, Merrick GS, Andreini H, et al. Prebiopsy PSA velocity not reliable predictor of prostate cancer diagnosis, gleason score, tumor location, or cancer volume after TTMB. Urology 2009;74(1): 171–6.

30. Shen PF, Zhu YC, Wei WR, et al. The results of transperineal versus transrectal prostate biopsy: A systematic review and meta-analysis. Asian J Androl 2012;14(2):310–5.

31. Rabbani F, Stroumbakis N, Kava BR, et al. Incidence and clinical significance of false-negative sextant prostate biopsies. J Urol 1998;159(4):1247–50.

32. Vis AN, Boerma MO, Ciatto S, et al. Detection of prostate cancer: a comparative study of the diagnostic efficacy of sextant transrectal versus sextant transperineal biopsy. Urology 2000;56(4):617–21.

33. Hossack T, Patel MI, Huo A, et al. Location and pathological characteristics of cancers in radical prostatectomy specimens identified by transperineal biopsy compared to transrectal biopsy. J Urol 2012;188(3):781–5.

34. Scott S, Samaratunga H, Chabert C, et al. Is transperineal prostate biopsy more accurate than transrectal biopsy in determining final Gleason score and clinical risk category? A comparative analysis. BJU Int 2015;116:26–30.

35. Takenaka A, Hara R, Ishimura T, et al. A prospective randomized comparison of diagnostic efficacy between transperineal and transrectal 12-core prostate biopsy. Prostate Cancer Prostatic Dis 2008;11(2):134–8.

36. Schouten MG, van der Leest M, Pokorny M, et al. Why and where do we miss significant prostate cancer with multi-parametric magnetic resonance imaging followed by magnetic resonance-guided and transrectal ultrasound-guided biopsy in biopsy-naïve men? Eur Urol 2017;71(6):896–903.

37. Sundi D, Kryvenko ON, Carter HB, et al. Pathological examination of radical prostatectomy specimens in men with very low risk disease at biopsy reveals distinct zonal distribution of cancer in black American men. J Urol 2014;191(1):60–6.

38. Faisal FA, Sundi D, Tosoian JJ, et al. Racial variations in prostate cancer molecular subtypes and androgen receptor signaling reflect anatomic tumor location. Eur Urol 2016;70(1):14–7.

39. Lu Z, Williamson SR, Carskadon S, et al. Clonal evaluation of early onset prostate cancer by expression profiling of ERG, SPINK1, ETV1, and ETV4 on whole-mount radical prostatectomy tissue. Prostate 2020;80(1):38–50.

40. McGrath S, Christidis D, Clarebrough E, et al. Transperineal prostate biopsy - tips for analgesia. BJU Int 2017;120(2):164–7.

41. Kum F, Elhage O, Maliyil J, et al. Initial outcomes of local anaesthetic freehand transperineal prostate biopsies in the outpatient setting. BJU Int 2020;125(2):244–52.

42. Marra G, Zhuang J, Marquis A, et al. Pain in men undergoing transperineal free-hand mpmri fusion-targeted biopsies under local anesthesia: outcomes and predictors from a multicenter study of 1,008 patients. J Urol 2020. https://doi.org/10.1097/JU.0000000000001234.

43. Ahmed HU, Hu Y, Carter T, et al. Characterizing clinically significant prostate cancer using template prostate mapping biopsy. J Urol 2011;186(2):458–64.

44. DiBianco JM, Mullins JK, Allaway M. Ultrasound guided, freehand transperineal prostate biopsy: an alternative to the transrectal approach. Urol Pract 2016;3(2):134–40.

45. Thurtle D, Starling L, Leonard K, et al. Improving the safety and tolerability of local anaesthetic outpatient transperineal prostate biopsies: a pilot study of the CAMbridge PROstate Biopsy (CAMPROBE) method. J Clin Urol 2018;11(3):192–9.

46. Gorin MA, Meyer AR, Zimmerman M, et al. Transperineal prostate biopsy with cognitive magnetic resonance imaging/biplanar ultrasound fusion: description of technique and early results. World J Urol 2020;38(8):1943–9.

47. Siddiqui MM, Rais-Bahrami S, Turkbey B, et al. Comparison of MR/ultrasound fusion-guided biopsy with ultrasound-guided biopsy for the diagnosis of prostate cancer. JAMA 2015;313(4):390–7.

48. Neale A, Stroman L, Kum F, et al. Targeted and systematic cognitive freehand-guided transperineal biopsy: is there still a role for systematic biopsy? BJU Int 2020;126(2):280–5.

49. Chang E, Jones TA, Natarajan S, et al. Value of tracking biopsy in men undergoing active surveillance of prostate cancer. J Urol 2018;199(1):98–105.

50. Kosarek CD, Mahmoud AM, Eyzaguirre EJ, et al. Initial series of magnetic resonance imaging (MRI)-fusion targeted prostate biopsy using the first transperineal targeted platform available in the USA. BJU Int 2018;122(5):909–12.

51. Calio B, Sidana A, Sugano D, et al. Changes in prostate cancer detection rate of MRI-TRUS fusion vs systematic biopsy over time: Evidence of a learning curve. Prostate Cancer Prostatic Dis 2017;20(4):436–41.

52. Meng X, Rosenkrantz AB, Huang R, et al. The institutional learning curve of magnetic resonance imaging-ultrasound fusion targeted prostate biopsy: temporal improvements in cancer detection in 4 years. J Urol 2018;200(5):1022–9.

53. Halstuch D, Baniel J, Lifshitz D, et al. Characterizing the learning curve of MRI-US fusion prostate biopsies. Prostate Cancer Prostatic Dis 2019;22(4):546–51.

54. Ho HSS, Mohan P, Lim ED, et al. Robotic ultrasound-guided prostate intervention device: system description and results from phantom studies. Int J Med Robot 2009;5(1):51–8.

55. Ho H, Yuen JS, Mohan P, et al. Robotic transperineal prostate biopsy: pilot clinical study. Urology 2011;78(5):1203–2120.

Historical Considerations and Surgical Quality Improvement in Robotic Prostatectomy

Danly O. Omil-Lima, MD[a],*, Karishma Gupta, MD[b], Adam C. Calaway, MD[b], Michael A. Zell, MD[b]

KEYWORDS

- Minimally invasive surgery • Prostate cancer • Robotic prostatectomy
- Surgical quality improvement

KEY POINTS

- Laparoscopic prostatectomy was technically challenging and not widely adopted.
- Robotics led to the widespread adoption of minimally invasive prostatectomy, which has been used heavily, supplanting the open and traditional laparoscopic approach.
- The benefits of robotic prostatectomy are disputed.
- Data suggest that robotic prostatectomy outcomes have improved over time.

INTRODUCTION

Robotic-assisted laparoscopic prostatectomy (RALP) is currently the most common modality for the treatment of clinically localized prostate cancer.[1–3] Initial critics of RALP cited lack of quality data on patient safety and outcomes as well as heavy dependance on low-quality direct-to-consumer marketing influencing the adoption of this modality.[4–6] Despite this, robotic prostatectomy has been widely adopted, with several randomized clinical trials (RCT) now suggesting it is both safe and effective.[7–10] Here, the authors examine the history of RALP with a focus on temporal improvements.

LAPAROSCOPIC SURGERY AND ROBOTICS IN UROLOGY

Initially popularized for its diagnostic capabilities, the use of laparoscopy as a therapeutic modality has revolutionized surgery. Urologists have always been at the forefront of minimally invasive surgery, with modern day laparoscopes originating from the first useable cystoscope developed in 1879 by German urologist Max Nitze; indeed, the first laparoscopic surgery used a rigid cystoscope as a lens.[11]

Schuessler and colleagues[12] were the first to perform laparoscopic radical prostatectomy (LRP) in the United States in 1991. Their initial experience demonstrated several shortcomings with this modality, echoed by other surgeons: prolonged operative times often greater than 9 hours, technical difficulty with traditional laparoscopic techniques/instruments, and a steep learning curve.[12,13] This initial work demonstrated that although the laparoscopic approach was feasible, it provided no additional benefit over what was then the standard of care: open retropubic radical prostatectomy (RRP). As a result of these shortcomings, LRP did not achieve widespread utilization even while the laparoscopic approach was

[a] Urology Institute, University Hospitals–Cleveland Medical Center, 11100 Euclid Avenue, Cleveland, OH 44106, USA; [b] Urology Institute–University Hospitals Cleveland Medical Center, Case Western Reserve University School of Medicine, Cleveland, OH, USA
* Corresponding author.
E-mail address: Danly.Omil-Lima@UHhospitals.org

Urol Clin N Am 48 (2021) 35–44
https://doi.org/10.1016/j.ucl.2020.09.015

adopted in treatment of other urologic diseases (eg, renal surgery).[14]

In 2000, the Food and Drug Administration (FDA) granted premarket approval to an Endoscopic Instrument Control System designed by Intuitive Surgical, Inc (Sunnyvale, CA, USA), which would ultimately become the Da Vinci surgical system (**Fig. 1**).[15] In 2001, the first robotic prostatectomy was performed by Pasticier and colleagues[16] (other sources credit Binder and colleagues[17] with this honor). In their series of 5 consecutive patients, the researchers noted operative times between 4 and 6 hours. Although they concluded that patient benefit remained unclear at that time, the surgeon's experience was markedly enhanced: noting improvements in ergonomics compared with traditional laparoscopy, visualization owing to incorporation of a binocular 3-dimensional camera system, motion scaling, and tremor filtration.[18] Owing to these improvements, which subjectively increased the ease of difficult surgical steps, such as the vesico-urethral anastomosis, Menon and colleagues[19] argued that, with the establishment of a structured robotics program, a surgeon with no laparoscopic experience could be trained in RALP such that he could achieve outcomes comparable to the "best in class values" for LRP.

Following these early reports, robotics in urology flourished, and urologists became the primary users of robotic assistance, at a rate 3 times greater than the next most frequent users (gynecology and endocrine surgery).[5]

SURGICAL SAFETY

As with any new technique, incorporation of RALP into modern urologic practice demonstrated a technical learning curve. The evolution of RALP technique in turn affected both long-term and short-term outcomes, including surgical safety.

Reporting on their first 5 years of experience with RALP, Hu and colleagues[20] demonstrated lower overall intraoperative complications (particularly bowel and vascular injury) among experienced surgeons performing RALP compared with LRP.

Using the National Inpatient Sample, Chughtai and colleagues[1] evaluated iatrogenic complications among patients undergoing RRP and RALP between 2001 and 2011. They noted that RALP was associated with a greater risk of iatrogenic complications, defined as accidental laceration or hemorrhage complication. In the early years, the risk of iatrogenic complication was noted to be 7.5% for RALP, almost 4 times the rate of complications observed in open RRP. However, the

investigators noted increasing safety of RALP, with the rate of iatrogenic complications decreasing to 1.3% for RALP after the first decade of experience, particularly at high-volume centers. In their series, the rate of complication for RRP remained equivalent throughout the study period (between 2.0% and 2.8%). Thus, with increasing experience, the rate of iatrogenic complication of RALP matched the open standard.

PERIOPERATIVE OUTCOMES AND COMPLICATIONS

In addition to feasibility and operative safety, several studies have demonstrated favorable perioperative morbidity and mortality in RALP.

Hu and colleagues[21] assessed outcomes in men undergoing radical prostatectomy from 2003 to 2005 using data from the Centers for Medicare and Medicaid Services (CMS). They identified 2702 men undergoing RALP, RRP, and perineal radical prostatectomy (PRP) and noted an increase in utilization of RALP among Medicare/Medicaid beneficiaries, such that greater than 30% of all procedures in 2005 were performed robotically. In comparison to RRP and PRP, men undergoing RALP (odds ratio [OR] 0.73) experienced fewer postoperative overall complications (a composite variable, including cardiac, respiratory, vascular, and wound-related complications among others). However, this report also identified a higher rate of vesicourethral anastomotic strictures in patients undergoing RALP as well as higher rates of need for salvage therapy within 6 months. In subgroup analysis, the investigators demonstrated that these adverse outcomes were mitigated at high-volume centers.

Using the National Surgical Quality Improvement Program (NSQIP) database, Liu and colleagues[22] assessed perioperative complications among patients undergoing RALP and RRP between 2005 and 2010. The researchers demonstrated prolonged operative time for RALP but noted that, compared with RRP, RALP was associated with decreased incidence of transfusion as well as decreased volume of transfused blood administered when required. Other major complications, including cardiovascular events, venous thromboembolism, and wound infection, were also reduced in RALP (5%) compared with open surgery (9%). The researchers also examined perioperative mortality. They noted mortality to be rare, but lower in incidence for RALP (0.05%) compared with RRP (0.4%).

Pilecki and colleagues[23] similarly used the NSQIP database to assess all patients undergoing radical prostatectomy in 2011. In that year, 80% of

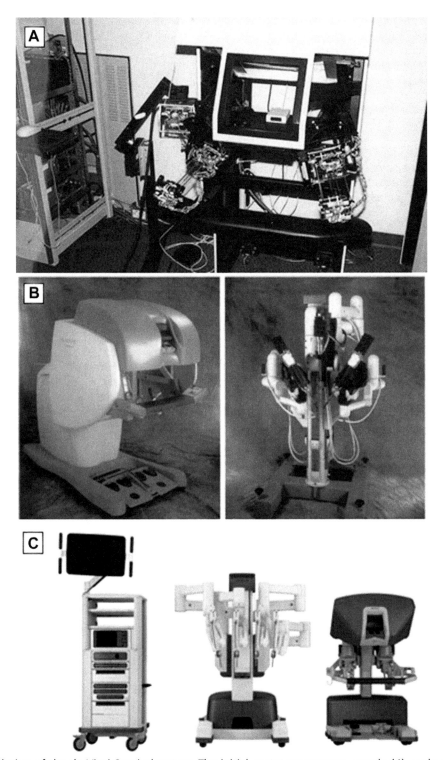

Fig. 1. Evolution of the da Vinci Surgical system. The initial prototype surgeon console (*A*), early commercial model (*B*), and the most recent model of the da Vinci Xi robot (*C*).

cases were performed with robotic assistance. In their retrospective database review, they demonstrated a higher rate of overall complications and higher rate of readmission in the cohort receiving RRP. No difference in mortality or reoperation was found between the 2 groups, although there was a greater percentage of unplanned readmission among patients undergoing RRP compared with RALP.

A 2012 metaanalysis of the literature by Novara and colleagues reviewed 110 studies from 2008 to 2011 and demonstrated blood loss (with a difference of almost 600 cc) and transfusion rate (OR 7.55) were higher in RRP. The mean complication rate of RALP was 9% with most low-grade complications (Clavien-Dindo grade I–III), with less than 1% grade IV or above.[24]

Assessing postoperative pain, Webster and colleagues[25] reported morphine equivalents used and postoperative pain scores (on a 10-point Likert scale) among patients undergoing RALP and RRP at a single institution between 2003 and 2004. Patients were treated on a postoperative care pathway using scheduled ketorolac, and as-needed narcotic (oxycodone) use was converted into morphine equivalents. In this study, patients reported low overall pain less than 3 on average. A statistically significant difference was seen on postoperative day 0, with lower pain scores in the group undergoing RALP (2.05) versus RRP (2.6). However, this difference (which did not carry over the remaining postoperative days) is of uncertain clinical significance, as patients' morphine equivalents were essentially the same when adjusted for hospital length of stay.

Dahl and colleagues[26] assessed return to work and sick leave following radical prostatectomy with a prospective survey-based study of men active in the workforce preoperatively. They demonstrated almost 30% of patients had declined work status after prostatectomy overall. Comparing the proportion of patients with a decline in work status following RALP (0.24) versus RRP (0.36) favored the robotic approach.

Overall, perioperative complication rates decreased with the introduction of RALP, following an initial learning curve. Specifically, RALP has been associated time and again with decreased intraoperative blood loss and need for postoperative transfusion, whereas other studies demonstrate other benefits of RALP. Some investigators report that as a result of these improvements in side-effect profile, surgeons have been able to offer radical prostatectomy to older patients with increasing comorbidities and higher-risk disease.[27]

LONG-TERM FUNCTIONAL OUTCOMES AND CONTEMPORARY UPDATES

The main long-term functional consequences of prostatectomy are urinary incontinence and sexual dysfunction. Whether RALP modifies these is uncertain. Management of clinically localized prostate cancer must balance the need for oncologic control, using a risk-stratified approach, with the burden of treatment versus overtreatment, as underscored by the controversy over prostate-specific antigen screening.[28,29]

A prospective trial by Haglind and colleagues[9] evaluated approximately 2500 men undergoing RALP or RRP at 14 European institutions between 2008 and 2011. There was no significant difference in continence among men undergoing RALP versus RRP, with 21.3% of patients reporting persistent incontinence at 12 months following RALP versus 20.2% for those undergoing RRP. This finding is somewhat higher than other studies, which report final postoperative incontinence rates between 2% and 15%.[30–32] To this end, Lee and colleagues describe the difficulty in quantifying postoperative continence following prostatectomy, as markers of dryness assessed by physicians (eg, pads per day) are not equivalent to complete urinary control as defined by patients. In fact, most men who report using zero pads per day still report some degree of daily leakage.[33] Several investigators have suggested techniques they think to be associated with improved continence and/or earlier return of continence following RALP. These techniques include preservation of the lateral prostatic fascia, athermal division and selective ligation of the dorsal venous complex, nerve sparing, and careful dissection of the prostatic apex to preserve urethral sphincter length, among others.[34–37]

Aside from urinary incontinence, the remainder of functional morbidity resulting from prostatectomy relates to sexual function. Resnick and others[38] reported that 78% of men at 2 years following prostatectomy thought their erections were insufficient for sexual intercourse, with 55% of men bothered by sexual dysfunction. Capogrosso and colleagues[39] evaluated a cohort of 2364 men treated with RALP or RRP between 2008 and 2015 and found no improvement in the last decade in terms of recovery of self-reported erectile function after prostatectomy associated with any modality. Thus, studies support noninferiority of RALP to RRP, but data are limited to determine whether advances in technology have improved functional outcomes for men treated with surgery for prostate cancer. In addition, updated studies are required to reevaluate outcomes in the current era of experienced robotic surgeons.

ONCOLOGIC OUTCOMES

Equally important as long-term functional outcomes are oncologic outcomes associated with RALP. However, robotic technology was largely adopted before data from RCT.

As previously mentioned, Hu and colleagues[21] demonstrated higher rates of salvage therapy needed for patients initially treated with RALP using CMS data between 2003 and 2005.

Scales and colleagues[40] also raised concerns regarding a greater frequency of positive surgical margins following RALP among 950 men undergoing surgery at a single center.

In contrast to these early studies, later studies reported decreased use of adjuvant therapy following RALP.[41] In a retrospective single-institutional study, Barocas and others demonstrated no difference in positive surgical margins among patients treated with RALP or RRP. Furthermore, they demonstrated no relationship between surgical approach and biochemical recurrence-free survival on multivariate analysis when correcting for pathologic features, such as Gleason grade and extraprostatic extension.[42]

The Swedish LAPPRO trial recruited a total of 4003 men with clinically localized prostate cancer who subsequently underwent treatment with either RALP or RRP at one of 14 Swedish centers between 2008 and 2011. Follow-up at 2 years, published in 2018, demonstrated no difference in recurrent or residual disease among those patients treated with either modality.[43]

Several other studies compared outcomes in RRP, LRP, and RALP, demonstrating no difference in surgical margin status, and biochemical recurrence-free survival at 12 months.[34,44,45] However, Chambers and colleagues[8] recommend caution interpreting oncologic outcomes of surgical clinical trials; reporting on their outcomes of an Australian RCT at 24-month follow-up, the investigators cited several limitations of such studies, including lack of standardization of postoperative management and contamination with other adjuvant and salvage treatment modalities.[8] In addition to these limitations, many trials represent single-surgeon, single-institutional studies with relatively short-term follow-up for a disease with a protracted natural history. Thus, although the available data suggest that RALP is equivalent to other surgical approaches, long-term data are lacking. For these reasons, Chambers and others recommend that clinicians and patients view the major benefits of RALP as derived from its minimally invasive nature, in lieu of any data suggesting superior oncologic control.

ENHANCED RECOVERY PATHWAYS AND PATIENT DISCHARGE

As discussed, RALP has been associated with decreased perioperative morbidity following the initial adoption period and associated learning curve. In addition, RALP has been shown to be associated with a shorter overall length of hospital stay.[46] These beneficial effects of minimally invasive surgery are supplemented by enhanced recovery after surgery (ERAS) pathways, which have gained popularity in parallel with robotic-assisted procedures. A study by Zhao and colleagues[47] demonstrated that utilization of ERAS pathways further decreased time to ambulation, flatus, bowel movement, and total length of stay among patients undergoing RALP. Another study by Trinh and colleagues[48] demonstrated that in the early years of RALP (2001–2007), patients experienced a 50% reduction in prolonged length of stay classified as greater than 3 days (decreased from 29% to 14%). Thus, owing to the success of RALP, new recovery pathways are being used, allowing for earlier patient discharges.

Several investigators have reported success with same-day discharge following RALP. Reporting on a small cohort of 11 men, Wolboldt and colleagues[49] demonstrated no reported complications or readmissions for patients receiving same-day discharge in their 2016 study. This series was hypothesis generating, albeit underpowered and subject to selection bias. A larger study by Abaza and colleagues[50] in 2019 reported results from a cohort of 246 men undergoing RALP discharged on the day of surgery. In his cohort, Abaza reports 1% of patients (5 patients) required an emergency department visit, and 1.6% (8 patients) required readmission. Same-day discharge at the study institution resulted in a savings of more than $500,000 over the 18 months of the study period. As experience and quality of surgery (increasing safety, decreasing complications) have improved, postoperative pathways may be tailored to decrease health care costs, potentially on an individual patient basis.

EFFECT ON TRAINING

The advent of new techniques and technologies necessitates changes in training paradigms in order to prepare surgeons to enter the workforce with the appropriate skills. The adoption of RALP necessitated one such paradigm shift, with RALP allowing for increasing resident involvement with, as primary surgeons surpassed their learning curve.[51]

The educational benefits of the robotic approach include improved visibility when compared with open surgery as well as the possibility for increasing resident involvement. Specifically, the resident benefits from graded responsibility, often starting as the bedside assistant before progressing to surgical console for parts or all of the procedure. As such, junior residents have an opportunity to visualize the steps of the procedure and learn alongside senior residents and the attending.[52] Several simulation packages are now available to assist in this transition, wherein residents can practice their robotic skills and engage in surgical planning before opportunities in the operating room.[53,54]

The American Urological Association (AUA) has published standard requirements in an attempt to guide institutions granting robotic surgery privileges.[55] However, these represent minimum requirements, and some investigators have suggested that even residency and fellowship training in minimally invasive surgery at high-volume centers do not negate the learning curve encountered as an attending.[56,57] Despite this, investigators have published on how junior attendings on their own learning curve while teaching can successfully incorporate RALP into residency and fellowship training programs, demonstrating improvements in both trainee and attending surgeon performance over time.[58,59]

There remains no consensus regarding a standardized robotics curriculum, although several formats have been recommended ranging from years-long structured residency didactics to week-long courses open to residents and practicing urologists.[52] Whatever the format, modern residency programs and fellowships must address education in robotic surgery in order to remain compliant with AUA requirements *and* remain competitive to applicants.

HOSPITAL COSTS

An initial complaint against utilization of RALP was the high associated hospital costs. Hofer and colleagues used the Nationwide Inpatient Sample to assess total hospital charges following RRP and RALP between 2002 and 2008. They noted mean total hospital charge for RALP was $46K in 2002 and $18K for RRP that same year. The investigators explain that increased equipment costs, including the robot itself and consumable equipment, as well as the cost of service contracts,

led to the increased cost of RALP. Throughout the years studied, however, the cost of RALP decreased to $34K in 2008. Interestingly, as the cost of RALP decreased, the cost of RRP increased to $32K in 2008, approaching the cost of RALP.[60]

A complex analysis of cost at a single institution was undertaken by researchers at the University of Texas Southwestern Medical Center. Analyzing the costs and payments to their hospital associated with radical prostatectomy between 2003 and 2008, Lotan and colleagues[61] showed that RRP resulted in a net profit, whereas both LRP and RALP resulted in net loss of revenue for their hospital between $2000 and $4,000, even as reimbursement for physician fees increased.

Scales and colleagues[40] performed sensitivity analysis in 2005 in order to identify characteristics of a practice in which RALP could become profitable. In their study, they state that in order to result in net positive revenue, a practice would need to perform 14 RALPs weekly with an average total length of stay less than 1.5 days. A study by Tyson and colleagues[62] demonstrated that as late as 2011, approximately 30% of institutions performing RALP performed less than 50 cases per year, whereas approximately 80% performed less than 250 per year. Thus, based on these findings, RALP was often performed at a cost to hospital systems given that most practices did not meet the required volume criteria.

A systematic review in 2017 by Schroeck and colleagues[63] concluded that the bulk of the literature supports the conclusion that RALP is costlier to payers and hospitals, and that initial costs of RALP were underestimated, as many studies published did not take into account selection bias for healthier patients initially offered RALP (which would tend to confound the ability of RALP to influence earlier patient discharge and other hospitals cost measures) as well as the upfront costs of acquiring the robot.

Given this, it can be concluded that adoption of the robotic approach was initially driven by market forces to attract patients and providers as well as a desire to advance surgical technology at the expense of short-term profits. Further multi-institutional studies are necessary to determine modern day RALP volume as well as the associated costs.

SUMMARY

Initially driven by market forces, utilization of the robotic approach has become the most commonly used tool for radical treatment of clinically localized prostate cancer. Data suggest that RALP has become a safer operation following an initial learning curve during what some investigators have dubbed the *era of dissemination*. Costs associated with RALP have also decreased, either because of increased subsidizing of the procedure by hospitals or because of changes in the structure of market contracts. Recovery/care pathways have also developed in parallel with robotic technology to hasten patient recovery and reduce health care costs to patients and hospital systems.

Overall, the benefits of RALP are predominantly related to reductions in perioperative blood loss and transfusion requirements compared with RRP, with some studies also pointing to a general improvement in the perioperative complication profile across the board. Long-term oncologic outcomes appear noninferior to RRP based on somewhat limited trial data available. Functional patient outcomes can also be considered noninferior when considering the aggregate data (although some series demonstrate modest improvements in potency and continence). Several investigators have made recommendations on how to adapt techniques using the robotic approach to further improve patient outcomes.

As with any other procedure, the surgeon's expertise will ultimately dictate the surgical modality most appropriate to treat the patient. To this end, it is interesting to note that most surgical volume has shifted toward RALP, and residents graduating from training programs today may have minimal, if any, exposure to RRP. Additional studies in the form of prospective trials are required to determine how to best optimize RALP as a treatment modality and a teaching tool for generations of patients and urologists to come.

FUTURE DIRECTIONS

Technological innovation continues to boom in minimally invasive urology. In 2018, the FDA approved a new robotic endoscopic system, the Da Vinci Single Port (SP) system (Intuitive Surgical, Inc).[64] This platform has already been applied to myriad urologic surgeries, including radical prostatectomy.[65,66] Proponents of SP RALP point to the ability to return to a retropubic or perineal approach such that the peritoneum is not violated, arguing that this leads to faster postoperative recovery with minimal use of narcotics.[67] To date, cohorts have been small, and further study is required to confirm the merits of SP RALP over traditional robotic surgery.

Increased market competition is also emerging in this sector; several competitors to the Da Vinci platform have entered the market seeking FDA approval.[68] Competition in the market has the potential to further drive down costs associated with robotic surgery as well as stimulate further innovation.

Considering the evolution and current status of robotics within urology, one thing remains clear: robotic-assisted surgery and RALP have proven themselves to be durable over the past 2 decades. These tools are unlikely to wane in popularity, and robotics will doubtlessly continue to shape the landscape of minimally invasive urology.

DISCLOSURE

None of the authors have any financial disclosures or conflicts of interest.

REFERENCES

1. Chughtai B, Isaacs AJ, Mao J, et al. Safety of robotic prostatectomy over time: a national study of in-hospital injury. J Endourol 2015;29(2):181–5.
2. Urológicas A, Junio E. Resumen Prostatectomia Radical Robótica: Revisión de Nuestra Curva de Aprendizaje Prostatectomía Radical Robótica. Revisión de Nuestra Curva de Aprendizaje.; 2007.
3. Mottrie A, De Naeyer G, Novara G, et al. Robotic radical prostatectomy: a critical analysis of the impact on cancer control. Curr Opin Urol 2011; 21(3):179–84.
4. Mirkin JN, Lowrance WT, Feifer AH, et al. Direct-to-consumer internet promotion of robotic prostatectomy exhibits varying quality of information. Health Aff 2012;31(4):760–9.
5. Juo Y-Y, Mantha A, Ahmad Abiri, et al. Diffusion of robotic-assisted laparoscopic technology across specialties: a national study from 2008 to 2013 and other interventional techniques. Surg Endosc 2018; 32:1405–13.
6. Parsons JK, Messer K, Palazzi K, et al. Diffusion of surgical innovations, patient safety, and minimally invasive radical prostatectomy. JAMA Surg 2014; 149(8):845–51.
7. Yaxley JW, Coughlin GD, Chambers SK, et al. Robot-assisted laparoscopic prostatectomy versus open radical retropubic prostatectomy: early outcomes from a randomised controlled phase 3 study. Lancet 2016;388(10049):1057–66.
8. Coughlin GD, Yaxley JW, Chambers SK, et al. Robot-assisted laparoscopic prostatectomy versus open radical retropubic prostatectomy: 24-month outcomes from a randomised controlled study. Lancet Oncol 2018;19(8):1051–60.
9. Haglind E, Carlsson S, Stranne J, et al. Urinary incontinence and erectile dysfunction after robotic versus open radical prostatectomy: a prospective, controlled, nonrandomised trial. Eur Urol 2015; 68(2):216–25.

10. Porpiglia F, Fiori C, Bertolo R, et al. Five-year outcomes for a prospective randomised controlled trial comparing laparoscopic and robot-assisted radical prostatectomy. Eur Urol Focus 2018;4(1):80–6.

11. Lau WY, Leow CK, Li AKC. History of endoscopic and laparoscopic surgery. World J Surg 1997; 21(4):444–53.

12. Schuessler WW, Schulam PG, Clayman RV, et al. Laparoscopic radical prostatectomy: initial short-term experience. Urology 1997;50(6):854–7.

13. Shuford MD. Robotically assisted laparoscopic radical prostatectomy: a brief review of outcomes. Proc (Bayl Univ Med Cent) 2007;20(4):354–6.

14. Cwach K, Kavoussi L. Past, present, and future of laparoscopic renal surgery. Investig Clin Urol 2016; 57(Suppl 2):S110–3.

15. U.S. Food and Drug Administration. 510(k) premarket notification. Available at: https://www. accessdata.fda.gov/scripts/cdrh/cfdocs/cfpmn/ pmn.cfm?start_search=1&Center=&Panel=& ProductCode=NAY&KNumber=&Applicant= INTUITIVE SURGICAL%2C INC.&DeviceName=& Type=&ThirdPartyReviewed=&ClinicalTrials=& Decision=&DecisionDateFrom=&DecisionDateTo= 08%2F11%2F2018&IVDProducts=& Redact510K=&CombinationProducts=& ZNumber=&PAGENUM=500. Accessed September 9, 2020.

16. Pasticier G, Rietbergen JBW, Guillonneau B, et al. Robotically assisted laparoscopic radical prostatectomy: feasibility study in men. Eur Urol 2001;40(1): 70–4.

17. Binder J, Kramer W. Robotically-assisted laparoscopic radical prostatectomy. BJU Int 2001;87(4): 408–10.

18. Kaul S, Shah NL, Menon M. Learning curve using robotic surgery. Curr Urol Rep 2006;7(2):125–9.

19. Menon M, Shrivastava A, Tewari A, et al. Laparoscopic and robot assisted radical prostatectomy: establishment of a structured program and preliminary analysis of outcomes. J Urol 2002;168(3). https://doi.org/10.1097/01.JU.0000023660.10494. 7D.

20. Hu JC, Nelson RA, Wilson TG, et al. Perioperative complications of laparoscopic and robotic assisted laparoscopic radical prostatectomy. J Urol 2006; 175(2):541–6.

21. Hu JC, Wang Q, Pashos CL, et al. Utilization and outcomes of minimally invasive radical prostatectomy. J Clin Oncol 2008;26(14):2278–84.

22. Liu JJ, Maxwell BG, Panousis P, et al. Perioperative outcomes for laparoscopic and robotic compared with open prostatectomy using the National Surgical Quality Improvement Program (NSQIP) database. Urology 2013;82(3):579–83.

23. Pilecki MA, Mcguire BB, Jain U, et al. National multi-institutional comparison of 30-day postoperative complication and readmission rates between open retropubic radical prostatectomy and robot-assisted laparoscopic prostatectomy using NSQIP. J Endourol 2014;28(4):430–6.

24. Novara G, Ficarra V, Rosen RC, et al. Systematic review and meta-analysis of perioperative outcomes and complications after robot-assisted radical prostatectomy. Eur Urol 2012;62(3):431–52.

25. Webster TM, Herrell SD, Chang SS, et al. Robotic assisted laparoscopic radical prostatectomy versus retropubic radical prostatectomy: a prospective assessment of postoperative pain. J Urol 2005;174(3):912–4.

26. Dahl S, Steinsvik EA, Dahl AA, et al. Return to work and sick leave after radical prostatectomy: a prospective clinical study. Acta Oncol 2014 Jun;53(6): 744–51. https://doi.org/10.3109/0284186X.2013. 844357.

27. Sathianathen NJ, Lamb AD, Lawrentschuk NL, et al. Changing face of robot-assisted radical prostatectomy in Melbourne over 12 years. ANZ J Surg 2018;88(3):E200–3.

28. Esserman L, Shieh Y, Thompson I. Rethinking screening for breast cancer and prostate cancer. JAMA 2009;302(15):1685–92.

29. Grossman DC, Curry SJ, Owens DK, et al. Screening for prostate cancer US Preventive Services Task Force recommendation statement. JAMA 2018;319(18):1901–13.

30. Walsh PC, Marschke P, Ricker D, et al. Patient-reported urinary continence and sexual function after anatomic radical prostatectomy. Urology 2000; 55(1):58–61.

31. Sacco E, Prayer-Galetti T, Pinto F, et al. Urinary incontinence after radical prostatectomy: incidence by definition, risk factors and temporal trend in a large series with a long-term follow-up. BJU Int 2006;97(6):1234–41.

32. Rassweiler J, Stolzenburg J, Sulser T, et al. Laparoscopic radical prostatectomy - the experience of the German Laparoscopic Working Group. Eur Urol 2006;49(1):113–9.

33. Lee SR, Kim HW, Lee JW, et al. Discrepancies in perception of urinary incontinence between patient and physician after robotic radical prostatectomy. Yonsei Med J 2010;51(6):883–7.

34. Walz J, Epstein JI, Ganzer R, et al. A critical analysis of the current knowledge of surgical anatomy of the prostate related to optimisation of cancer control and preservation of continence and erection in candidates for radical prostatectomy: an update. Eur Urol 2016;70(2):301–11.

35. Lei Y, Alemozaffar M, Williams SB, et al. Athermal division and selective suture ligation of the dorsal vein complex during robot-assisted laparoscopic radical prostatectomy: description of technique and outcomes. Eur Urol 2011;59(2):235–43.

36. Choi WW, Freire MP, Soukup JR, et al. Nerve-sparing technique and urinary control after robot-assisted laparoscopic prostatectomy. World J Urol 2011; 29(1):21–7.

37. van der Poel HG, de Blok W, Joshi N, et al. Preservation of lateral prostatic fascia is associated with urine continence after robotic-assisted prostatectomy. Eur Urol 2009;55(4):892–901.

38. Resnick MJ, Koyama T, Fan K-H, et al. Long-term functional outcomes after treatment for localized prostate cancer. N Engl J Med 2013;368(5):436–45.

39. Capogrosso P, Vertosick EA, Benfante NE, et al. Are we improving erectile function recovery after radical prostatectomy? Analysis of patients treated over the last decade. Eur Urol 2019;75(2):221–8.

40. Scales CD, Jones PJ, Eisenstein EL, et al. Local cost structures and the economics of robot assisted radical prostatectomy. J Urol 2005;174(6):2323–9.

41. Hu JC, O'Malley P, Chughtai B, et al. Comparative effectiveness of cancer control and survival after robot-assisted versus open radical prostatectomy. J Urol 2017;197(1):115–21.

42. Barocas DA, Salem S, Kordan Y, et al. Robotic assisted laparoscopic prostatectomy versus radical retropubic prostatectomy for clinically localized prostate cancer: comparison of short-term biochemical recurrence-free survival. J Urol 2010;183(3):990–6.

43. Nyberg M, Hugosson J, Wiklund P, et al. Functional and oncologic outcomes between open and robotic radical prostatectomy at 24-month follow-up in the Swedish LAPPRO trial. Eur Urol Oncol 2018;1(5): 353–60.

44. Porpiglia F, Morra I, Lucci Chiarissi M, et al. Randomized controlled trial comparing laparoscopic and robot-assisted radical prostatectomy. J Endourol 2013;27(2):120–1.

45. Asimakopoulos AD, Pereira Fraga CT, Annino F, et al. Randomized comparison between laparoscopic and robot-assisted nerve-sparing radical prostatectomy. J Sex Med 2011;8(5):1503–12.

46. Cao L, Yang Z, Qi L, et al. Robot-assisted and laparoscopic vs open radical prostatectomy in clinically localized prostate cancer. Medicine (Baltimore) 2019;98(22):e15770.

47. Zhao Y, Zhang S, Liu B, et al. Clinical efficacy of enhanced recovery after surgery (ERAS) program in patients undergoing radical prostatectomy: a systematic review and meta-analysis. World J Surg Oncol 2020;18(1):131.

48. Trinh QD, Bianchi M, Sun M, et al. Discharge patterns after radical prostatectomy in the United States of America. Urol Oncol 2013;31(7):1022–32.

49. Wolboldt M, Saltzman B, Tenbrink P, et al. Same-day discharge for patients undergoing robot-assisted laparoscopic radical prostatectomy is safe and feasible: results of a pilot study. J Endourol 2016; 30(12):1296–300.

50. Abaza R, Martinez O, Ferroni MC, et al. Same day discharge after robotic radical prostatectomy. J Urol 2019;202(5):959–63.

51. Ahmed F, Rhee J, Sutherland D, et al. Surgical complications after robot-assisted laparoscopic radical prostatectomy: the initial 1000 cases stratified by the Clavien classification system. J Endourol 2012; 26(2):135–9.

52. Guzzo TJ, Gonzalgo ML. Robotic surgical training of the urologic oncologist. Urol Oncol 2009;27(2): 214–7.

53. Cimen HI, Atik YT, Gul D, et al. Serving as a bedside surgeon before performing robotic radical prostatectomy improves surgical outcomes. Int Braz J Urol 2019;45(6):1122–8.

54. Sun LW, Van Meer F, Schmid J, et al. Advanced da Vinci surgical system simulator for surgeon training and operation planning. Int J Med Robot 2007; 3(3):245–51.

55. Robotic Surgery (Urologic) Standard Operating Procedure (SOP) - American Urological Association. Available at: https://www.auanet.org/guidelines/robotic-surgery-(urologic)-sop. Accessed September 14, 2020.

56. Brown JA, Sajadi KP. Laparoscopic radical prostatectomy: six months of fellowship training doesn't prevent the learning curve when incorporating into a lower volume practice. Urol Oncol 2009;27(2): 144–8.

57. Davis JW, Kreaden US, Gabbert J, et al. Learning curve assessment of robot-assisted radical prostatectomy compared with open-surgery controls from the Premier Perspective Database. J Endourol 2014;28(5):560–6.

58. Thiel DD, Francis P, Heckman MG, et al. Prospective evaluation of factors affecting operating time in a residency/fellowship training program incorporating robot-assisted laparoscopic prostatectomy. J Endourol 2008;22(6):1331–8.

59. Rocha R, Fiorelli RKA, Buogo G, et al. Robotic-assisted laparoscopic prostatectomy (RALP): a new way to training. J Robot Surg 2016;10(1):19–25.

60. Hofer MD, Meeks JJ, Cashy J, et al. Impact of increasing prevalence of minimally invasive prostatectomy on open prostatectomy observed in the National Inpatient Sample and National Surgical Quality Improvement Program. J Endourol 2013;27(1):102–7.

61. Lotan Y, Bolenz C, Gupta A, et al. The effect of the approach to radical prostatectomy on the profitability of hospitals and surgeons. BJU Int 2010; 105(11):1531–5.

62. Tyson MD, Andrews PE, Ferrigni RF, et al. Radical prostatectomy trends in the United States: 1998 to 2011. Mayo Clin Proc 2016;91(1):10–6.

63. Schroeck FR, Jacobs BL, Bhayani SB, et al. Cost of new technologies in prostate cancer treatment: systematic review of costs and cost effectiveness of

robotic-assisted laparoscopic prostatectomy, intensity-modulated radiotherapy, and proton beam therapy. Eur Urol 2017;72(5):712–35.

64. Lai A, Dobbs RW, Talamini S, et al. Single port robotic radical prostatectomy: a systematic review. Transl Androl Urol 2020;9(2):898–905.

65. Dobbs RW, Halgrimson WR, Madueke I, et al. Single-port robot-assisted laparoscopic radical prostatectomy: initial experience and technique with the da Vinci® SP platform. BJU Int 2019;124(6):1022–7.

66. Kaouk J, Valero R, Sawczyn G, et al. Extraperitoneal single-port robot-assisted radical prostatectomy: initial experience and description of technique. BJU Int 2020;125(1):182–9.

67. Kaouk JH, Haber GP, Autorino R, et al. A novel robotic system for single-port urologic surgery: first clinical investigation. Eur Urol 2014;66(6):1033–43.

68. Brodie A, Vasdev N. The future of robotic surgery. Ann R Coll Surg Engl 2018;100(Suppl 7):4–13.

Robotic Radical Cystectomy in the Contemporary Management of Bladder Cancer

Peter Y. Cai, MD, Aleem I. Khan, BS, Douglas S. Scherr, MD*, Jonathan E. Shoag, MD, MS

KEYWORDS

- Bladder cancer • Robotic surgery • Minimally invasive surgery • Radical cystectomy

KEY POINTS

- Robotic approaches are increasingly being used for radical cystectomy.
- There are no absolute contraindications to robotic cystectomy.
- High-quality evidence suggests the robotic approach is associated with shorter hospital stays.
- Less-experienced surgeons (who have performed <20–30 cases) should be supervised by an experienced mentor and only offer ileal conduit reconstructions.
- Surgical approach is only one aspect of optimizing care for patients undergoing radical cystectomy

BACKGROUND

In 2019, the United States will have more than 80,000 new bladder cancer diagnoses and 17,000 deaths from the disease.[1] Approximately 75% of newly diagnosed bladder cancer will be nonmuscle invasive at diagnosis and the remaining 25% will present with muscle invasion.[2] Untreated muscle-invasive bladder cancer is associated with 38% rate of developing metastatic disease at 6 months and 86% cancer-specific mortality at 5 years.[3] Because of its aggressive nature, current consensus guidelines for nonmetastatic muscle-invasive bladder cancer recommend using cisplatin-based neoadjuvant chemotherapy in eligible patients immediately followed by radical cystectomy (RC).[4] RC is also recommended for some patients with high-risk non–muscle invasive bladder cancer.[5]

Traditionally, RC is performed using an open approach through a lower abdominal midline incision. Laparoscopic cystectomy was first described in the early 1990s,[6,7] and the robotic approach was subsequently described using the DaVinci surgical system and a 6-port transperitoneal approach.[8] Between 2004 and 2010, utilization of the robotic approach to perform RC in the United States increased from 0.6% to 12.8%.[9] This trend has continued, with more recent data from 2013 suggesting that the minimally invasive approach was used in almost 40% of cystectomy surgeries.[10] Robotic-assisted radical cystectomy (RARC) has become an important skill that many urologic oncologists now offer patients.

PATIENT SELECTION

There are no major differences in evaluating patients for either the robotic or open approaches for RC.[11] Recent consensus guidelines from expert cystectomy surgeons caution against the robotic approach for patients with body mass index (BMI) greater than 30, extravesical disease, bulky lymphadenopathy, previous vascular

Department of Urology, New York Presbyterian – Weill Cornell Medicine, 525 East 68th Street, Starr 900, New York, NY 10065, USA
* Corresponding author.
E-mail address: dss2001@med.cornell.edu

surgery, pelvic radiation, distal colorectal surgery, pelvic trauma, or preexisting cardiopulmonary disease that is compromised with positioning.[12] Although these all may make surgery more challenging, the authors emphasize that these contraindications are relative, and many expert robotic surgeons feel comfortable operating in these contexts.

PERIOPERATIVE MANAGEMENT

Mechanical and antibiotic bowel preparation were previously considered standard of care under the assumption that this would reduce the risk of infections and anastomotic leaks. However, data have not demonstrated any significant advantage to these measures with no differences seen in gastrointestinal complications.[13,14] There is now evidence to suggest in reconstruction using ileum, bowel preparation is associated with more, rather than fewer, infections (urinary tract and *Clostridium difficile*).[15] Because of this, bowel preparation is thought to be unnecessary, unless the colon is going to be used for reconstruction, if a single dose of a second- or third-generation cephalosporin is given before skin incision and less than 1 hour before surgery.[11]

More recently, alvimopan (Entereg), a μ-opioid antagonist that targets the side effects of opioid analgesics on bowel motility has been used in patients undergoing bowel resections and anastomosis, as it has been shown to accelerate gastrointestinal recovery and shorten length of hospitalization.[16,17] The drug is administered initially as a single 12 mg dose between 30 minutes and 5 hours before surgery starts and subsequently continued 2 times a day for a maximum of 7 days for a total of 15 in-hospital doses.

Another important consideration in patients with RC is venous thromboembolism (VTE) prophylaxis. The short-term incidence of symptomatic VTE is reported to be between 3% and 11.6% with more than half of these cases occurring after discharge.[18] A double-blind randomized clinical trial data have shown that extended enoxaparin in patients with gastrointestinal, genitourinary, or gynecologic malignancy undergoing surgery significantly reduces the rate of VTE.[19] In patients with RC, extended outpatient chemoprophylaxis significantly reduces VTE rates (~5%) and has been shown to be superior to inpatient subcutaneous heparin at preventing VTE (12%–17%).[20,21] At the same time, the risk of bleeding necessitating reoperation was only 0.3% in a meta-analysis of extended prophylaxis.[18] Currently, a 4-week period of VTE prophylaxis postoperatively is consistently recommended across different

urologic associations and consensus guidelines internationally.[11]

The use of each of the above medications and other interventions has been incorporated into enhanced recovery after surgery (ERAS) pathway protocols.[22] In colorectal surgery, such protocols have provided level 1 evidence for reducing complications and length of hospital stay and improving return of bowel function.[23] Subsequent studies in patients with RC have also shown a statistically significant lower rates of complications and shorter length of hospitalization after surgery[24] when these pathways are implemented. Although multiple such pathways exist, many include interventions such as early oral nutrition after surgery, chewing gum, early mobilization, postoperative analgesia using epidural or other nonnarcotic analgesia, incentive spirometry, and avoiding overhydration by optimizing fluid balance based on targeting cardiac output.[22]

SURGICAL EXPERIENCE

Database cohorts predominantly consisting of origin recognition complex (ORC) have shown an inverse relationship between surgeon volume (≥28 cases annually) and 90-day complication rates and direct hospital costs.[25] During a similar time interval (2003–2004), trainees at urology residency programs performed a median of 3 continent urinary diversions and 4 incontinent urinary diversions.[26] An international consortium used a prospectively maintained database to determine that an acceptable level of proficiency for the robotic approach is reached by the 30th case.[27] Expert consensus recommends surgeons performing the first 20 to 30 cases to be supervised by an experienced mentor and only offer ileal conduit reconstructions and eventually after reaching 100 cases to perform neobladder or continent reconstruction in 25% to 50% of cases.[11]

LENGTH OF SURGERY

Although initial studies evaluating RARC operative times compared with ORC demonstrated longer operative times,[28–30] studies assessing the learning curve in RARC indicate progressively decreasing mean operative times as surgeon experience increases. As Schumacher and colleagues demonstrated in a cohort study of 45 patients undergoing RARC with total intracorporeal urinary diversion, mean operative time decreased from 532 to 434 minutes across the first 45 patients.[28] In the RAZOR study, the largest randomized, multicenter noninferiority phase 3 trial to date comparing RARC with ORC outcomes, mean operative time for RARC was 422 minutes versus 361 minutes for open cystectomy (P = .0005),[31] with operative time in this trial defined as time from patient entry to exit from the operating theater.[32]

PERIOPERATIVE TRANSFUSION

Most of the literature supports lower transfusion rates in RARC, with estimates suggesting a relative risk of 0.58 (95% confidence interval [CI] 0.43–0.80) or 193 fewer transfusions per 1000 participants (95% CI 262–92 fewer), as compared with ORC, which reflects similar effects seen from laparoscopic or robotic-assisted radical prostatectomy.[33–35] The general consensus remains that there is significantly less blood loss in RARC than ORC, with nearly all trials that have included blood loss data indicating an average decrease of approximately 400 mL of blood loss in patients undergoing RARC as compared with open surgery.[31,33] Similarly, when the RAZOR trial stratified perioperative transfusions by timepoint, ORC was associated with increased transfusion requirement both intra- and postoperatively.[31,36]

LENGTH OF HOSPITAL STAY/READMISSIONS

RARC has also been associated with shorter hospital stay than ORC,[33] with median length of stay for the robotic approach estimated to be 2.5 days shorter (P<.0001).[37] It is important to recognize that there is some conflicting data regarding the degree to which hospital stay is shortened,[38,39] which may reflect the increasing adoption of the ERAS protocols.[40] It is difficult to truly determine whether the cause of decreased length of stay is the result of using a minimally invasive approach, a reduction in perioperative transfusion requirements, or even a reflection of surgical proficiency. In the RAZOR trial, perioperative parameters (blood loss, transfusion rates, length of stay, and surgery duration) and open conversion rate (3%) were all compared favorably with previous studies, which suggests that in the hands of highly proficient robotic surgeons, the robotic approach is associated with shorter hospital stay.[31]

ONCOLOGIC OUTCOMES

RARC and ORC have been associated with similar oncologic outcomes, with no significant difference in time to recurrence, cancer-specific survival, or overall survival.[33,41–43] For example, in the RAZOR trial, RARC was noninferior to ORC for progression-free survival at 2 years in the primary endpoint analysis.[31] SEER-Medicare data also suggest that RARC provides similar overall (hazard ratio 0.88, 95% CI 0.74–1.05) and cancer-specific (hazard ratio 0.91, 95% CI 0.66–1.26) survival at median follow-up of 44 months compared with the open approach.[44] Data from the National Cancer Database analysis suggests RARC was associated with significantly greater rates of pelvic lymph node dissection and greater median lymph node count as compared with ORC (17 vs 12, P<.001).[45]

Although no difference in survival outcomes has been observed, there remains concern that the pattern and location of recurrences differ between approaches. A retrospective review of 383 patients showed that although the number of distant recurrences did not differ, a higher proportion of extrapelvic lymph node recurrences (23% vs 15%) and peritoneal carcinomatosis (21% vs 8%) occurred in RARC patients compared to ORC patients.[46] On the other hand, Bochner and colleagues demonstrated a greater proportion of distant recurrences and extrapelvic lymph nodes for first site recurrences in ORC patients, whereas RARC patients had a greater proportion of local recurrences.[41] Both of these studies suffered from limited sample sizes and were insufficiently powered to definitively demonstrate differences in long-term recurrence patterns.

COMPLICATION RATES

A recent meta-analysis performed by Kimuera and colleagues found no significant difference in complication rates between RARC and ORC within 90 days both in randomized and nonrandomized comparative studies. In addition, postoperative quality-of-life scores did not significantly differ between RARC and ORC patients 3 or 6 months postprocedure.[47] Although complications have been reported at similar rates between RARC and ORC, there are studies that demonstrate RARC results in fewer major (Clavien grade 3–5) complications (31% vs 17%, P = .03).[37] However, no studies have demonstrated significant differences in occurrence of postoperative ileus, perioperative urinary tract infections, or thrombosis.[29,33,38,47] It should be noted, however, that there is a growing body of evidence demonstrating RARC has a higher incidence of ureteroenteric strictures compared with ORC (hazard ratio 1.70, 95% CI 1.28–2.26).[48]

COST-EFFECTIVENESS

In some studies, RARC has been shown to be more expensive than ORC, ranging from 16% to

19% higher cost.[49–51] Although associated with higher cost of materials, some data suggest that the robotic approach actually diminishes costs due to a shorter length of hospital stay.[52] An analysis examining factors associated with the cost of RARC found that RARC became more expensive than ORC when operative time exceeded 361 minutes, the length of stay extended beyond 6.6 days, or the robotic supply cost exceeded $5853. If the procedure remained within these constraints then RARC was associated with a 38% cost advantage as compared with ORC.[51]

CONCLUSIONS

RARC has been shown to have equivalent oncologic outcomes with shorter hospital stay and fewer perioperative transfusions. This relatively new technology has become increasingly adopted by the urologic oncology community. Consensus meetings and guidelines have been published to provide guidance on all aspects of how to implement the robotic approach in the urologic oncology clinic. These include being mindful of relative contraindications (BMI>30, bulky lymphadenopathy, prior vascular surgery, pelvic radiation, distal colorectal surgery, pelvic trauma or preexisting cardiopulmonary disease that is compromised with positioning), using bowel preparation only if colon is to be used for reconstruction, abiding by an ERAS pathway, using extended outpatient thromboprophylaxis, and having supervision by an experienced mentor in the first 20 to 30 cases.

DISCLOSURE

Supported by The Frederick J. and Theresa Dow Wallace Fund of the New York Community Trust (JES).

REFERENCES

1. Siegel RL, Miller KD, Jemal A. Cancer statistics, 2019. CA Cancer J Clin 2019;69(1):7–34.
2. Burger M, Catto J, Dalbagni G, et al. Epidemiology and risk factors of urothelial bladder cancer. Eur Urol 2013;63(2):234–41.
3. Martini A, Sfakianos JP, Renström-Koskela L, et al. The natural history of untreated muscle-invasive bladder cancer. BJU Int 2020;125(2):270–5.
4. Chang SS, Bochner BH, Chou R, et al. Treatment of non-metastatic muscle-invasive bladder cancer: AUA/ASCO/ASTRO/ SUO guideline. J Urol 2017; 198(3):552–9.
5. Woldu SL, Bagrodia A, Lotan Y. Guideline of guidelines: non-muscle-invasive bladder cancer. BJU Int 2017;119(3):371–80.
6. Sanchez de Badajoz E, Gallego Perales JL, Reche Rosado A, et al. Radical cystectomy and laparoscopic ileal conduit. Arch Esp Urol 1993;46(7): 621–4.
7. Parra RO, Andrus CH, Jones JP, et al. Laparoscopic cystectomy: initial report on a new treatment for the retained bladder. J Urol 1992;148(4):1140–4.
8. Menon M, Hemal AK, Tewari A, et al. Nerve-sparing robot-assisted radical cystoprostatectomy and urinary diversion. BJU Int 2003;92(3):232–6.
9. Leow JJ, Reese SW, Jiang W, et al. Propensity-matched comparison of morbidity and costs of open and robot-assisted radical cystectomies: a contemporary populationbased analysis in the United States. Eur Urol 2014;66(3):569–76.
10. Bachman AG, Parker AA, Shaw MD, et al. Minimally invasive versus open approach for cystectomy: trends in the utilization and demographic or clinical predictors using the national cancer database. Urology 2017;103:99–105.
11. Wilson TG, Guru K, Rosen RC, et al. Best practices in robot-assisted radical cystectomy and urinary reconstruction: recommendations of the Pasadena Consensus Panel. Eur Urol 2015;67(3):363–75.
12. Chan KG, Guru K, Wiklund P, et al. Robot-assisted radical cystectomy and urinary diversion: technical recommendations from the Pasadena Consensus Panel. Eur Urol 2015;67(3):423–31.
13. Raynor MC, Lavien G, Nielsen M, et al. Elimination of preoperative mechanical bowel preparation in patients undergoing cystectomy and urinary diversion. Urol Oncol 2013;31(1):32–5.
14. Guenaga KF, Matos D, Wille-Jorgensen P. Mechanical bowel preparation for elective colorectal surgery. Cochrane Database Syst Rev 2011;9:CD001544.
15. Large MC, Kiriluk KJ, DeCastro J, et al. The impact of mechanical bowel preparation on postoperative complications for patients undergoing cystectomy and urinary diversion. J Urol 2012;188(5):1801–5.
16. Wang S, Shah N, Philip J, et al. Role of alvimopan (entereg) in gastrointestinal recovery and hospital length of stay after bowel resection. PT 2012;37(9): 518–25.
17. Lee CT, Chang SS, Kamat AM, et al. Alvimopan accelerates gastrointestinal recovery after radical cystectomy: a multicenter randomized placebo-controlled trial. Eur Urol 2014;66(2):265–72.
18. Klaassen Z, Arora K, Goldberg H, et al. Extended venous thromboembolism prophylaxis after radical cystectomy: a call for adherence to current guidelines. J Urol 2018;199(4):906–14.
19. Bergqvist D, Agnelli G, Cohen AT, et al. Duration of prophylaxis against venous thromboembolism with enoxaparin after surgery for cancer. N Engl J Med 2002;346(13):975–80.
20. Schomburg J, Krishna S, Soubra A, et al. Extended outpatient chemoprophylaxis reduces venous

thromboembolism after radical cystectomy. Urol Oncol 2018;36(2). 77.e9–13.

21. Pariser JJ, Pearce SM, Anderson BB, et al. Extended duration enoxaparin decreases the rate of venous thromboembolic events after radical cystectomy compared to inpatient only subcutaneous heparin. J Urol 2017;197(2):302–7.

22. Cerantola Y, Valerio M, Persson B, et al. Guidelines for perioperative care after radical cystectomy for bladder cancer: (ERAS((R))) society recommendations. Clin Nutr 2013;32(6):879–87.

23. Varadhan KK, Neal KR, Dejong CH, et al. The enhanced recovery after surgery (ERAS) pathway for patients undergoing major elective open colorectal surgery: a metaanalysis of randomized controlled trials. Clin Nutr 2010;29(4):434–40.

24. Tyson MD, Chang SS. Enhanced recovery pathways versus standard care after cystectomy: a metaanalysis of the effect on perioperative outcomes. Eur Urol 2016;70(6):995–1003.

25. Leow JJ, Reese S, Trinh QD, et al. Impact of surgeon volume on the morbidity and costs of radical cystectomy in the USA: a contemporary population-based analysis. BJU Int 2015;115(5):713–21.

26. Chang SS, Smith JA Jr, Herrell SD, et al. Assessing urinary diversion experience in urologic residency programs-are we adequately training the next generation? J Urol 2006;176(2):691–3.

27. Hayn MH, Hussain A, Mansour AM, et al. The learning curve of robot-assisted radical cystectomy: results from the International Robotic Cystectomy Consortium. Eur Urol 2010;58(2):197–202.

28. Schumacher MC, Jonsson MN, Hosseini A, et al. Surgery-related complications of robot-assisted radical cystectomy with intracorporeal urinary diversion. Urology 2011;77(4):871–6.

29. Smith AB, Raynor M, Amling CL, et al. Multi-institutional analysis of robotic radical cystectomy for bladder cancer: perioperative outcomes and complications in 227 patients. J Laparoendosc Adv Surg Tech A 2012;22(1):17–21.

30. Nix J, Smith A, Kurpad R, et al. Prospective randomized controlled trial of robotic versus open radical cystectomy for bladder cancer: perioperative and pathologic results. Eur Urol 2010;57(2): 196–201.

31. Parekh DJ, Reis IM, Castle EP, et al. Robot-assisted radical cystectomy versus open radical cystectomy in patients with bladder cancer (RAZOR): an open-label, randomised, phase 3, non-inferiority trial. Lancet 2018;391(10139):2525–36.

32. Parekh DJ, Venkatramani V. on behalf ofRAZOR trial authors. Robot-assisted versus open cystectomy in the RAZOR trial - authors' reply. Lancet 2019; 393(10172):645–6.

33. Rai BP, Bondad J, Vasdev N, et al. Robotic versus open radical cystectomy for bladder cancer in

adults. Cochrane Database Syst Rev 2019;4: CD011903.

34. Sathianathen NJ, Kalapara A, Frydenberg M, et al. Robotic assisted radical cystectomy vs open radical cystectomy: systematic review and meta-analysis. J Urol 2019;201(4):715–20.

35. Ilic D, Evans SM, Allan CA, et al. Laparoscopic and robotic-assisted versus open radical prostatectomy for the treatment of localised prostate cancer. Cochrane Database Syst Rev 2017;9:CD009625.

36. Parekh DJ, Messer J, Fitzgerald J, et al. Perioperative outcomes and oncologic efficacy from a pilot prospective randomized clinical trial of open versus robotic assisted radical cystectomy. J Urol 2013; 189(2):474–9.

37. Ng CK, Kauffman EC, Lee MM, et al. A comparison of postoperative complications in open versus robotic cystectomy. Eur Urol 2010;57(2):274–81.

38. Bochner BH, Sjoberg DD, Laudone VP, et al. A randomized trial of robotassisted laparoscopic radical cystectomy. N Engl J Med 2014;371(4):389–90.

39. Bochner BH, Dalbagni G, Sjoberg DD, et al. Comparing open radical cystectomy and robot-assisted laparoscopic radical cystectomy: a randomized clinical trial. Eur Urol 2015;67(6):1042–50.

40. Pang KH, Groves R, Venugopal S, et al. Prospective implementation of enhanced recovery after surgery protocols to radical cystectomy. Eur Urol 2018; 73(3):363–71.

41. Bochner BH, Dalbagni G, Marzouk KH, et al. Randomized trial comparing open radical cystectomy and robot-assisted laparoscopic radical cystectomy: oncologic outcomes. Eur Urol 2018;74(4): 465–71.

42. Davis RB, Farber NJ, Tabakin AL, et al. Open versus robotic cystectomy: comparison of outcomes. Investig Clin Urol 2016;57(Suppl 1):S36–43.

43. Brassetti A, Cacciamani G, Anceschi U, et al. Long-term oncologic outcomes of robot-assisted radical cystectomy (RARC) with totally intracorporeal urinary diversion (ICUD): a multi-center study. World J Urol 2020;38(4):837–43.

44. Hu JC, Chughtai B, O'Malley P, et al. Perioperative outcomes, health care costs, and survival after robotic-assisted versus open radical cystectomy: a national comparative effectiveness study. Eur Urol 2016;70(1):195–202.

45. Hanna N, Leow JL, Sun M, et al. Comparative effectiveness of robot assisted vs. open radical cystectomy. Urol Oncol 2018;36(3):88 e1–9.

46. Nguyen DP, Al Hussein Al Awamlh B, Wu X, et al. Recurrence patterns after open and robot-assisted radical cystectomy for bladder cancer. Eur Urol 2015;68(3):399–405.

47. Kimura S, Iwata T, Foerster B, et al. Comparison of perioperative complications and health-related quality of life between robot-assisted and open radical

cystectomy: a systematic review and meta-analysis. Int J Urol 2019;26(8):760–74.

48. Goh AC, Belarmino A, Patel NA, et al. A population-based study of ureteroenteric strictures after open and robot-assisted radical cystectomy. Urology 2020;135:57–65.

49. Bansal SS, Dogra T, Smith PW, et al. Cost analysis of open radical cystectomy versus robot-assisted radical cystectomy. BJU Int 2018;121(3):437–44.

50. Michels CTJ, Wijburg CJ, Leijte E, et al. A cost-effectiveness modeling study of robot-assisted (RARC) versus open radical cystectomy (ORC) for bladder cancer to inform future research. Eur Urol Focus 2019;5(6):1058–65.

51. Martin AD, Nunez RN, Castle EP. Robot-assisted radical cystectomy versus open radical cystectomy: a complete cost analysis. Urology 2011;77(3):621–5.

52. Lee R, Ng CK, Shariat SF, et al. The economics of robotic cystectomy: cost comparison of open versus robotic cystectomy. BJU Int 2011;108(11):1886–92.

Intracorporeal Urinary Diversion in Robotic Radical Cystectomy

Prithvi B. Murthy, MD*, Rebecca A. Campbell, MD, Byron H. Lee, MD, PhD[1]

KEYWORDS

- Minimally invasive surgery • Bladder cancer • Intracorporeal • Urinary diversion

KEY POINTS

- Intracorporeal urinary diversion can minimize the morbidity burden of radical cystectomy through decreased operative times, intraoperative blood loss, blood transfusion rates, and length of stay without compromising long-term oncologic outcomes.
- Coordinated efforts between the surgeon/operating room team are required to overcome the learning curve of intracorporeal diversion, which is likely a minimum of 30 cases for intraoperative oncologic parameters and more than 100 to decrease long-term technically related complications.
- Multiple techniques have been described for intracorporeal ileal conduit, continent cutaneous diversion, and neobladder.
- Enhanced Recovery After Surgery Protocols specific to intracorporeal diversion are published and can further assist in decreasing morbidity.

INTRODUCTION

Robotic-assisted radical cystectomy (RARC) has been widely adopted over the past decade.[1] RARC initially entailed excision of the bladder and lymph nodes robotically, with the urinary diversion performed extracorporeally. Several technical modifications have allowed for the performance of intracorporeal urinary diversion (ICUD), with some high-volume cystectomists adopting this technique.[2]

In light of the technical challenges associated ICUD, initial studies showed higher complication rates when compared with extracorporeal urinary diversion (ECUD).[2,3] As experience increased, ICUD has been associated with decreased operative time, and lower intraoperative blood loss and blood transfusion rates as compared with ECUD and ORC.[2,4,5] In this review we highlight technical points, oncologic outcomes, and complications specific to each form of ICUD (ileal conduit,

continent cutaneous diversion, neobladder). We also describe the learning curve and the future of intracorporeal diversion.

ROBOTIC CYSTECTOMY

Before discussion of ICUD, it is important to note that the literature to date suggests that RARC does not compromise oncologic outcomes when compared with ORC, irrespective of diversion. Initial concerns with RARC related to increased positive surgical margin rates as well as higher a proportion of local, abdominal, and peritoneal recurrences.[6,7] However, subsequent analyses from retrospective studies and randomized controlled trials have suggested that tumor biology, not surgical approach, influences overall oncologic outcomes.[8,9]

Although level 1b evidence is currently being accumulated with regards to RARC with ICUD versus ORC (iROC Trial), several large volume

---

Department of Urology, Glickman Urological & Kidney Institute, Cleveland Clinic, 9500 Euclid Avenue, Cleveland, OH 44195, USA

[1] Senior author.

* Corresponding author.

E-mail address: murthyp@ccf.org

Urol Clin N Am 48 (2021) 51–70

https://doi.org/10.1016/j.ucl.2020.09.005

retrospective reviews and multi-institutional studies demonstrate similar oncologic outcomes and complications outcomes between the two techniques.[5,10–13] The largest volume long-term outcomes series is the 10-year data of 446 patients in the International Robotic Cystectomy Consortium (IRCC).[10] Forty percent of these patients underwent ICUD, and the entire cohort demonstrated a 5-year cancer-specific survival of 71%. Simone and colleagues[5] showed comparable 4-year CSS rates of 86.4% and 85.3% in a propensity matched cohort of patients undergoing RARC with intracorporeal neobladder versus ORC with neobladder, respectively. In their retrospective review of 94 ORC and 90 RARC with ICUD, Tan and colleagues[12] did not find surgical technique to influence recurrence-free, disease-specific or overall survival. It should be noted that their RARC group was a more contemporary series with a higher proportion of patients receiving neoadjuvant chemotherapy. Brassetti and colleagues[13] noted 5-year CSS rates of 61% in a retrospective review of 113 patients undergoing RARC with ICUD. More detailed comparative outcomes are displayed in **Table 1**.

TECHNICAL POINTS FOR ALL FORMS OF INTRACORPOREAL URINARY DIVERSION
Patient Selection and Preoperative Planning

Given that prior abdominal surgical history has been associated with a higher rate of postoperative complications following RARC, surgeons early in ICUD adoption may elect to operate on patients without prior abdominal surgery.[2] Preoperative mechanical bowel preparation is not required for intracorporeal ileal conduit or neobladder, but may be use for continent cutaneous diversion.[14–17] Adding and colleagues[18] also suggest that patients avoid vegetable consumption the day before surgery. Solids can be consumed up to 6 hours before surgery. Several Enhanced Recovery After Surgery (ERAS) protocols recommend preoperative nutrition with a carbohydrate dense clear liquid in the 2 to 3 hours preceding induction of anesthesia.[18–20]

Positioning and Port Placement

Optimal patient positioning and port placement are critical to operative success. When using the DaVinci Si robot (Intuitive Surgical, Sunnyvale, CA), patients are required to be in dorsal lithotomy position.[21,22] The DaVinci Xi robot permits side docking and allows patients to be in supine position, greatly reducing the risk of lower extremity neuropathy. Moderate Trendelenburg position is still required to facilitate bowel manipulation, regardless of robot model. Although the Pasadena Consensus Panel has previously recommended 30° of Trendelenburg, we use a more conservative angle between 23 to 24° at our institution.[23]

In general, ports are placed more cranially when compared with robotic prostatectomy to permit bowel manipulation and node dissection. We use a combination of measurements and anatomic landmarks for a 5-port technique, as depicted in **Table 2**. The 8-mm camera port is placed supraumbilically in line with the tip of the 11th rib. Two 8-mm robotic ports are placed 4.5 cm inferior and 7 cm lateral to the camera port. A third 8 mm robotic port is placed in line with the camera port on the left hand side an additional 7 to 10 cm

Table 1
Comparison of oncologic outcomes among ICUD cohorts

Series	Tan et al. (2 y)		Simone et al. (4 y)		Brassetti et al. (5 y)	IRCC (10 y, 40% ICUD)
Diversion type	*Open (n = 94)*	Robotic (n = 90)	*Open (n = 46)*	Robotic (n = 64)	Robotic (n = 113)	Robotic (n = 446)
Overall survival, %	73.5	83.8	79.6	82.1	54	35
Cancer-specific survival, %	80.9	84.4	85.3	86.4	61	65
Recurrence-free survival, %	69.5	78.8	73.4	79.3	58	59
Positive surgical margin rate, %	19.3	8.2	0	0	8	7
≥ pT3	41.4	30	35	36	42	43

Abbreviations: ICUD, intracorporeal urinary diversion; IRCC, International Robotic Cystectomy Consortium.
  Data from Refs.[5,10,12,13]

Table 2
Technical variations in RARC with ICUD

Institute	Port Configuration	Assistant Ports	Ureterointestinal Anastomosis	Stent Type
Cleveland Clinic R – Robot 8 mm C – Camera 8 mm A – Assistant 12 mm		1	Bricker Continuous 4-0 Vicryl (Ethicon, Sommerville, NJ, USA)	Double-J via right most assistant port
USC[a]	 Fig. 1 – Trocar configuration. The camera port and three robotic ports were placed at positions 1, 2, 3, and 4, respectively. Additionally, 15-mm and 12-mm assistant ports were used at positions 5 and 6.	2	Bricker Continuous 4-0 Vicryl (Ethicon)	Single-J via 2 mm suprapubic "mini" port
Karolinska[b]	 ○ 15 mm ● 12 mm ○ 12 mm (right) ○ 8 mm (robot) Fig. 1 – (a) Patient position; (b) port placement.	2	Wallace ureter-to-ureter 4-0 Biosyn (Covidien) uretero-enteral 3-0 Quill (barbed, Surgical Specialties Corporation, Reading, PA, USA)	Single-J via lower abdominal 4-mm incisions

(continued on next page)

Table 2
(continued)

Institute	Port Configuration	Assistant Ports	Ureterointestinal Anastomosis	Stent Type
Roswell Park[c]	2	2	Bricker Interrupted 4-0 Vicryl or PDS (Ethicon)	Single-J via assistant lap suction device (**Fig. 6**)
City of Hope[d]	Fig. 2 – City of Hope port placement. A = assistant, 12 mm; C = camera, 12 mm; R = robot, 8 mm.	2	Bricker varied practices	-

Abbreviations: ICUD, intracorporeal urinary diversion; RARC, Robotic-assisted radical cystectomy.
  [a] *From* Goh AC, Gill IS, Lee DJ, et al. Robotic Intracorporeal Orthotopic Ileal Neobladder: Replicating Open Surgical Principles. *European Urology.* 2012;62(5):891-901. https://doi.org/10.1016/j.eururo.2012.07.052.
  [b] *From* Collins JW, Tyritzis S, Nyberg T, et al. Robot-assisted radical cystectomy: description of an evolved approach to radical cystectomy. *Eur Urol.* 2013;64(4):654-663. https://doi.org/10.1016/j.eururo.2013.05.020.
  [c] *From* Guru KA, Mansour AM, Nyquist J. Robot-assisted intracorporeal ileal conduit "Marionette" technique. *BJU Int.* 2010;106(9):1404-1420. https://doi.org/10.1111/j.1464-410X.2010.09772.x.
  [d] *From* Chan KG, Guru K, Wiklund P, et al. Robot-assisted Radical Cystectomy and Urinary Diversion: Technical Recommendations from the Pasadena Consensus Panel. *European Urology.* 2015;67(3):423-431. https://doi.org/10.1016/j.eururo.2014.12.027; with permission.

lateral to the robotic port. A 12-mm port is placed just inferior to the costal margin on the right side, and more medial relative the third robotic port on the left hand side. The positioning of the assistant port in this manner allows the bedside assistant to facilitate bowel manipulation without the placement of additional ports.

Numerous additional docking techniques have been described, see **Table 2**. The University of Southern California (USC) group uses a 6-port technique, with 1 assistant port at the level of the umbilicus.[24] An additional 12-mm assistant port is placed superior to the camera port and medial to the first robotic port.

At the Karolinska Institute, all ports are placed near the level of the umbilicus apart from the camera port. The lateral left-most 15-mm port is placed just superiorly and medially to anterior superior iliac spine. This permits laparoscopic stapling by the assistant, as well as robotic use via the port-in-port technique.[25] At City of Hope, all ports are positioned in relation to the pubic symphysis, with the camera port 25 cm away and robotic and assistant ports 20 to 23 cm away.[23]

Bowel Division and Anastomosis

Regardless of diversion technique, ICUD requires bowel division and establishing recontinuity with reliance on robust staple lines. Improvement in endoscopic stapling devices that allow for articulation and variable staple height selection have permitted the safe execution of ICUD. We use Covidien (Medtronic Minimally Invasive Therapies) Endo GIA staplers (Medtronic, Dublin, Ireland). The ileal loop is created by introducing the stapler through the assistant port, and dividing the proximal and distal bowel and adjacent mesenteric segments with a 60-mm "tan" load. Additional mesenteric length is obtained at the distal end by division with a harmonic scalpel or robotic vessel sealer. In obtaining mesenteric length, it is critical to divide the mesentery perpendicular to the orientation of the bowel. Medial deviation may result in division of a larger vascular branch and cause distal bowel ischemia. Though not used at our institution, visualization of mesenteric vasculature with indocyanine green (ICG) may be a useful tool. Manny and Hemal[26] have previously described successful mesenteric angiography with ICG in 8 of 8 patients undergoing intracorporeal ileal conduit at a median time of less than 1 minute after intravenous injection (**Fig. 1**).

Following isolation of the bowel segment for diversion, bowel continuity is established by first placing stay stitches to orient the proximal and distal ileal limbs. After sharply incising the corner of the staple line at the anti-mesenteric border, a side-to-side anastomosis is created with two 60-mm "tan" loads. A third "purple" load, used for thicker tissues, is used transversely to close the defect. Our technique of bowel division and reanastomosis is shown in **Fig. 2**.

Although this serves as a general outline, there are some notable institutional variations. Some favor placing an additional 12-mm suprapubic port to perform all laparoscopic stapling, while others use a left-sided assistant port for ergonomic preference.[27,28] A robotic stapling device can also be used if the surgeon prefers. Of note, bowel recontinuity can also be performed after the ureteroenteric anastomoses (UEA).[27]

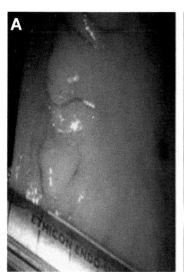
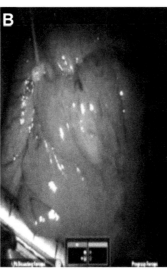

Fig. 1. Mesenteric angiography after intravenous injection of indocyanine green. (A) Distal ileum under white light, (B) distal ileum under near infrared fluorescence (color version available online). (From Manny TB, Hemal AK. Fluorescence-enhanced Robotic Radical Cystectomy Using Unconjugated Indocyanine Green for Pelvic Lymphangiography, Tumor Marking, and Mesenteric Angiography: The Initial Clinical Experience. Urology. 2014;83(4):824-830. https://doi.org/10.1016/i.uroloav.2013.11.042; with permission.)

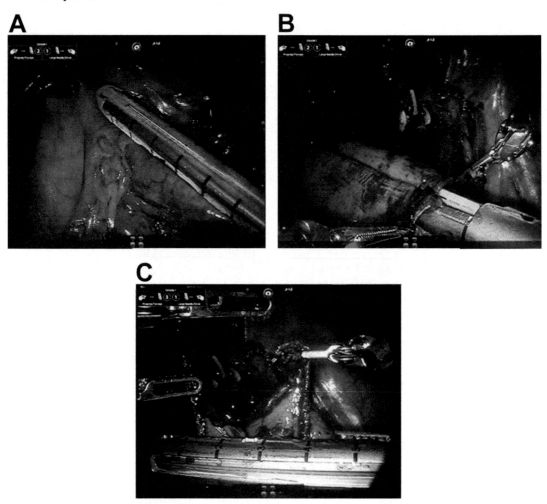

Fig. 2. Bowel division and anastomosis. (*A*) Division of distal bowel with 60 mm "tan" EndoGIA Stapler (Medtronic, Dublin, Ireland). (*B*) Side-to-side bowel anastomosis with "tan" stapler load. (*C*) Transverse bowel closure with "purple" load to complete establishing recontinuity.

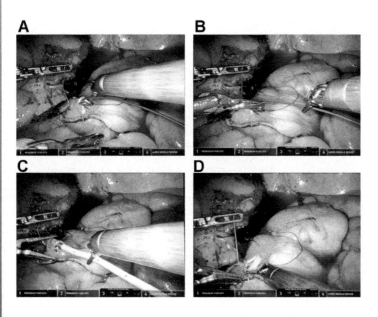

Fig. 3. Retrograde insertion of ureteral stent during intracorporeal ileal conduit. (*A*) Passage of glidewire from assistant port through spatulated ureter. (*B*) Further passage until resistance is met in renal pelvis. (*C*) Retrograde passage of 8 Fr × 30 cm double-J ureteral stent. (*D*) Glidewire is removed and distal coil is placed directly into ileal conduit.

Ureteral Isolation, Ureteroenteric Anastomosis, and Stent Placement

Before the radical cystectomy, the peritoneum overlying the ureters is incised. The ureters are dissected distal to the level of the superior vesical artery, at which point a Hem-o-lock (Teleflex, Wayne, PA) clip is placed on the bladder side of the ureter, and the ureter is transected. The ureter is then mobilized proximally with great care taken to preserve the peri-ureteral tissue. A length similar to that required for ORC is obtained. The ureters are then clipped distally with Hem-o-lock clips, and ureteral margins are sent for frozen section. The remainder of the radical cystectomy and pelvic lymphadenectomy are then performed. On completion, a tunnel is created underneath the mesentery of the sigmoid colon with electrocautery, and the left ureter is passed through the tunnel to the right side of the abdomen. The bowel isolation and anastomoses are then completed.

As with open diversion, ureteroenteric anastomoses can be performed using either a Bricker or Wallace technique. Definitive evidence to support one or the other is not available for ICUD. We use a Bricker approach. The ureters are spatulated for ~1 cm and we continuously run two 4 to 0 Vicryl sutures, one dyed and one undyed, for each ureteral wall starting from the apex of the spatulated ureter. The use of interrupted sutures and monofilament sutures have also been reported.[27,28] We use 8Fr × 30 cm double-J ureteral stents, though single-J stenting has also been reported.

Double-J stenting is performed by passing a glidewire through the 12-mm assistant port directly into the ureter after completion of the posterior wall and half of the anterior wall of the UEA, with subsequent retrograde stent placement into the renal pelvis and direct placement of the distal coil into the diversion, as shown in **Fig. 3**. If the stents have not auto-displaced by 1 month, office-based endoscopy is performed to retrieve them. The USC group uses a suprapubic 2-mm mini-port to pass in single-J stents, and Jonsson and colleagues[24] similarly pass single-J stents just above the suprapubic region percutaneously through 4-mm incisions.

Of note, Ahmed and colleagues[29] demonstrated that longer resected right ureteral length (22 mm vs 15 mm) was associated with lower rates of UEA stricture after RARC (hazard ratio [HR] 0.66, $P<.01$). Therefore, it is critical to adequately trim the distal ureter to avoid potential ischemia or kinking. This can also be addressed with the use of intraoperative ICG, which permits real-time visualization of ureteral vascularity as shown in **Fig. 4**. In their assessment of ICG use and ureteroenteric strictures following RARC, Ahmadi and colleagues[30] noted that ICG use promoted long segment ureteral resection (>5 cm). They also showed that no patients in their ICG cohort of 47 patients developed strictures compared with a 6.6% per ureter stricture rate in the non-ICG group of 132 patients. The ICG solution was prepared by mixing 25 mg ICG in 10 mL water. All 10 mL was administered before ureteral spatulation to assess perfusion. Shen and colleagues[31] had a similar experience with ICG and noted a 0% versus 7.5% stricture rate between the ICG group (93 ureters) and non-ICG group (93 ureters). In addition, 34% of ureters in the ICG group had poor distal perfusion requiring more proximal resection.

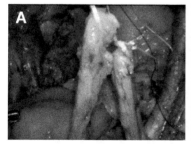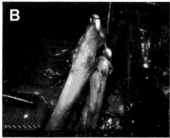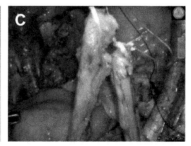

Fig. 4. Identical images obtained of bilateral distal ureters. (A) White light view with no visual cues of poor perfusion. (B) Firefly view with excellent uptake of tracer up to the distal clip. (C) PINPOINT view showing poor distal perfusion of left ureter. (From Shen JK, Jamnagerwalla J, Yuh BE, et al. Real-time indocyanine green angiography with the SPY fluorescence imaging platform decreases benign ureteroenteric strictures in urinary diversions performed during radical cystectomy. Therapeutic Advances in Urology. 2019;11:1756287219839631. https://doi.org/10.1177/1756287219839631; this figure is reproduced in an unmodified format according to the following Creative Commons License: https://creativecommons.Org/licenses/bv-nc/4.0/legalcode

RESERVOIR-SPECIFIC TECHNICAL POINTS, OUTCOMES, AND COMPLICATIONS DATA
Ileal Conduit

Technical points

There are a variety of methods for performing intracorporeal ileal conduit (ICIC), and the previously described methods of bowel division, ureteroenteric anastomosis and stent placement are broadly applicable to ICIC. In addition, the Roswell Park group has described the unique "Marionette" technique (**Fig. 5**) whereby a silk suture is brought through the anterior abdominal wall on a Keith needle then attached to the distal end of the conduit.[32] The suture is not tied but is rather held by one of the robotic instruments, which then controls this end of the conduit like a marionette. In this fashion, the bowel can be maneuvered as needed for stapling and creation of the UEA. Of note, the Roswell Park group establishes bowel recontinuity after performing the ureteroenteric anastomosis. In addition, single-J ureteral stents are advanced to the UEA site retrograde through the conduit. After creating an enterotomy in the distal aspect of the conduit, a laparoscopic suction tip is passed from the assistant port through the enterotomy and to the UEA site, at which point the stent is passed (**Fig. 6**).[27,32]

Outcomes

The Roswell Park group has published outcomes of their first 100 consecutive robotic cystectomy with ICIC. They found mean operative times of 352 minutes with a diversion time of 123 minutes. Other outcomes included mean EBL of 300 mL and median length of stay of 9 days.[33] When comparing outcomes between 13 consecutive ICUD to 13 consecutive ECUD patients, they found no difference in diversion time or EBL.[27] Tan and colleagues examined 59 cases of ICIC and found a mean operative time of 330 minutes and mean EBL of 300 mL, similar to Azzouni and colleagues.[4] The Karolinska group noted median operative time of 292 minutes, median EBL of 200 mL and median length of stay (LOS) 9 days in 43 patients undergoing ICIC, of whom 1 patient required conversion to open surgery.[25] For oncologic outcomes specifically, studies have shown mean lymph node yields of 17 to 24 and positive surgical margin rates of 4% to 8.5% after RARC with ICIC.[4,25,33]

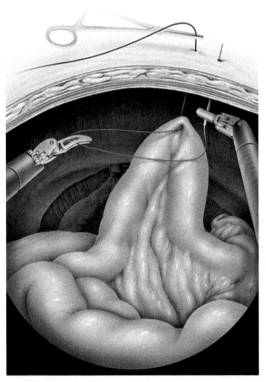

Fig. 5. "Marionette" stitch. (*From* Guru KA, Mansour AM, NyquistJ. Robot-assisted intracorporeal ileal conduit "Marionette" technique. BJU Int. 2010;106(9):1404-1420. https://doi.org/10.1111/i.l464-410X.2010.09772.x; with permission.)

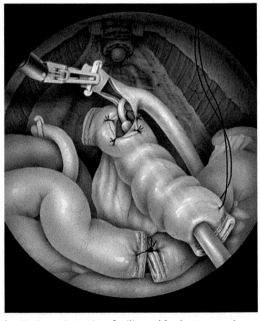

Fig. 6. Stent insertion facilitated by laparoscopic suction. (*From* Guru KA, Mansour AM, NyquistJ . Robot-assisted intracorporeal ileal conduit "Marionette" technique. BJU Int. 2010;106(9):1404-1420. https://doi.org/10.1111/i.l464-   410X.2010.09772.x;   with permission.)

Complications

The Roswell Park group found overall 90-day complication rates of 81% including 19% that were high grade (Clavien 3–5).[33] Infectious complications were the most common, representing 31%. Tan and colleagues[34] reported on complications in 100 patients who underwent ICIC at University College London from 2011 to 2015. They found a 90-day complication rate of 68% with 21% major complications. The 90-day mortality was 3%. Blood transfusion requirements and male gender were both associated with 90-day major complications ($P = .002$ and $P = .0015$, respectively). The same group subsequently examined 59 patients who underwent ICIC from 2015 to 2017 and found 30-day complication rate of 48.4% with 8.1% of these being high grade; 30-day to 90-day complication rates were 16.2% with 11.6% of these high-grade. The 90-day mortality rate in this later series was 0%. UEA stricture rates were 3.2%.[4]

A total of 37 early (<30 day) and 10 late (>30 day) complications were observed in a series of 43 patients who underwent ICIC in the Karolinska group.[25] This included 21 high-grade early complications; notably, all 10 late complications were high-grade. The most common early complication was ureteroileal leakage requiring nephrostomy tube placement (9 patients, 20.9%). The most common late complication was parastomal hernia in 3 patients (6.9%) requiring reoperation. As a whole, complication rates decrease with time, and are comparable to those encountered after ORC.[35]

Continent Cutaneous Diversion

Technical points

Only a few small series exist in the literature that report on technique, outcomes and complications for intracorporeal continent cutaneous diversion (ICCCD). Goh and colleagues[17] initially described the technique. The robot is undocked after completion of the cystectomy and the patient is taken out of steep Trendelenburg and dorsal lithotomy. Three additional ports are placed to gain access to the right colon, including one at the site of the future stoma. The patient is transitioned to a modified lateral position and the robot is redocked over the patient's right side. The pouch is created from cecum and 30 cm of detubularized ascending colon. The ureters are implanted into the posterior plate of the colon with the Bricker technique. Two 7 Fr single-J stents are placed though a 2 mm port used exclusively for stent placement. The catheterizable channel is created from 10 cm of distal ileum, which is tapered over a 14-Fr catheter by externalizing the ileal segment via the extraction site. It is then delivered through the stoma site and the stoma matured.

Desai and colleagues[36] described a series of 10 patients who underwent ICCCD. In their technique, the terminal ileum and cecum are mobilized before repositioning the patient for pouch creation. The robot is then undocked, 3 additional ports are placed and 1 port is upsized, and the patient is then moved to modified right lateral position if using the DaVinci Si. If using the DaVinci Xi in men or when vaginal extraction is not being performed in women, the entire procedure can be performed in the supine position although the robot still needs to be undocked and redocked after the new ports are placed. After repositioning, the right and transverse colon are mobilized. A Bricker UEA is performed into the posterior plate of the colon over 6 Fr × 28 cm double-J ureteral stents. The ileum is tapered by externalizing it through the umbilical extraction site and which is also the stomal site. Matulewicz and colleagues[37] published a video detailing this technique for intracorporeal Indiana Pouch creation. They describe the addition of an ileal chimney to the colonic reservoir using an additional 10 cm of ileum proximal to the segment used for the afferent limb (**Fig. 7**). This may facilitate UEA given its similarities to intracorporeal ileal conduit, which is a more familiar technique for those performing ICUD. The UEA is completed with a Bricker technique over single-J ureteral stents.

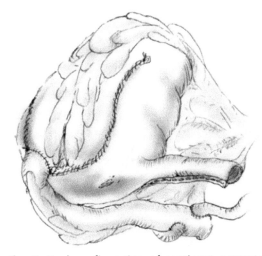

Fig. 7. Final configuration of continent cutaneous diversion with addition of ileal chimney. (*From* Matulewicz RS, Chesnut GT, Huang CC, Bochner BH, Goh AC. Evolution in technique of robotic intracorporeal continent catheterizable pouch after cystectomy. Urol Video J. 2019;4. https://doi.org/10.1016/i. urolvi. 2019.100020; with permission.)

Outcomes

Desai and colleagues[36] reported a median operative time of 6 hours, mean diversion time of 3.5 hours, median EBL of 200 mL and mean LOS of 10 days. Oncologic outcomes in this study were similar to others in the RARC literature, with median lymph node yield of 22 and no positive surgical margins. Importantly, 9 of 10 patients included in their study were completely continent at a median follow-up of 13.7 months. In the series by Matulewicz and colleagues[37] of 11 patients, mean EBL was 235 mL, mean operative time was 8.5 hours and mean LOS was 7.2 days. They had zero conversions to open surgery; 100% of patients were continent at last follow-up of 3 months.

Complications

In the series by Desai and colleagues,[36] the 30-day complication rate was 60%, although none were high grade. The 31-day to 90-day complication rate was 20% and included 2 high-grade complications that were UEA strictures. One stricture was treated successfully with a robotic re-implant and the other was managed with chronic ureteral stents. Matulewicz and colleagues[37] reported a 30-day major complication rate of 9% and readmission rate of 9%. There were no urine leaks, bowel leaks, stomal stenosis, or UEA stricture.

Neobladder

Technical points

The various techniques for intracorporeal neobladder (ICN) are more widely reported when compared with ICIC and ICCCD. Tan and colleagues[38] at of University College of London describe a "Pyramid Neobladder" technique in which stay sutures are placed between each distal ureter and the anterior abdominal wall to make them easily identifiable. A 50-cm ileal segment, at least 15 cm from the ileocecal valve is then identified. The urethro-ileal anastomosis is then created in the midline of the ileal segment over a 16 Fr catheter. A stay suture is placed 25 cm from the urethro-ileal anastomosis in either direction and this ileal segment is isolated with staplers. The small bowel is then detubularized with monopolar scissors starting at the dependent apical portion and moving outwards with the exclusion of 2 cm from the staple line on either side. The patient is then repositioned to zero degrees to enable the small bowel to move into the pelvis. The posterior plate is closed with barbed suture. The anterior plate is closed by suturing the bowel together in the midline from the urethro-ileal anastomosis cranially for 10 cm. The lateral bowel is then folded to the midline and closed from lateral to medial to complete closure of the neobladder. The ureters are anastomosed to the 2-cm ileal segments on either side of the neobladder using the Bricker technique over single-J ureteral stents or 8 Fr feeding tubes.

The USC group completes their neobladder using the same principles applied to creation of the Studer pouch in open surgery.[24,39] They isolate 44 cm of distal ileum for the neobladder with an additional 15 cm for the afferent limb. The distal ileum is detubularized and two 22-cm segments of ileum are positioned adjacent to each other after creating the posterior plate, which is then closed. The posterior plate is then rotated 90° counter clockwise and the urethro-ileal anastomosis is performed at the midline of the rotated segment (Fig. 8). The anterior closure is performed by cross-folding the bowel and the UEAs are implanted into the afferent limb with the Bricker technique.

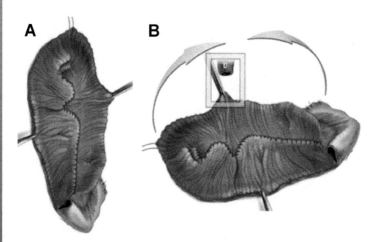

Fig. 8. (A) Posterior wall reconstruction. (B) Rotation of punch 90° counterclockwise with alignment for the urethroenteric anastomosis (yellow box). Blue arrows depict second folding of the bowl segment to create a globular configuration. U = urethra. (From Goh AC, Gill IS, Lee Di, et al. Robotic Intracorporeal Orthotopic Ileal Neobladder: Replicating Open Surgical Principles. European Urology. 2012;62(5) .891-901. doi:l0.1016/i.eururo.2012.07.052: with permission.)

The Karolinska group positions the patient at 10 to 15° Trendelenburg following the extirpative portion of the procedure and begins with the urethro-ileal anastomosis.[40] They isolate a 55-60 cm segment of terminal ileum (Part A) and detubularize along the anti-mesenteric border with 12-14 cm preserved at the proximal end for the afferent limb (Part B). The ureters are anastomosed to the afferent limb through the Wallace technique (Part E) (**Fig. 9**).[41]

The University of Florence group has described construction of a "neo-trigone" with "orthotopic" UEA, deemed the Florence robotic intracorporeal neobladder (FloRIN).[42] They isolate 50 cm of ileum and created the urethro-ileal anastomosis in an asymmetrical "U"-shape with 30 cm distal and 20 cm proximal to the anastomosis. After detubularization, the posterior wall is configured in an "L", which creates a neo-trigone. The bladder neck is reconfigured anteriorly and the posterior bladder is folded anteriorly to close the neobladder. Finally, the ureters are then reimplanted on the neo-trigone in orthotopic position.

At our institution, we use a 55-cm segment of ileum located 15 cm proximal to the ileocecal valve. The proximal 15 cm of the bowel segment is used as an ileal chimney and the distal 40 cm is used for the urinary reservoir. The distal 40 cm are detubularized and the posterior bowel plate is anchored to the posterior urethral plate. The posterior neobladder wall is closed with a running 3 to 0 V-loc suture. Nearly the entire anterior wall of

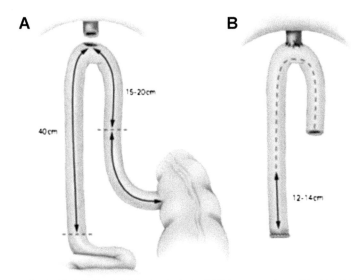
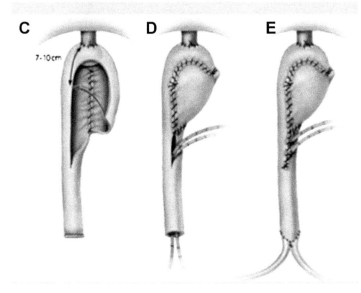

Fig. 9. Karolinska modified intracorporeal Studer neobladder. (*From* Wiklund NP, Poulakis V. Robotic neobladder. BJU Int. 2011;107(9):1514-1537.https://doi:org/10.11ll/i.l464410X.2011.10307. x; with permission.)

the neobladder is similarly closed, though a space is left to facilitate suprapubic catheter placement. The ureteroenteric anastomosis and stent placement are then performed as previously described on the proximal ileal chimney. The urethro-ileal anastomosis is performed with a running 2 to 0 Monocryl suture. An additional 12 mm suprapubic port is then inserted under direct vision, and a 20Fr Malecot suprapubic catheter is inserted and incorporated into the closure of the remainder of the anterior neobladder wall. Full details have been previously reported.[43]

It is critical to obtain a tension-free urethro-ileal anastomosis, and failure to do so may result in anastomotic urine leak or stricture. Our group has previously published our techniques to overcome challenging urethro-ileal anastomoses, which include the following maneuvers.[43]

- Maximizing urethral length at the prostatic apex
- Removing sigmoid colon from the pelvis to create room for the ileal loop
- Careful selection of an ileal segment with the longest possible mesentery
- Reducing pneumoperitoneum and Trendelenburg during suturing of the anastomosis with application of perineal pressure
- Use of barbed suture
- Detubularization of the ileal loop closer to the mesentery, lengthening the posterior plate

If the previous maneuvers fail to create a tension-free set-up, then incision of the peritoneum overlying the mesentery and releasing mesenteric fat can provide additional length. To stage the urethro-ileal anastomosis for success, we anchor the posterior bowel/neobladder to the posterior urethral plate before loop detubularization.[43]

Outcomes
Many studies have reported on both operative and oncologic outcomes for ICN. Median or mean operative times have ranged from 330 to 594 minutes depending on the series, with estimated blood loss ranging from 225 to 550 mL.[24,25,42–45] Average LOS has varied from 5 to 14 days, though most reports found medians in the 7-day to 9-day range.[24,25,42–45] Median or mean lymph node yields range from 19 to 25 and positive surgical margin rates are 0% to 3.7%.[24,25,28,40,45,46]

An initial series from the Karolinska Institute of 36 patients receiving ICN demonstrated continence rates of 97% and 83% for daytime and nighttime, respectively with a mean follow-up time of 25 months.[28] Of 20 patients who had a nerve-sparing surgery, 15 reported potency with

or without use of phosphodiesterase-5 inhibitors. Updated overall continence outcomes in their 70-patient cohort was 74% for men, and 67% for women at 1 year with potency reported in 26 of 41 men undergoing nerve-sparing surgery.[47] Porreca and colleagues[48] noted 90.2% and 70.6% daytime and nighttime continence at a median of 14 months, respectively in a cohort of 51 patients undergoing ICN. Canda and colleagues[45] reported on 27 cases and found 73% had full daytime continence with mean follow-up of 6.3 months. Nighttime continence was described as "good" in 20% of patients, "fair" in 26%, and "poor" in 53%. These functional outcomes compare favorably with historical continence outcomes in open neobladder series.[49]

Complications
Consistent with most literature on cystectomy and urinary diversion procedures, there a high incidence of early and late complications. The series by Canda and colleagues[45] of 27 patients showed 9 low-grade (33%, Clavien grade 1–2) and 4 high-grade (15%, Clavien grade 3–5) complications at 30 days. High-grade complications included the following: right external iliac vein injury with 7L EBL and conversion to open surgery, pulmonary issue requiring bronchoscopy, urinary leak, and death. The USC group has reported 30-day complication rates for their first series of 8 neobladder patients, which included 5 (63%) low-grade complications and 2 (25%) high-grade complications, with 2 additional high-grade complications at 90 days.[24] Early complications were infectious, and late complications related to urinary fistula or ureteral leak. The Karolinska group demonstrated a 31% rate of high-grade complications occurring by 30 days in their 70 patient series.[47] The most common complications were urosepsis (8.6%), lymphocele (5.7%), ureteroileal leakage (4.3%), and abdominal abscess (4.3%). In comparison, at 90 days, they identified a 21.4% incidence of high-grade complications with the most common being UTI (7.0%), hydronephrosis (4.3%), and ureteroileal stricture (4.3%). Tan and colleagues[34] reported a 90-day complication rate of 82.4% including 20.6% high-grade complications in 34 patients undergoing ICN. Across series, open conversion rates have been reported between 0% to 5.7% with 90-day mortality rates up to 2.9%.[24,34,43,47] It is clear that the morbidity burden following intracorporeal neobladder is high up to 90 days and almost certainly extends beyond this period. Complications relating to both infectious and technical etiologies persist throughout this time frame.

LEARNING CURVE

Progression through the learning curve of ICUD and complication rates following the procedure are inversely related. Even in the most experienced hands, up to 73% of patients experience some degree of complication following ORC, and 90-day mortality has been reported to be as high as 6.9%.[10,50] Complication rates following ICUD are similar to that reported for ORC and findings from series with ≥100 patients are highlighted in **Table 3**.

A clear number of cases to establish competency is harder to define. For robotic cystectomy in general, it has been suggested that 30 RARCs are needed to consistently obtain a minimum of 20 lymph nodes and cumulative positive surgical margin rate less than 5%.[51] Although this estimate of the learning curve accounts for intraoperative oncologic parameters, it does not account for surgery-related complications. For ICUD in particular, the learning curve is even less well defined. Based on an in-depth retrospective review of ICUD complications, such as urinary leak, ureteral stricture, wound dehiscence, incisional hernia and bleeding following ICUD by 2 experienced surgeons, Tan and colleagues[34] suggest that the learning curve may be closer to 100 cases or beyond, even for experienced surgeons.

Regardless of the true number of cases required to be proficient, ICUD use increased dramatically in IRCC surgeons from 9% in 2005, to 97% in 2015, of which 81% were ileal conduits.[2] In concordance, aggregate data of 1094 ICUD performed over a 10-year period demonstrate a decline in high-grade complications, from 25% in 2005 to 6% in 2015.[2] Clearly, a dedicated effort over time is required to master ICUD, and several have reported on their experiences overcoming the learning curve.

At an institutional level, Schumacher and colleagues[3] evaluated 45 consecutive patients undergoing RARC with ICUD, divided into 3 groups of 15. They noted a significant decrease in operative time, LOS, and greater than 30-day complication rate in the later groups. Of note, early Clavien grade III and greater complications did not change between groups. Desai and colleagues[46] similarly identified a decrease in LOS and operative time in a consecutive series of 132 intracorporeal neobladder.

In addition to individual experience, learning from expert surgeons can also assist in overcoming the learning curve. For example, Porreca and colleagues[48] reported a decrease in 30-day to 90-day complication rates and operative times after attending a training program at a referral center. The program consisted of theoretic didactics, video-based instruction, and step-by-step intraoperative training. Collins and colleagues[52] described how mentorship may allow a junior surgeon to abbreviate the learning curve. In prospectively evaluating 67 RARC with intracorporeal neobladder, the mentor surgeon experienced statistically significant improvements in operative time, early and late complications and a decreased conversion rate to open surgery over 47 consecutive patients. The mentee surgeon did not experience the same relative improvements over 20 cases, but both surgeons had statistically similar outcome endpoints on overall cohort analysis. This implies that the mentor surgeon's experience in overcoming the learning curve directly translated to the mentee surgeon.

Our institution uses a similar mentorship model to that described by Collins and colleagues.[52]

Table 3
Comparison of complications among ICUD cohorts

Series	Tan WS et al. (n = 134)	Desai et al. (n = 132)	Porreca et al. (n = 100)	Hussein et al. IRCC (n = 1094)
Number of institutions	Single	Multiple (2)	Single	Multiple (26)
0–30 day ≤ Clavien 3, %	38.9	31.8	25	-
30–90 day ≤ Clavien 3, %	50.8	14.4	18.8	-
0–30 day ≥ Clavien 3, %	14.9	15.2	9	31
30–90 day ≥ Clavien 3, %	20.9	12.9	10	5
Blood transfusion, %	21.6 (within 90 d)	4.5 (intraop)	14 (intraop)	5 (intraop)
90-d mortality, %	3	1.5	2	3
≥ pT3, %	41.4	35	36	42

Abbreviations: ICUD, intracorporeal urinary diversion; intraop, intraoperative.
Data from Refs.[2,34,46,48]

The mentee surgeon benefits from oversight by the mentor surgeon in their initial 15 to 20 cases, and they function as co-surgeons for the operation. We also "centralize" RARC with ICUD as follows:

- RARC with ICUD are performed on the same days of the week, each week, allowing for a consistent operative team
- Surgeries take place in adjacent rooms, permitting open communication and operative assistance between surgeons, if required.

DIRECT COMPARISON OF INTRACORPOREAL URINARY DIVERSION WITH EXTRACORPOREAL URINARY DIVERSION

Although many are comfortable using robotic assistance to perform the extirpative component of radical cystectomy, hesitancy with the technical components of ICUD result in ECUD being selected. Some data suggest that ICUD is associated with enhanced bowel recovery due to limited peritoneal cavity exposure to air, shorter operative times and less intraoperative blood loss when compared with ECUD.[4] Comparative perioperative outcomes between ICUD and ECUD series are shown in **Table 4**.

In the largest multi-institutional comparison of ICUD and ECUD, the IRCC retrospectively evaluated 1094 ICUD and 1031 ECUD between 2005 and 2016.[2] Patients undergoing ICUD were more likely to have American Society of Anesthesiologists (ASA) score less than 3 (odds ratio [OR] 1.75, $P<.01$) and undergo surgery in the most recent 3 years of the study (2013–2016 vs earlier – OR 68, $P<.01$). ICUD was associated with shorter operative times (357 min vs 400 min), less blood loss (300 mL vs 350 mL) and blood transfusion rate (5% vs 13%, all $P<.01$). Though the cohorts were similar with regard to prior abdominal surgical history, radiation history, presentation with cT3 or greater and final pT3 or greater, the ICUD group was more likely to have higher-grade complications (13% vs 10% $P = .02$) and have poorer overall survival (49% vs 58% at 5 years, log-rank test $P = .05$). The investigators attribute this to more severe complications occurring early in adopting ICUD, as high-grade complications decreased from 25% in 2005 to 6% in 2015. The same trend was not observed in ECUD, as complications were 13% in 2005 and 14% in 2015. Despite the number of patients in the study, findings must be interpreted cautiously as data were submitted from 26 institutions, each with varying surgical volumes and practice patterns.

At a single-institution level, Tan TW and colleagues[4] described their transition from extracorporeal (n = 68) to intracorporeal (n = 59) ileal conduit following RARC. They noted lower 30-day complication rates (48.4% vs 71.4%), decreased blood loss (300 mL vs 425 mL) and operative times (330 min. vs 375 min) in the ICUD group compared with ECUD.[4] In addition, operative times were significantly lower in the latter half of patients undergoing ICUD compared with the first half (300 vs 360 minutes).

Bertolo and colleagues[53] compared diversion outcomes between 2 experienced RARC surgeons at a single institution during the same time period: one surgeon who only performed ICUD and another that only performed ECUD. Apart from ICUD patients being younger, no other differences in preoperative demographic or pathology were noted. Patients undergoing ECUD had shorter overall operative times (6 hours vs 7 hours, $P<.01$), though no differences in complications or other perioperative outcomes were identified.

In a large, contemporary single-institution study, Zhang and colleagues[35] compared outcomes between ORC, RARC/ICUD, and RARC/ECUD, in 272, 301, and 375 (total n = 948) patients who did not differ in preoperative demographics or final pathology. Of note, nearly 85% of patients underwent ileal conduit in the ICUD group, compared with 71% and 75% in the ECUD and ORC groups, respectively. They identified ICUD to be associated with lower estimated blood loss and shorter LOS than ECUD or ORC (300 mL vs 400 mL vs 700 mL and 6 days vs 7 days vs 8 days, respectively, both $P<.001$). In addition, the ICUD group experienced lower 30-day and 90-day major complications when compared with ECUD or ORC (90-day Clavien 3–5 complication rates: 16.9% vs 24.8% vs 26.1%, respectively, $P = .015$) and ICUD was independently associated with reduced 90-day Clavien 3 to 5 complication rates on multivariable analysis (OR 0.58, $P = .037$).

Ultimately, definitive benefits of ICUD over ECUD cannot be generalized given the influence of the early surgical learning curve on initial perioperative outcomes and differences in diversion type by surgical approach. Despite these limitations, retrospective literature has demonstrated that ICUD can offer benefits with regards to convalescence with decreased complication rates, though this will likely only manifest at higher volume cystectomy centers.

ENHANCED RECOVERY AFTER SURGERY

ICUD itself can decrease the morbidity of radical cystectomy, though the benefits may not be

Table 4
Comparison of perioperative outcomes between intracorporeal urinary diversion (ICUD) and extracorporeal urinary diversion (ECUD)

Series	Zhang et al,[35] 2020		Lenfant et al. (2018)		Bertolo et al,[53] 2019		Tan et al,[4] 2019		Hussein et al,[2] (2018) IRCC	
Diversion type	ECUD (n = 375)	ICUD (n = 301)	ECUD (n = 34)	ICUD (n = 74)	ECUD (n = 66)	ICUD (n = 60)	ECUD (n = 68)	ICUD (n = 59)	ECUD (n = 1031)	ICUD (n = 1094)
Operative time (min)	421	396	285	320	360	420	375	330	400	357
Estimated blood loss (mL)	400	300	500	400	350	380	425	300	350	300
Length of stay (days)	7	6	12	14	8	7	8	8	8	9
90-d Clavien 3–5 complication rate, %	24.8	16.9	17.6	12.2	0	1.6	9.1	11.6	4	5
Blood transfusion requirement, %	24.3 (intraop)	16.9 (intraop)	23.5[a] (periop)	5.4[a] (periop)	9.1 (intraop)	13.3 (intraop)	NR	NR	13[a]	5[a]

Abbreviations: intraop, intraoperative; NR, not reported; periop, perioperative.
[a] Time course not specified.

Data from Zhang JH, Ericson KJ, Thomas LJ, et al. Large Single Institution Comparison of Perioperative Outcomes and Complications of Open Radical Cystectomy, Intracorporeal Robot-Assisted Radical Cystectomy and Robotic Extracorporeal Approach. *J Urol.* 2020;203(3):512-521. https://doi.org/10.1097/JU.0000000000000570; Lenfant L, Verhoest G, Campi R, et al. Perioperative outcomes and complications of intracorporeal vs extracorporeal urinary diversion after robot-assisted radical cystectomy for bladder cancer: a real-life, multi-institutional french study. *World Journal of Urology.* 2018;36(11):1711-1718. https://doi.org/10.1007/s00345-018-2313-8; Bertolo R, Agudelo J, Garisto J, Armanyous S, Fergany A, Kaouk J. Perioperative Outcomes and Complications after Robotic Radical Cystectomy With Intracorporeal or Extracorporeal Ileal Conduit Urinary Diversion: Head-to-head Comparison From a Single-Institutional Prospective Study. *Urology.* 2019;129:98-105. https://doi.org/10.1016/j.urology.2018.11.059; Tan TW, Nair R, Saad S, Thurairaja R, Khan MS. Safe transition from extracorporeal to intracorporeal urinary diversion following robot-assisted cystectomy: a recipe for reducing operative time, blood loss and complication rates. *World J Urol.* 2019;37(2):367-372. https://doi.org/10.1007/s00345-018-2386-4; Hussein AA, May PR, Jing Z, et al. Outcomes of Intracorporeal Urinary Diversion after Robot-Assisted Radical Cystectomy: Results from the International Robotic Cystectomy Consortium. *The Journal of Urology.* 2018;199(5):1302-1311. https://doi.org/10.1016/j.juro.2017.12.045.

actualized unless the surgeon commits to overcoming the learning curve. In the overall morbidity scheme of RC, however, ICUD remains a single factor. Other care paradigms can help minimize morbidity, along with ICUD. These multi-modal care pathways to expedite convalescence and decrease complications have collectively come to be known as Enhanced Recovery After Surgery, or ERAS.

Tan and colleagues[54] described their experience comparing ORC, RARC/ICUD without ERAS, and RARC/ICUD with an ERAS protocol. They found that when compared with the ICUD group without ERAS, the ICUD group with ERAS experienced statistically significant improvements in 90-day readmission rates (7.5% vs 25%), 30-day gastrointestinal complications (20% vs 45%) and 90-day all complications (45% vs 75%).

Koupparis and colleagues[20] also noted a LOS decrease of 5 days favoring their RARC/ICUD with ERAS cohort compared with ORC with ERAS. The Karolinska Institute demonstrated that despite increasing age, higher ASA grade, and higher T-stage in their ERAS cohort, there were no differences in 30-day complication rates, 90-day mortality rates, or overall readmission rates with a lower median LOS (8 days vs 9 days, $P<.01$).

The European Association of Urology Robotic Urology Section published a working group policy for ERAS in RARC.[15] Eighty-five percent of the group agreed that epidural analgesia could routinely be omitted in ICUD. Although not ICUD specific, other notable ERAS features included the following:

- Avoiding intraoperative overhydration
- Minimizing intraoperative narcotics
- Removal of nasogastric tube (NGT) in the recovery unit
- Prokinetic medication use to prevent ileus
- Limited postoperative narcotic use
- Mobilization within 24 hours of surgery
- Early feeding

In their assessment of 35 consecutive patients following an ERAS protocol undergoing RARC with intracorporeal ileal conduit, Tamhankar and colleagues[19] specify that goal directed fluids are 1 L for every 6 hours of surgery. They also emphasize the importance of a consistent surgical team and use a urethral foley catheter as a surgical drain.

In addition to the aforementioned policies, we administer alvimopan, a peripherally acting mu-opioid receptor antagonist that has been shown to decrease time to first bowel movement (5.5 vs 6.8 days, $P<.01$) and LOS (7.4 vs 10.1 days, $P<.01$) in a randomized double-blind placebo controlled trial (NCT00708201).[55] Alvimopan is administered preoperatively and continued until the patient has returned to flatus. We also schedule intravenous and oral acetaminophen with ketorolac, as this limits but does not eliminate narcotic use.

UPCOMING ADVANCES AND FUTURE RESEARCH IN INTRACORPOREAL DIVERSION

Although significant progress has been made in ICUD since its initial technical description, further evaluation is necessary to optimize its use. Though patient benefits remain to be seen, single port surgery has the potential to further decrease operative morbidity. In the initial description of intracorporeal ileal conduit using the DaVinci SP Surgical System, Kaouk and colleagues[56] were able to successfully perform the procedure in 3 (2 men and 1 woman) of 4 patients. One female patient was converted to ECUD given significant bowel adhesive burden. In female patients, a transvaginal 12-mm assistant port is placed after specimen extraction and vaginal closure to permit laparoscopic stapling for bowel isolation. Diversion times were 90, 76, and 67 minutes and overall operative times were 496, 420, and 425 minutes. These times are consistent with initial descriptions of RARC with ICUD using a conventional robotic platform by Karolinska (477 minutes for ileal conduit/neobladder), USC (450 minutes for ileal conduit/neobladder), Roswell Park (391 minutes, ileal conduit only), and Cleveland Clinic (486 minutes neobladder only).[24,27,28,43] Further cases will be required to establish any benefits when compared with multi-arm ICUD.

In assessing ERAS protocols, The European Association of Urology Robotic Urology Section identified several areas warranting additional research.[15] This includes standardizing anesthetic protocols and identifying optimal timing of ureteral stent removal and urethral foley catheter after neobladder. In addition, a multicenter prospective randomized trial comparing ORC with RARC with ICUD (NCT03049410), the iROC trial, will provide the current highest level of evidence in order to elucidate differences between these 2 approaches.[11]

With the increasing use of robotics in urologic oncology, ICUD may see further adoption given that urologists may have more exposure to this technically challenging procedure during their training. Over time, national-database comparisons may help highlight outcomes aside from those generated from large single-center and multi-institutional reports. On the other hand,

Clinics care points	
Preoperative	• Avoid routine bowel preparation
	• Oral intake recommendations:
	○ Solids up to 6 hours prior
	○ Clear liquids up to 2 hours prior
	• Consider clear liquid carbohydrate loading 2–3 hours prior
	• Epidural analgesia can be safely avoided
Intraoperative	• Select patients with lower ASA scores and absence of prior abdominal surgery early in learning curve, as these factors are associated with a higher risk of postoperative complications
	• Ensure adequate ureteral resection length to avoid postoperative ureteroenteral anastomotic stricture
	○ Safe minimum 1.5-cm resection
	• Consider indocyanine green use to identify mesenteric vasculature before bowel resection and to assess distal ureteral perfusion
	• Either Bricker or Wallace ureteral anastomotic technique is suitable
	• Either single-J or double-J ureteral stenting is suitable
Postoperative	• The nasogastric tube can be removed immediately postoperatively
	• Early ambulation and early feeding within 24 hours postoperatively are encouraged
	• Limit narcotic use and include acetaminophen for baseline pain control
	• One dose of alvimopan administered preoperatively (12 mg 30 minutes to 5 hours before anesthesia induction) and continued until discharge (12 mg twice daily, max 15 doses) is associated with a faster return to stooling and shorter hospital stay
	• Optimal timing for ureteral stent removal has not been determined but has been safely performed from 5 to 14+ days.
	• Optimal timing for Foley catheter removal after neobladder has not been determined, but most suggest a 14-day minimum.

given that ICUD may take longer to perform without appreciable patient benefits outside of high-volume centers, it may not become a part of routine urologic practice in the future.

SUMMARY

Intracorporeal urinary diversion following RARC has been increasingly adopted among high-volume cystectomists in the past decade. The procedure is technically challenging, and requires a committed effort between the surgeon and operative team to overcome the learning curve. ICUD can potentially provide patient-related benefits with regard to intraoperative blood loss, transfusion rates, operative times, and overall complication rates without sacrificing long-term oncologic outcomes when compared with ORC or ECUD. Numerous technical modifications have been described to facilitate the procedure and help diminish morbidity, while enhanced recovery protocols and standardization of postoperative care may further improve patient outcomes. In summary, ICUD provides a promising alternative to ECUD, and should be more widely adopted among high-volume cystectomists.

DISCLOSURE

None of the authors have any financial disclosures or conflicts of interest.

REFERENCES

1. Zamboni S, Soria F, Mathieu R, et al. Differences in trends in the use of robot-assisted and open radical cystectomy and changes over time in peri-operative outcomes among selected centres in North America and Europe: an international multicentre collaboration. BJU Int 2019;124(4):656–64.
2. Hussein AA, May PR, Jing Z, et al. Outcomes of intracorporeal urinary diversion after robot-assisted radical cystectomy: results from the International

Robotic Cystectomy Consortium. J Urol 2018; 199(5):1302–11.

3. Schumacher MC, Jonsson MN, Hosseini A, et al. Surgery-related complications of robot-assisted radical cystectomy with intracorporeal urinary diversion. Urology 2011;77(4):871–6.

4. Tan TW, Nair R, Saad S, et al. Safe transition from extracorporeal to intracorporeal urinary diversion following robot-assisted cystectomy: a recipe for reducing operative time, blood loss and complication rates. World J Urol 2019;37(2):367–72.

5. Simone G, Tuderti G, Misuraca L, et al. Perioperative and mid-term oncologic outcomes of robotic assisted radical cystectomy with totally intracorporeal neobladder: Results of a propensity score matched comparison with open cohort from a single-centre series. Eur J Surg Oncol 2018;44(9):1432–8.

6. Bochner BH, Dalbagni G, Marzouk KH, et al. Randomized trial comparing open radical cystectomy and robot-assisted laparoscopic radical cystectomy: oncologic outcomes. Eur Urol 2018;74(4):465–71.

7. Nguyen DP, Al Hussein Al Awamlh B, Wu X, et al. Recurrence patterns after open and robot-assisted radical cystectomy for bladder cancer. Eur Urol 2015;68(3):399–405.

8. Venkatramani V, Reis Isildinha M, Castle Erik P, et al. Predictors of recurrence, and progression-free and overall survival following open versus robotic radical cystectomy: analysis from the RAZOR trial with a 3-year followup. J Urol 2020;203(3):522–9.

9. Nguyen DP, Al Hussein Al Awamlh B, O'Malley P, et al. Factors impacting the occurrence of local, distant and atypical recurrences after robot-assisted radical cystectomy: a detailed analysis of 310 patients. J Urol 2016;196(5):1390–6.

10. Hussein AA, Elsayed AS, Aldhaam NA, et al. Ten-year oncologic outcomes following robot-assisted radical cystectomy: results from the international robotic cystectomy consortium. J Urol 2019;202(5):927–35.

11. Catto JWF, Khetrapal P, Ambler G, et al. Robot-assisted radical cystectomy with intracorporeal urinary diversion versus open radical cystectomy (iROC): protocol for a randomised controlled trial with internal feasibility study. BMJ Open 2018;8(8):e020500.

12. Tan WS, Sridhar A, Ellis G, et al. Analysis of open and intracorporeal robotic assisted radical cystectomy shows no significant difference in recurrence patterns and oncological outcomes. Urol Oncol 2016;34(6):257.e1-9.

13. Brassetti A, Cacciamani G, Anceschi U, et al. Long-term oncologic outcomes of robot-assisted radical cystectomy (RARC) with totally intracorporeal urinary diversion (ICUD): a multi-center study. World J Urol 2019. https://doi.org/10.1007/s00345-019-02842-3.

14. Wilson TG, Guru K, Rosen RC, et al. Best practices in robot-assisted radical cystectomy and urinary reconstruction: recommendations of the pasadena consensus panel. Eur Urol 2015;67(3):363–75.

15. Collins JW, Patel H, Adding C, et al. Enhanced recovery after robot-assisted radical cystectomy: EAU Robotic Urology Section Scientific Working Group Consensus View. Eur Urol 2016;70(4):649–60.

16. Large MC, Kiriluk KJ, DeCastro GJ, et al. The impact of mechanical bowel preparation on postoperative complications for patients undergoing cystectomy and urinary diversion. J Urol 2012;188(5):1801–5.

17. Goh AC, Aghazadeh MA, Krasnow RE, et al. Robotic intracorporeal continent cutaneous urinary diversion: primary description. J Endourol 2015;29(11):1217–20.

18. Adding C, Collins JW, Laurin O, et al. Enhanced recovery protocols (ERP) in robotic cystectomy surgery. Review of current status and trends. Curr Urol Rep 2015;16(5):32.

19. Tamhankar AS, Ahluwalia P, Patil SR, et al. Implementation of ERAS protocol in robot-assisted radical cystectomy with intracorporeal ileal conduit urinary diversion: An outcome analysis beyond the learning curve. Indian J Urol 2020;36(1):37–43.

20. Koupparis A, Villeda-Sandoval C, Weale N, et al. Robot-assisted radical cystectomy with intracorporeal urinary diversion: impact on an established enhanced recovery protocol. BJU Int 2015;116(6):924–31.

21. Maerz DA, Beck LN, Sim AJ, et al. Complications of robotic-assisted laparoscopic surgery distant from the surgical site. Br J Anaesth 2017;118(4):492–503.

22. Warner MA, Warner DO, Harper CM, et al. Lower extremity neuropathies associated with lithotomy positions. Anesthesiology 2000;93(4):938–42.

23. Chan KG, Guru K, Wiklund P, et al. Robot-assisted radical cystectomy and urinary diversion: technical recommendations from the pasadena consensus panel. Eur Urol 2015;67(3):423–31.

24. Goh AC, Gill IS, Lee DJ, et al. Robotic intracorporeal orthotopic ileal neobladder: replicating open surgical principles. Eur Urol 2012;62(5):891–901.

25. Collins JW, Tyritzis S, Nyberg T, et al. Robot-assisted radical cystectomy: description of an evolved approach to radical cystectomy. Eur Urol 2013;64(4):654–63.

26. Manny TB, Hemal AK. Fluorescence-enhanced robotic radical cystectomy using unconjugated indocyanine green for pelvic lymphangiography, tumor marking, and mesenteric angiography: the initial clinical experience. Urology 2014;83(4):824–30.

27. Guru K, Seixas-Mikelus SA, Hussain A, et al. Robot-assisted intracorporeal ileal conduit: marionette technique and initial experience at Roswell Park Cancer Institute. Urology 2010;76(4):866–71.

28. Jonsson MN, Adding LC, Hosseini A, et al. Robot-assisted radical cystectomy with intracorporeal urinary diversion in patients with transitional cell carcinoma of the bladder. Eur Urol 2011;60(5):1066–73.

29. Ahmed YE, Hussein AA, May PR, et al. Natural history, predictors and management of ureteroenteric strictures after robot assisted radical cystectomy. J Urol 2017;198(3):567–74.

30. Ahmadi N, Ashrafi AN, Hartman N, et al. Use of indocyanine green to minimise uretero-enteric strictures after robotic radical cystectomy. BJU Int 2019;124(2):302–7.

31. Shen JK, Jamnagerwalla J, Yuh BE, et al. Real-time indocyanine green angiography with the SPY fluorescence imaging platform decreases benign ureteroenteric strictures in urinary diversions performed during radical cystectomy. Ther Adv Urol 2019;11. 1756287219839631.

32. Guru KA, Mansour AM, Nyquist J. Robot-assisted intracorporeal ileal conduit "Marionette" technique. BJU Int 2010;106(9):1404–20.

33. Azzouni FS, Din R, Rehman S, et al. The first 100 consecutive, robot-assisted, intracorporeal ileal conduits: evolution of technique and 90-day outcomes. Eur Urol 2013;63(4):637–43.

34. Tan WS, Lamb BW, Tan M-Y, et al. In-depth critical analysis of complications following robot-assisted radical cystectomy with intracorporeal urinary diversion. Eur Urol Focus 2017;3(2):273–9. https://doi.org/10.1016/j.euf.2016.06.002.

35. Zhang JH, Ericson KJ, Thomas LJ, et al. Large single institution comparison of perioperative outcomes and complications of open radical cystectomy, intracorporeal robot-assisted radical cystectomy and robotic extracorporeal approach. J Urol 2020;203(3):512–21.

36. Desai MM, Simone G, de Castro Abreu AL, et al. Robotic intracorporeal continent cutaneous diversion. J Urol 2017;198(2):436–44.

37. Matulewicz RS, Chesnut GT, Huang CC, et al. Evolution in technique of robotic intracorporeal continent catheterizable pouch after cystectomy. Urol Video J 2019;4. https://doi.org/10.1016/j.urolvj.2019.100020.

38. Tan WS, Sridhar A, Goldstraw M, et al. Robot-assisted intracorporeal pyramid neobladder. BJU Int 2015;116(5):771–9.

39. Abreu AL de C, Chopra S, Azhar RA, et al. Robotic radical cystectomy and intracorporeal urinary diversion: The USC technique. Indian J Urol 2014;30(3):300–6.

40. Collins JW, Sooriakumaran P, Sanchez-Salas R, et al. Robot-assisted radical cystectomy with intracorporeal neobladder diversion: The Karolinska experience. Indian J Urol 2014;30(3):307–13.

41. Wiklund NP, Poulakis V. Robotic neobladder. BJU Int 2011;107(9):1514–37.

42. Minervini A, Vanacore D, Vittori G, et al. Florence robotic intracorporeal neobladder (FloRIN): a new reconfiguration strategy developed following the IDEAL guidelines. BJU Int 2018;121(2):313–7.

43. Almassi N, Zargar H, Ganesan V, et al. Management of challenging urethro-ileal anastomosis during robotic assisted radical cystectomy with intracorporeal neobladder formation. Eur Urol 2016;69(4):704–9.

44. Pruthi RS, Nix J, McRackan D, et al. Robotic-assisted laparoscopic intracorporeal urinary diversion. Eur Urol 2010;57(6):1013–21.

45. Canda AE, Atmaca AF, Altinova S, et al. Robot-assisted nerve-sparing radical cystectomy with bilateral extended pelvic lymph node dissection (PLND) and intracorporeal urinary diversion for bladder cancer: initial experience in 27 cases. BJU Int 2012;110(3):434–44.

46. Desai Mihir M, Gill Inderbir S, de Castro Abreu Andre Luis, et al. Robotic intracorporeal orthotopic neobladder during radical cystectomy in 132 patients. J Urol 2014;192(6):1734–40.

47. Tyritzis SI, Hosseini A, Collins J, et al. Oncologic, functional, and complications outcomes of robot-assisted radical cystectomy with totally intracorporeal neobladder diversion. Eur Urol 2013;64(5):734–41.

48. Porreca A, Mineo Bianchi F, Romagnoli D, et al. Robot-assisted radical cystectomy with totally intracorporeal urinary diversion: surgical and early functional outcomes through the learning curve in a single high-volume center. J Robot Surg 2019. https://doi.org/10.1007/s11701-019-00977-4.

49. Tan WS, Lamb BW, Kelly JD. Evolution of the neobladder: a critical review of open and intracorporeal neobladder reconstruction techniques. Scand J Urol 2016;50(2):95–103.

50. Moschini M, Simone G, Stenzl A, et al. Critical review of outcomes from radical cystectomy: can complications from radical cystectomy be reduced by surgical volume and robotic surgery? Eur Urol Focus 2016;2(1):19–20.

51. Hayn MH, Hussain A, Mansour AM, et al. The learning curve of robot-assisted radical cystectomy: results from the International Robotic Cystectomy Consortium. Eur Urol 2010;58(2):197–202.

52. Collins JW, Tyritzis S, Nyberg T, et al. Robot-assisted radical cystectomy (RARC) with intracorporeal neobladder – what is the effect of the learning curve on outcomes? BJU Int 2014;113(1):100–7.

53. Bertolo R, Agudelo J, Garisto J, et al. Perioperative outcomes and complications after robotic radical cystectomy with intracorporeal or extracorporeal ileal conduit urinary diversion: head-to-head comparison from a single-institutional prospective study. Urology 2019;129:98–105.

54. Tan WS, Tan M-Y, Lamb BW, et al. Intracorporeal robot-assisted radical cystectomy, together with an enhanced recovery programme, improves postoperative outcomes by aggregating marginal gains. BJU Int 2018;121(4):632–9.

55. Lee CT, Chang SS, Kamat AM, et al. Alvimopan accelerates gastrointestinal recovery after radical cystectomy: a multicenter randomized placebo-controlled trial. Eur Urol 2014;66(2):265–72.

56. Kaouk J, Garisto J, Eltemamy M, et al. Single-port robotic intracorporeal ileal conduit urinary diversion during radical cystectomy using the SP surgical system: step-by-step technique. Urology 2019;130: 196–200.

Robot-Assisted Surgery for Upper Tract Urothelial Carcinoma

Eric M. Lo, BS[a], Hyung L. Kim, MD[b],*

KEYWORDS

- Cancer • Transitional cell carcinoma • Urothelial carcinoma • Upper tract • Robotic surgery
- Ureterectomy

KEY POINTS

- Upper tract transitional cell carcinoma is a rare malignancy for which surgery is the only definitive treatment.
- Robot-assisted surgery provides a minimally invasive approach and has become more popular in recent years.
- Robot-assisted techniques for upper tract urothelial carcinoma seem to have similar outcomes to open and laparoscopic approaches.
- For select ureteral cancers, the involved kidney can be spared by performing robot-assisted distal ureterectomy or segmental ureterectomy.

INTRODUCTION AND BACKGROUND

Upper tract urothelial carcinoma (UC), also referred to as upper tract transitional cell carcinoma, is a rare disease that makes up approximately 5% of all UCs and less than 5% to 7% of all renal tumors.[1] Upper tract UC is two times more common in men than in women and is commonly diagnosed in the eighth decade of life.[2] The disease is often multifocal at presentation because the entire urothelial surface has been exposed to urinary carcinogens resulting in a "field cancerization" effect.[3] Staging of upper tract UC is based on the tumor, node, metastasis (TNM) system.[4] In the eighth edition of the staging system, stage IV cancers have metastasized to the lymph nodes or distant sites.[5] Lower stages are categorized by the invasiveness of the primary tumor. Stage 0a and 0is refer to tumors that are papillary and noninvasive carcinoma (Ta), and carcinoma in situ (Tis), respectively. Stages 1 to 3 correspond to T1, T2, and T3 tumor

categories, with each category representing an increase in tumor invasiveness. Survival correlates with tumor stage at diagnosis, with 5-year survival rates of 100% for stage Ta and Tis versus 41% for stage T3 disease.[6] Surgery is considered the only definitive treatment for upper tract UC. Historically, open nephroureterectomy was considered the treatment of choice. However, technological developments have ushered in newer, minimally invasive techniques, such as laparoscopic nephroureterectomy and robot-assisted laparoscopic nephroureterectomy. Clayman and colleagues described the first laparoscopic nephroureterectomy in 1991, and subsequent reports demonstrated comparable oncologic outcomes with reduced morbidity when compared with open surgery.[7,8,9] The first robot-assisted nephrectomy was reported in 2000, and the robotic platform rapidly grew in popularity for numerous urologic procedures in the following two decades.[10,11] Robot-assisted nephroureterectomies demonstrated comparable

[a] Baylor College of Medicine, 1 Baylor Plaza, Houston, TX 77030, USA; [b] Cedars-Sinai Medical Center, 8635 West Third Street, Los Angeles, CA 90048, USA
* Corresponding author.
E-mail address: kimhl@csmc.edu

Urol Clin N Am 48 (2021) 71–80
https://doi.org/10.1016/j.ucl.2020.09.011

clinical outcomes to laparoscopic and open approaches, and were also associated with the shortest hospital stays.[12] Increased use of robot-assisted surgeries can be attributed to improved dexterity provided by the da Vinci surgical system (Intuitive Surgical, Sunnyvale, CA), increased use of minimally invasive techniques in training programs, and increased availability of the robot platform.[13] Techniques, such as distal ureterectomy with ureteral reimplant, which has the advantage of sparing both kidneys, can be performed using the robotic platform. Segmental ureterectomy with primary ureteroureterostomy is an additional method of managing upper tract UC and also can be performed robotically. Compared with open surgery, robot-assisted surgery offers the advantage of improved cosmesis and shorter recovery.[14]

OUTCOMES

Historically, open radical nephroureterectomy was considered the gold standard for definitive treatment of upper tract UC.[15] Technological developments led to laparoscopic and robot-assisted techniques in the management of upper tract UC. With the increased dexterity offered by the da Vinci surgical system, minimally invasive approaches have become more widely available. Although the robotic approach has not been evaluated in prospective, randomized trials, retrospective data show cancer control outcomes that are similar to open and laparoscopic approaches. Clements and colleagues[12] performed a comparative survival analysis of 3801 patients undergoing robot-assisted versus laparoscopic or open surgery for upper tract UC and found that robotic surgery was associated with the shortest length of hospital stay with no difference in readmission rates, overall, or cancer-specific survival (CSS) rates. De Groote and colleagues[16] performed a retrospective review from three high-volume centers for robotic surgery and assessed perioperative, pathologic, and oncologic outcomes. They concluded that robot-assisted nephroureterectomy is safe and feasible, has low postoperative morbidity, is rarely associated with major complications, and has acceptable oncologic outcomes.[16] Lenis and colleagues[17] identified 3116 patients in the National Cancer Database and evaluated whether choice of surgical approach had any effect on decision to perform lymph node dissection, lymph node yield, and overall survival. The authors concluded that compared with open nephroureterectomy, robot-assisted nephroureterectomy did not compromise performance of a lymphadenectomy and that robot-assisted nephroureterectomy may actually be associated with improved lymph node yield.[17]

Robotic surgery provides dexterity to perform minimally invasive reconstructive surgeries that can preserve the kidney. Therefore, it is relevant to review the data supporting the safety and efficacy of kidney-sparing surgeries, such as distal ureterectomy with ureteral reimplant and segmental ureterectomy with primary ureteroureterostomy. Fukushima and colleagues[18] retrospectively reviewed a multi-institution database of 1329 patients treated for upper tract UC and found that there was no statistically significant difference in CSS and recurrence-free survival between the distal ureterectomy and nephroureterectomy, even when patients were stratified by tumor stage. Dalpiaz and colleagues[19] performed a retrospective chart review of 49 patients who underwent distal ureterectomy and 42 patients who underwent radical nephroureterectomy. Notably, both high- and low-grade cancers were represented in both treatment groups. The authors found that CSS and recurrence-free survival at 5 years did not differ significantly between the two groups. Jeldres and colleagues[20] compared the outcomes of segmental ureterectomy with nephroureterectomy in an analysis of 2044 patients and found no significant differences in cancer-specific mortality rates at 5 years. Seisen and colleagues[21] performed a meta-analysis comparing segmental ureterectomy with nephroureterectomy and found no significant differences in CSS between the two groups at 3 years, 5 years, or last follow-up.

PREOPERATIVE WORK-UP

Patients with upper tract UC often present with hematuria as the first clinical sign of disease, with gross or microscopic hematuria found in 70% to 80% of patients at time of diagnosis. Flank pain secondary to ureteral obstruction caused by a mass is another common presenting symptom and occurs in approximately 20% of patients.[22] Physical examination may reveal a flank mass in a rare cases. Imaging is critical to diagnosing upper tract UC. Computed tomography urography is the most accurate imaging technique for diagnosing upper tract UC with a reported sensitivity of 0.97 and specificity of 0.93.[23] In patients who cannot undergo computed tomography, MRI can be performed. The sensitivity of magnetic resonance urography is 0.75 for detecting tumors less than 2 cm.[22] Urine cytology and cystoscopy provide additional means of evaluating the urothelium. Positive urine cytology with negative cystoscopy is highly suggestive of upper tract UC and further evaluation with upper tract imaging is critical. However, it is important to keep in mind that cytology from the bladder is less sensitive for upper tract UC when compared with UC of the bladder, and Messer and colleagues[24] recommended that when upper tract UC is suspected, cytology be performed using samples obtained directly from the renal cavities. Fluorescence in situ hybridization is commonly used in the diagnosis of bladder cancer, but like urine cytology, has a limited role in upper tract UC. Diagnostic ureteroscopy provides direct visualization and allows for sampling from the renal pelvis for urine cytology. Furthermore, flexible ureteroscopy allows biopsies to be taken from suspicious lesions and is critical in diagnosing upper tract UC. When considering kidney-sparing surgery for ureteral cancer, it is critical to visually inspect the upper tract and ensure that there is no visible disease in the portion of the urothelial being spared.

Following appropriate clinical assessment and diagnosis, the urologist must decide on the optimal treatment strategy. Surgery is the only definitive treatment for nonmetastatic upper tract UC and open, laparoscopic, and robot-assisted approaches have all been found to be equally effective for controlling the cancer.[12] Although not the focus of this article, ablative therapies are appropriate for some small UCs. Compared with open surgery, minimally invasive techniques result in lower morbidity, but the use of these techniques ultimately depends on surgeon expertise. Nephroureterectomy has long been the gold standard. However, in carefully selected patients with disease localized to the ureter, segmental ureterectomy is a viable alternative.[20] Distal ureterectomy with reimplantation of the ureter is ideal for patients with low-grade disease in the distal ureter. Overall, kidney-sparing surgery should be strongly considered in patients with normally functioning kidneys with low-grade disease, or in patients with solitary kidney and/or impaired renal function.

Ureteral stents can promote periureteral inflammation, making surgery more challenging. Therefore, if a ureteral stent is present, it can be removed 3 to 7 days before the procedure; however, in patients with symptomatic ureteral obstruction this may not be possible. A urine culture should be strongly considered preoperatively and culture-specific antibiotics given at least 3 to 5 days before surgery, because these patients are more susceptible to becoming septic during the perioperative period. Historically, bowel preparation to decompress the colon was routinely performed; however, the surgery can be safely performed without a formal bowel preparation.

The role of neoadjuvant and adjuvant chemotherapy has not been definitively defined for upper tract UC. For stage II-IIIa bladder cancer, neoadjuvant chemotherapy has been shown to improve survival.[25,26] Therefore, it is reasonable to consider neoadjuvant chemotherapy in select patients with high-grade upper tract disease, particularly if imaging suggests at least stage II disease. Another important consideration is the benefit of neoadjuvant chemotherapy for bladder cancer that has been associated with cisplatin-based chemotherapy, which requires adequate renal function. Therefore, some patients may have adequate renal function to tolerate neoadjuvant chemotherapy but not adjuvant chemotherapy.

ROBOT-ASSISTED NEPHROURETERECTOMY

Radical nephroureterectomy involves removal of the kidney and ureter along with bladder cuff excision and is recommended for UC of the renal pelvis and upper ureter. The patient is positioned in a lateral decubitus position with the umbilicus at the level of kidney rest. The surgical table is partly flexed to open the space between the thorax and hip. An axillary role is placed two fingerbreadths below the axilla. A gel roll is placed against the back to keep patients in a 45° to 90° flank position. Three-inch cloth tape may be strapped across the upper chest and hip to help secure the patient (**Fig. 1**). The contralateral, lower arm should be placed on an arm board, supported by foam and loosely secured to the arm board with tape. The ipsilateral arm should be loosely secured with tape to an arm rest, which may be composed of pillows stacked on top of the lower arm. After the patient has been secured to the operating table, the abdomen and flank are shaved, prepared, and draped in standard sterile fashion.

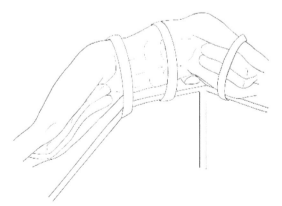

Fig. 1. Positioning of patient on table for robot-assisted nephroureterectomy.

The robot provides the greatest advantage when performing the distal ureterectomy and bladder repair. With older generations of the da Vinci robot, such as the da Vinci S and Si, it was often necessary to dock the robot separately for the nephrectomy and the distal ureterectomy. To avoid having to dock twice, it was often simpler to perform the nephrectomy laparoscopically and dock the robot for the distal ureterectomy. However, with the da Vinci Xi, it is possible to dock the robot once because the robotic arms have greater mobility.

Pneumoperitoneum is established using any variety of techniques. **Fig. 2** shows the port placement for a left nephroureterectomy using the da Vinci Xi. It is often helpful to plan port placement after establishing pneumoperitoneum, which can distend the abdominal wall. The camera port should be placed superior to the umbilicus and immediately lateral to the rectus muscle. The fourth arm is the inferior-most port and care should be taken to avoid inadvertently entering the bladder. A 12-mm assistant port is required. All trocars should be placed under vision if possible. For a right-sided nephroureterectomy, an additional 5-mm port is placed in the midline, just below the xyphoid and used to retract the liver (**Fig. 2**).

Access to the retroperitoneum is gained via incision lateral to the colon along the white line of Toldt.[27] Excision of this avascular tissue lateral to the colon allows the colon to then be reflected medially, providing access to the retroperitoneum. Depending on the laterality of the nephroureterectomy, either the spleen or the liver must then be manipulated. For a left-sided nephroureterectomy, the spleen is mobilized after excision of its lateral attachments. If the spleen is sufficiently mobilized, it will remain off the kidney during the remaining dissection without having to apply any instruments to the spleen. For a right-sided nephroureterectomy a blunt, locking grasper is inserted through the 5-mm trocar below the xyphoid to lift the liver and lock onto the abdominal wall near the lateral attachment of the liver. The duodenum is also mobilized and deflected medially to provide exposure to the inferior vena cava and renal hilum.

Attention is then directed toward the lower pole of the kidney where the ureter and gonadal vein can be readily identified (**Fig. 3**). The ureter should be identified as early as possible so that a locking clip can be placed below the tumor to prevent distal seeding of cancer during manipulation of the kidney. The ureter is superiorly retracted as the dissection is continued to the hilum. The renal vein should be clearly identified and separated from tissue posterior to the vein, which is expected to contain the renal artery. A laparoscopic vascular stapler can be used to staple and cut the artery and vein separately (**Fig. 4**). Using this approach, it is not necessary to completely mobilize and visualize the renal artery as long as the renal vein has been lifted off the structures immediately posterior to it and hilar tissue containing the artery has been thinned out sufficiently to accommodate the laparoscopic vascular stapler. The adrenal gland should be spared. On the left, the adrenal vein should be visualized, and care should be taken to divide the renal vein distal to the adrenal vein.

The importance of performing a retroperitoneal lymph node dissection (RPLND) has not been established. However, it is likely that an RPLND will improve nodal staging and help determine prognosis.[28] During an RPLND, bulky nodes and nodes visible on preoperative imaging should be prioritized for removal. A complete nodal dissection may include the retroperitoneal package extending from the crus of the diaphragm down

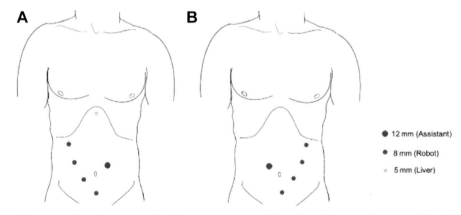

Fig. 2. Port placement for robot-assisted nephroureterectomy. (*A*) Right-sided port placement. (*B*) Left-sided port placement.

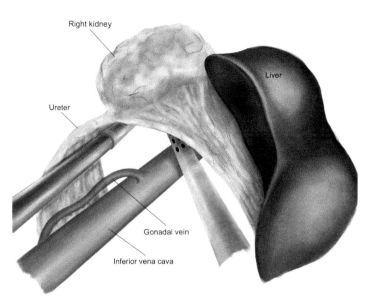

Fig. 3. Identification of ureter and gonadal vein at lower pole of kidney during a right-sided nephroureterectomy.

to pelvic nodes. However, the template can be modified based on the location of the tumor. For a left renal pelvis tumor, our practice is to perform an RPLND using the following structures to define the template: crus of the diaphragm, the left ureter, the aortic bifurcation, and the vena cava. For a right renal pelvis tumor, the following structures define our template: crus of the diaphragm, the right ureter, bifurcation of the vena cava, and aorta. Patients undergoing RPLND are at risk for developing a chyle leak. Therefore, all lymphatic vessels should be clipped using metal clips before

being divided. The assistant can apply the clips using a multifire laparoscopic clip applier.

The goal is to remove kidney, ureter, and bladder cuff en bloc. To complete the distal ureterectomy and bladder cuff excision, the ureter is traced down to its entry into the bladder. Before doing this, it is helpful to move the three working robotic trocars from the top three 8-mm trocars to the bottom three 8-mm trocars. While tracing the ureter, the vas deferens should be ligated where it crosses the ureter anteriorly. As dissection of the ureter is continued distally, the

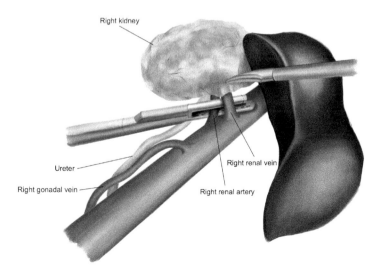

Fig. 4. Exposure of vessels of renal hilum during robot-assisted nephroureterectomy.

obliterated umbilical artery and bladder pedicles are encountered lateral and perpendicular to the course of the ureter (**Fig. 5**). These structures should be divided between Hem-o-lok clips to facilitate the ureteral dissection. When the detrusor is encountered, 2-cm incisions are made at the 12- and 6-o'clock positions. This should expose the underlying mucosal layer. A full-thickness apical stitch is placed at the top of this incision. The mucosal layer can be pulled into the surgical field by gently pulling on the ureter. This facilitates resection of the bladder cuff and helps identify the mucosal layer for the subsequent bladder closure (**Fig. 6**). Care should be taken to avoid damaging the contralateral ureter. The bladder is closed in two layers with a 2–0 polyglactin 910 barbed stitch placed in a running fashion. A leak test is performed through a urethral catheter. A Foley catheter should remain in place for approximately 1 week; however, if the patient passes the intraoperative leak test, some surgeons remove the Foley catheter as early as postoperative Day 1. The 12-mm assist port may be used to insert a specimen bag and the specimen may be removed through a Pfannenstiel incision. It should be noted that the distal ureterectomy and bladder repair can be performed before the nephrectomy and this provides the advantage of keeping the kidney and upper ureter in their orthotopic position, allowing more tension to be applied to the ureter.

ROBOT-ASSISTED DISTAL URETERECTOMY WITH REIMPLANT

Although nephroureterectomy is considered the gold standard for treatment of upper tract UC, kidney-sparing surgery may be considered in patients with distal ureteral tumors, particularly when renal function is compromised. The preoperative evaluation must include ureteroscopy of the proximal collecting system that will be preserved to ensure that this portion of the urothelium is free of visible cancer. Uberoi and colleagues[29] first described the robot-assisted distal ureterectomy with ureteral reimplantation and since then, various retrospective studies have compared distal ureterectomy with nephroureterectomy, and identified similar outcomes.

For surgery, the patient is placed supine and near-maximum Trendelenburg position. Foam pads should be placed under all pressure points and the surgeon should verify that the patient is secured to the operating table. A urinary catheter is inserted into the bladder, which is drained after the balloon is inflated. Once positioned, the abdomen is shaved, prepared, and draped in standard sterile fashion. Pneumoperitoneum is achieved with Veress needle. Five to six robotic

Fig. 5. Exposure of distal ureter during nephroureterectomy.

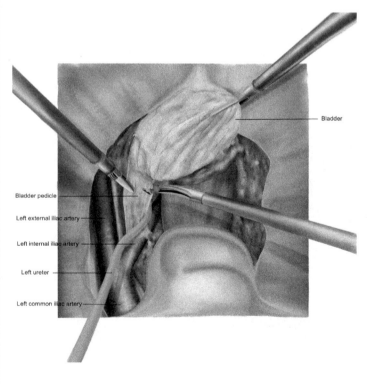

Bladder

Bladder pedicle

Left external iliac artery

Left internal iliac artery

Left ureter

Left common iliac artery

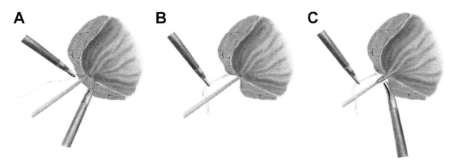

Fig. 6. Bladder cuff excision during nephroureterectomy. (*A, B*) Placement of a holding stitch into the detrusor muscle. (*C*) Tenting of the bladder mucosa before incision.

arm ports are placed (**Fig. 7**). The robot is then docked along the side of the bed.

In most cases, the ureteral tumor should be identifiable based on a bulging appearance. Preoperative imaging should provide additional guidance on location of the tumor. However, for smaller masses where no appreciable mass may be detected via the robotic scope, a ureteroscope may be used. In these cases, a guidewire is placed cystoscopically and advanced to the renal pelvis before docking. During the robotic portion of the case, a ureteroscope is introduced and advanced over the guidewire to the level of the tumor. At this point, the light from the ureteroscope should be visible laparoscopically and help the surgeon localize the tumor.[30]

Once the robot is fully docked, the surgeon should mobilize the colon to access the retroperitoneum. The ureter should be identified, and the distal ureter should be dissected along with a cuff of bladder. The ureteral lesion should be identified, and the ureter tied off or clipped proximal and distal to the tumor to prevent tumor spillage. When dissecting the distal ureter, the vas deferens

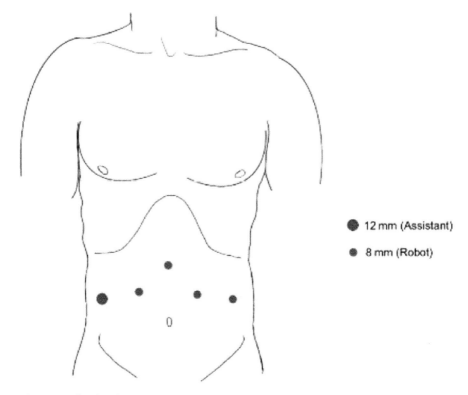

12 mm (Assistant)

8 mm (Robot)

Fig. 7. Port placement for distal ureterectomy.

(round ligament in women), obliterated umbilical artery, and bladder pedicle are divided between Hem-o-lok clips. The bladder detrusor is then incised and opened adjacent to the ureter. A retracting stitch can be placed in the bulging mucosa, just inside the detrusor, or in the full thickness of the bladder to help provide traction during subsequent bladder closure. The bladder cuff is excised circumferentially around the ureteral orifice. The ureter is divided proximal to the ureteral tumor and the proximal margin of the ureter is sent for frozen section analysis. Because of the small size of most ureteral tumors, a specimen retrieval bag is usually not required. The specimen may be removed through a trocar, but if the trocar needs to be removed to enlarge the incision, a specimen bag should be used to prevent tumor spillage and port-site seeding by tumor. The bladder is then closed with a 2–0 polyglactin 910 barbed suture. A pelvic lymph node dissection is performed within the borders of the genitofemoral nerve, aortic bifurcation, obturator nerve, and lymph node of Cloquet. Following confirmation from frozen section analysis that the proximal ureteral margin is negative, the surgeon can prepare for ureter reimplantation.

The surgeon first removes the previously placed clip on the ureter and then proceeds to spatulate the ureter for approximately 1.5 cm using robotic Potts scissors. Next, the bladder is dropped from the abdominal wall by incising the peritoneum lateral to the obliterated umbilical ligaments and dividing the obliterated urachal structures. The contralateral bladder pedicle should be preserved because the ipsilateral bladder pedicles will have been divided while mobilizing the ureter. On adequate mobilization of the bladder, a psoas hitch or a Boari flap can be performed to allow for a tension-free ureterovesical anastomosis.

For a psoas hitch, 2–0 polyglactin 910 suture is used to hitch the bladder superiorly to the psoas tendon with special care taken to avoid the genitofemoral and ilioinguinal nerves. Once the bladder is appropriately fixed, the surgeon proceeds to ureteral reimplantation, using either running or interrupted sutures. A 1.5-cm incision is made through the bladder muscle and mucosa. Once half of the anastomosis is complete, a double-J ureteral stent is placed. A guidewire is placed through the assistant's trocar and up the ureter. The proximal end of the stent is advanced up the ureter using robotic arms. The guidewire is then removed and the robotic arms are used to insert the distal end of the stent into the bladder without need for a guidewire. The anastomosis is then completed (**Fig. 8**). Anastomosis patency can be tested by filling the bladder.

ROBOT-ASSISTED SEGMENTAL URETERECTOMY WITH PRIMARY URETEROURETEROSTOMY

Robot-assisted segmental ureterectomy with ureteroureterostomy is considered for mid-ureteral tumors. Ideal candidates have low-grade, mid-ureteral tumors that are not amenable to endoscopic ablation.[31] High-grade tumors are treated with this approach when there is a solitary kidney or poor renal function, and distal ureterectomy is not technically feasible. The preoperative evaluation must include ureteroscopy of the collecting system, which is preserved to ensure that the urothelium is free of visible cancer.

The patient is positioned on the operating table in lateral decubitus position with ipsilateral side up.[32] Patient positioning and trocar placement is the same as described for robotic nephroureterectomy. A urinary catheter is inserted into the bladder. On entry into the abdomen, the colon should be mobilized and the white line of Toldt incised to expose the retroperitoneum. The ureter should be visualized, and the tumor may be located based on its bulging appearance. However, if tumor location is not completely clear, a ureteroscope may be advanced over a guidewire to locate the ureteral tumor as described for robotic distal ureterectomy. The surgeon should then be able to identify the location of the ureteral tumor laparoscopically from the light emitted by the ureteroscope. Once the ureter has been sufficiently mobilized to completely excise the tumor and perform a tension-free anastomosis, the ureter can be clipped above and below the tumor to minimize the risk of tumor spillage. Proximal and distal margins are sent for frozen section before proceeding with ureteroureterostomy. The surgeon ensures that the ureteral ends may be anastomosed in a tension-free manner. Ureteral resections larger than 2 cm may require a more complex reconstruction, such as ileal interposition.[32] A segmental ureterectomy may be the best option for a small high-grade ureteral tumor with a solitary kidney; lymphadenectomy in the draining lymph area is performed for high-grade tumors. For the primary ureteroureterostomy, the proximal and distal ends of the divided ureter should be spatulated on opposing sides by 1 cm and stay sutures should be placed on each end. Care must be taken to avoid twisting the ureteral ends during this process. The ureteral ends are then positioned so that the spatulated side of one ureter is sewn to the unspatulated side of the other ureteral end. A stent is placed after the first side of the anastomosis is complete, the ureter is flipped, and the anastomosis is completed.

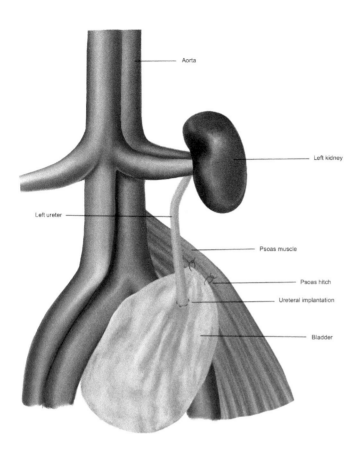

Aorta

Left kidney

Left ureter

Psoas muscle

Psoas hitch

Ureteral implantation

Bladder

Fig. 8. Reimplantation of ureter onto bladder with psoas hitch following distal ureterectomy.

SUMMARY

Upper tract UC is a rare malignancy for which surgery provides definitive management. Open radical nephroureterectomy was the gold standard treatment, but laparoscopic and robot-assisted approaches are alternative options. Kidney-sparing approaches are feasible for carefully selected patients with ureteral cancer.

DISCLOSURES

The authors have no disclosures to make.

REFERENCES

1. Jemal A, Siegel R, Ward E, et al. Cancer statistics, 2009. CA Cancer J Clin 2009;59(4):225–49.
2. Raman JD, Messer J, Sielatycki JA, et al. Incidence and survival of patients with carcinoma of the ureter and renal pelvis in the USA, 1973–2005. BJU Int 2011;107(7):1059–64.
3. Kakizoe T. Development and progression of urothelial carcinoma. Cancer Sci 2006;97(9):821–8.
4. Honda Y, Nakamura Y, Teishima J, et al. Clinical staging of upper urinary tract urothelial carcinoma for T staging: review and pictorial essay. Int J Urol 2019;26(11):1024–32.
5. Amin MB, Edge SB. AJCC cancer staging manual. New York: Springer; 2017.
6. Hall MC, Womack S, Sagalowsky AI, et al. Prognostic factors, recurrence, and survival in transitional cell carcinoma of the upper urinary tract: a 30-year experience in 252 patients. Urology 1998; 52(4):594–601.
7. Clayman RV, Kavoussi LR, Figenshau RS, et al. Laparoscopic nephroureterectomy: initial clinical case report. J Laparoendosc Surg 1991;1(6):343–9.
8. Ni S, Tao W, Chen Q, et al. Laparoscopic versus open nephroureterectomy for the treatment of upper urinary tract urothelial carcinoma: a systematic review and cumulative analysis of comparative studies. Eur Urol 2012;61(6):1142–53.
9. Margulis V, Shariat SF, Matin SF, et al. Outcomes of radical nephroureterectomy: a series from the upper tract urothelial carcinoma collaboration. Cancer 2009;115(6):1224–33.
10. Klingler DW, Hemstreet GP, Balaji K. Feasibility of robotic radical nephrectomy: initial results of single-institution pilot study. Urology 2005;65(6): 1086–9.

11. Ludwig WW, Gorin MA, Pierorazio PM, et al. Frontiers in robot-assisted retroperitoneal oncological surgery. Nat Rev Urol 2017;14(12):731–41.

12. Clements MB, Krupski TL, Culp SH. Robotic-assisted surgery for upper tract urothelial carcinoma: a comparative survival analysis. Ann Surg Oncol 2018;25(9):2550–62.

13. Rodriguez JF, Packiam VT, Boysen WR, et al. Utilization and outcomes of nephroureterectomy for upper tract urothelial carcinoma by surgical approach. J Endourol 2017;31(7):661–5.

14. Hemal AK, Nayyar R, Gupta NP, et al. Experience with robot assisted laparoscopic surgery for upper and lower benign and malignant ureteral pathologies. Urology 2010;76(6):1387–93.

15. Rouprêt M, Babjuk M, Comperat E, et al. European guidelines on upper tract urothelial carcinomas: 2013 update. Eur Urol 2013;63(6):1059–71.

16. De Groote R, Decaestecker K, Larcher A, et al. Robot-assisted nephroureterectomy for upper tract urothelial carcinoma: results from three high-volume robotic surgery institutions. J Robot Surg 2020;14(1):211–9.

17. Lenis AT, Donin NM, Faiena I, et al. Role of surgical approach on lymph node dissection yield and survival in patients with upper tract urothelial carcinoma. Paper presented at: Urologic Oncology: Seminars and Original Investigations, 2018.

18. Fukushima H, Saito K, Ishioka J, et al. Equivalent survival and improved preservation of renal function after distal ureterectomy compared with nephroureterectomy in patients with urothelial carcinoma of the distal ureter: a propensity score-matched multicenter study. Int J Urol 2014;21(11):1098–104.

19. Dalpiaz O, Ehrlich G, Quehenberger F, et al. Distal ureterectomy is a safe surgical option in patients with urothelial carcinoma of the distal ureter. Paper presented at: Urologic Oncology: Seminars and Original Investigations, 2014.

20. Jeldres C, Lughezzani G, Sun M, et al. Segmental ureterectomy can safely be performed in patients with transitional cell carcinoma of the ureter. J Urol 2010;183(4):1324–9.

21. Seisen T, Peyronnet B, Dominguez-Escrig JL, et al. Oncologic outcomes of kidney-sparing surgery versus radical nephroureterectomy for upper tract urothelial carcinoma: a systematic review by the EAU non-muscle invasive bladder cancer guidelines panel. Eur Urol 2016;70(6):1052–68.

22. Rouprêt M, Babjuk M, Compérat E, et al. European Association of Urology guidelines on upper urinary tract urothelial carcinoma: 2017 update. Eur Urol 2018;73(1):111–22.

23. Cowan NC, Turney BW, Taylor NJ, et al. Multidetector computed tomography urography for diagnosing upper urinary tract urothelial tumour. BJU Int 2007; 99(6):1363–70.

24. Messer J, Shariat SF, Brien JC, et al. Urinary cytology has a poor performance for predicting invasive or high-grade upper-tract urothelial carcinoma. BJU Int 2011;108(5):701–5.

25. Grossman HB, Natale RB, Tangen CM, et al. Neoadjuvant chemotherapy plus cystectomy compared with cystectomy alone for locally advanced bladder cancer. N Engl J Med 2003;349(9):859–66.

26. International Collaboration of Trialists. International phase III trial assessing neoadjuvant cisplatin, methotrexate, and vinblastine chemotherapy for muscle-invasive bladder cancer: long-term results of the BA06 30894 trial. J Clin Oncol 2011;29(16):2171.

27. Taylor BL, Scherr DS. Robotic nephroureterectomy. Urol Clin 2018;45(2):189–97.

28. Chapman TN, Sharma S, Zhang S, et al. Laparoscopic lymph node dissection in clinically node-negative patients undergoing laparoscopic nephrectomy for renal carcinoma. Urology 2008; 71(2):287–91.

29. Uberoi J, Harnisch B, Sethi AS, et al. Robot-assisted laparoscopic distal ureterectomy and ureteral reimplantation with psoas hitch. J Endourol 2007;21(4): 368–73.

30. Glinianski M, Guru KA, Zimmerman G, et al. Robot-assisted ureterectomy and ureteral reconstruction for urothelial carcinoma. J Endourol 2009;23(1): 97–100.

31. McClain PD, Mufarrij PW, Hemal AK. Robot-assisted reconstructive surgery for ureteral malignancy: analysis of efficacy and oncologic outcomes. J Endourol 2012;26(12):1614–7.

32. Aboumohamed AA, Ghavamian R. Distal and segmental ureterectomy. In: Urothelial malignancies of the upper urinary tract. New York: Springer; 2018. p. 171–7.

Robotic Partial Nephrectomy
Update on Techniques

Laura Bukavina, MD, MPH[a], Kirtishri Mishra, MD[a], Adam Calaway, MD, MPH[a], Lee Ponsky, MD[b,*]

KEYWORDS

- Partial nephrectomy • Single site surgery • Renal cell carcinoma • Robotic partial nephrectomy
- Selective artery clamping

KEY POINTS

- Advances in imaging technology, coupled with innovation in surgical approach have enabled surgeons to consider partial nephrectomy in complex renal tumors.
- There are short-term and long-term differences in renal function seen in off clamp and selective artery clamping during partial nephrectomy.
- Robotic platform offers a variety of surgical approaches for partial nephrectomy, with transperitoneal being the most common. Single site offers an opportunity to further evaluate retroperitoneal approach in partial nephrectomy.

INTRODUCTION

It is estimated that there will be 73,750 new cases of kidney cancer diagnosed in 2020 according to American Cancer Society.[1] There has been a steady increase in kidney cancer diagnosis since the 1990s, with levels slowly leveling off over the past several years.[2] Most renal masses are now diagnosed at an early stage due to the widespread use of cross-sectional imaging.[3] In fact, the average size of renal mass at diagnosis has decreased from 7.0 to 3.5 cm[2]. As a result, the clinical management of small renal masses has dramatically changed.[4,5] Although radical nephrectomy has historically been considered the treatment of choice for all renal masses, partial nephrectomy (PN) is now accepted as standard of care, especially for treating T1a and T1b renal tumors amenable for nephron-sparing procedures.[6,7] The idea of nephron-sparing surgery has been the primary impetus for increased adoption of PN.[8,9] Although previous indications for PN such as solitary kidney or bilateral renal masses continue to be indications for a partial, they are no longer the only indications for a PN.[10] There is an abundance of retrospective studies showing equivalent oncologic outcomes, improved renal function preservation, and decreased risk of future development of cardiovascular disease in PN patients.[11–13]

Advances in imaging technology, coupled with innovation in surgical approaches have enabled surgeons to consider PN in patients previously thought to be impossible. Recent efforts have focused on integrating the anatomy of the renal masses and its vasculature to aid in surgical planning, amalgamation of imaging and hilar clamping techniques, and introduction of single-port robotic platform (SP).

[a] University Hospitals Cleveland Medical Center, Urology Institute, Case Western Reserve University School of Medicine, Cleveland, OH, USA; [b] Urology Institute, University Hospitals Cleveland Medical Center, Case Western Reserve University School of Medicine, 11100 Euclid Avenue, Suite 411, Cleveland, OH 44106, USA
* Corresponding author.
E-mail address: Lee.Ponsky@UHhospitals.org

Urol Clin N Am 48 (2021) 81–90
https://doi.org/10.1016/j.ucl.2020.09.013
0094-0143/21/© 2020 Elsevier Inc. All rights reserved.

Robotic PN is an evolving field. The purpose of this article was to provide contemporary overview of recent advances in robotic PN, including overview of novel imaging and planning approaches, novel vascular and renorrhaphy techniques impacting post-PN function, and an introduction to single-port platform in PN.

PARTIAL NEPHRECTOMY PLANNING

Despite improvement in techniques and advancement in technology used for robotic PN, the management of complex tumors with intraparenchymal component remains a controversial issue. Intrarenal tumors present a technical challenge during PN because these lesions cannot be visualized on the surface of the kidneys.[14] Similarly, posteriorly located tumors are unable to be visualized without rotation of the kidney with extensive defatting. This can be a challenge when the kidney is surrounded by "sticky" and densely adherent adipose tissue.[15] Given the increasing surgeon comfort and widespread adoption of the robotic platform, there has been a steady rise in the utilization of PN in the management of complex tumors.[10] To date, positive surgical margins (PSM), historically reported as 0% to 7% in PN, can be as high as 18% in these complex masses.[16]

The clinical implications of PSMs have been extensively debated. Sutherland and colleagues, among other retrospective studies, have reported no difference in relapse in patients with PSM.[17,18] This was in contrast to a study by Shah and colleagues,[19,20] which evaluated a large multi-institutional database. They concluded that patients with PSM did in fact experience twofold increased risk of local recurrence ($P = .03$).

To that end, with an increase in complexity and understand of tumor anatomy, different imaging tools have been adopted to improving the quality of PN, and intraoperative surgical navigation.[21] At this time, there are 2 specific categories for PN imaging, real-time intraoperative imaging and preoperative surgical planning.

Intraoperative Imaging of Renal Tumors and Vascular System

Among the most commonly used techniques is the intraoperative robotic ultrasonography for tumor identification.[22,23] Recent ultrasonographic include the use of Doppler modes, contrast-enhanced ultrasonography (CE-US), and FireFly (Firefly; Intuitive Surgical, Sunnyvale, CA) fluorescent imaging with indocyanine green for the improved visualization of kidney tumors.[24,25]

Both Doppler and CE-US can be used to assist in selective ischemia, where CE-US has the added advantage of minimizing movement artifacts.[25] CE-US is a novel intraoperative imaging technique that combines the microbubble technology of contrast media with complementary ultrasound technology. The duration of enhancement via microbubble technology enhances the kidney for about 2 minutes in real time, although this can be variable in patients with chronic kidney disease. CE-US is most useful with selective artery clamping.[24]

Both options come with laparoscopic ultrasound probes that can be used in vivo at the time of robotic PN. Ultrasound images are projected onto the console screen so the surgeon has the ability to implement and alter the course of surgery from the surgical console without having to leave to see images on an external screen.[26,27] The added benefits of CE-US is increased tissue penetration, as well as tissue resolution. This allows for improved tumor localization, improved accuracy in differentiation of tumor from normal kidney, as well as the ability to assess surgical cavity and margins of the resected specimen.[26] Tumors generally have good vascularity, a feature that can enhance the quality of the signals detected with CE-US when compared with other ultrasound modalities such as power Doppler. When combining selective occlusion angiography with CE-US, CE-US was more useful in assessing the regions of ischemia and perfusion. A study by Alenezi and Karim[24] evaluating use of CE-US in complex renal lesions, reported improved vascular visualization and decreased global ischemia in selective clamping compare to standard on clamp PN (warm ischemia time [WIT] 17.1 vs 21.4, respectively, $P = .01$). (see **Table 1**).

A relatively novel approach in renal cancer surgery is the use of intraoperative fluorescence imaging. First introduced in 2009 by Hoda and Popken,[28] the study reported a 94% sensitivity, and a 95% specificity for renal cell carcinoma (RCC) uptake of fluorescence dye. Further research has focused on near the infrared range (NIR) since penetration is significantly improved, with indocyanine green (ICG) as the agent of choice.[26,29–33] In addition, ICG has the potential to differentiate the tumor from normal kidney parenchyma, because RCC appears hypofluorescent compared with normal kidney parenchyma.[33] Successful differentiation of tumor tissue from normal parenchyma ranges from 73% to 100% in a recent meta-analysis composed of 7 studies with 287 PNs.[26,33–35] ICG imaging has limited utility in endophytic tumors, because of the visual obstruction from the overlying normal parenchyma. Although results of ICG studies are encouraging, a recent analysis showed a positive predictive value of 84% and negative predictive value of 57%, certainly lacking the precision and reliability necessary in PN of complex renal tumors[34] (Table 1).

One of the major drawbacks of ICG and NIR is the limited tissue penetration; this is especially relevant for endophytic tumors. Gamma radiation, on the contrary, has very high tissue penetration, thus it can be useful for intraoperative localization of these tumors via the utilization of a gamma probe in combination with ICG.[41,42] A recent study showed that this dual modality imaging is feasible and a clinical trial is under way.[26]

Preoperative Surgical Planning and Ex Vivo Reconstruction

With the limitations imposed by ultrasound and ICG, as well as a desire to have a precise understanding of the patient anatomy specific to the case, there has been a shift toward the concept of "precision surgery".[43] Recent advancements in 3-dimensional (3D) technology and virtual models have been evaluated as a part of "augmented reality" (AR), where preoperative images are superimposed onto the surgical field. This can only be useful to the surgeon if the overlay is precise, accurate and easy to use.[44] Recent retrospective analysis by Porpiglia and colleagues[43] evaluated AR as an intraoperative tool in complex renal tumors. They concluded that the use of 3D AR improved the ability to correctly identify the lesion and intraparenchymal structure with a more accurate perception of the location and nature of different structures, including aberrant vessels when compared with standard 2D ultrasound. This translated to a lower rate of global ischemia (45.8% vs 69.7%, $P = .03$), higher rate of enucleation (62.5% vs 37.5%, $P = .02$) and lower rate of collecting system violation (0.4% vs 45.5%, $P = .003$). There was a short follow-up in the study, thus long-term outcomes on oncologic outcomes and renal function are limited.

One of the biggest drawbacks of AR is the organ movements and tissue deformation. In fact, some segmented branches of the renal artery can be shifted at much as 11 mm comparing supine

Table 1
Summary of imaging techniques

Imaging Technique	Strength	Weakness	Results
In Vivo US	• Widely available • Established efficacy	• Contact with tissue required at all times • Tissue/Tumor penetration	• WIT 17.9 min, OR time 205.7 min • 95% endophytic tumors (0%PSM)[36]
CE-US	• Dynamic imaging • Useful for selective clamping • Improved tissue penetration/visualization	• Contrast agent required • Not readily available • Short enhancement time (2 min)	• In combination with selective clamping, ↓WIT (21.4 vs 17.1) • May increase total OR time[25,37,38]
AR	• No contrast needed • Accurate visualization of tumor and vessels • More precise tumor vessel/segmental artery clamping	• Tissue deformation currently limits approach • Complex set up	• Feasibility studies showing WIT/OR time 19.8 and 81.8, respectively[39]
ICG/FireFly	• Real-time imaging before, during, and after PN[29] • Tumor specific	• Lag time between injection and fluorescence • Injection required • Not suitable for endophytic tumors[26]	• No difference[a] (in OR time 8.12 (−22.46, 6.23), EBL −7.74(−35.97, 20.50), Complications 0.66(0.32, 1.34), PSM 0.79(0.2, 3.08) • ↓ WIT −1.46(−2.32, −0.60)[40]

Abbreviations: AR, augmented reality; CE-US, contrast-enhanced ultrasound technology; EBL, estimated blood loss; ICG, indocyanine green with infrared technology; OR, operating room; PSM, positive surgical margins; WIT, warm ischemia time.
[a] Odds Ratio.

positioning of preoperative imaging to intraoperative flank position.[45] Ways to minimize this interference includes application of organ trackers to correct for real-time movements as well as real-time intraoperative imaging with cone beam CT (CBCT).[46] The major disadvantage in the current era of robotic surgery is the interference of the C-arm of the CBCT with the robot, and the need to disconnect the robot at the time of surgery. Furthermore, this also requires the use of a hybrid operating room and dedicated imaging technology.[45]

All of the described techniques have their own benefits and limitations, and no standard approach can be used across all patients. Preferably, a thorough evaluation should address patient-specific factors and potential challenges before surgery. PN of low complexity tumors will unlikely require further intraoperative imaging, aside from 2D ultrasound. As the complexity of the lesion and patients increases, the planning for additional intraoperative imaging, or aid of AR or ICG maybe beneficial.

SURGICAL APPROACH

Aside from achieving oncologic cure during PN, another factor to consider is to maximize the preservation of renal function. The 3 main drivers of post-PN functional recovery, in order of importance, are pre-PN function, remnant vascularized renal parenchyma, and prolonged ischemia time.[11,47] From a surgical perspective, the remaining healthy parenchyma and ischemia time are intercorrelated and potentially modifiable (**Fig. 1**).

Although the quality of the kidney preserved during PN is patient-dependent due to patient's age, comorbidities, and baseline renal function, the quantity can be maximized with several techniques aimed to

1. Minimize excisional volume
2. Establish an anatomic minimal margin
3. Reduce renal ischemia
4. Minimize devascularization of the spared parenchyma via optimal renorrhaphy techniques[48–50]

Renal artery clamping has been a standard of care in PN surgery, with the aim not only to deliver a controlled, bloodless field for precise tumor resection and negative margins, but also with the long-term goal for maximal preservation of remaining parenchyma and adequate renorrhaphy.[50] Ischemia to a healthy, uninvolved parenchyma is a an undesirable sequala of main renal artery clamping, when prolonged, is an independent risk factor of acute kidney injury and late-

stage onset chronic kidney disease.[47] Techniques to minimize ischemia of the healthy parenchyma are as follows: off clamp, selective/super-selective clamping, and early unclamping.

Control of Hilum

Off clamp is defined as the entire PN performed without any hilar clamping. The hilum maybe dissected in the event that emergent hilar control becomes necessary. Studies evaluating off clamp data, reported a higher estimated blood loss (weighted mean difference [WMD]: 47.84, $P = .004$) between off clamp and on clamp.[51] While the off clamp group experienced higher blood loss, there was no difference in transfusion rate, open conversion rate, hospital length of stay and most importantly surgical margins. As expected, renal functional outcomes were superior in the off clamp PN group, with absolute estimated glomerular filtration rate (eGFR) difference (WMD 16.05, $P = .06$), % short-term change (WMG: 7.02, $P<.00001$), long-term absolute GFR difference (WMD: 6.59, $P = .02$), and long-term % change in GFR (WMD:4.09, $P = .005$).[50,52,53] Cumulative analysis of 7 studies evaluating off clamp PN as compared with on clamp PN revealed similar findings. There were differences in tumor complexity among the 2 groups, largely due to higher Preoperative Aspects and Dimensions Used for an Anatomic Classification (PADUA) and radius exophytic/endophytic nearness anterior/posterior location scoring (RENAL) scores in off clamp group.[54,55] Off clamp minimally invasive PN may be aided by prior imaging, and AR reconstruction in select cases, as well as preoperative super-selective embolization of tumor specific arteries and prior radiofrequency ablation.[52,56] Although results are promising, clinically, off clamp PN might be a more feasible option in tumors with favorable anatomic features (small size, exophytic lesion, low nephrometry score).

In patients whose tumor complexity precludes an off clamp PN, segmental renal artery clamping maybe an option. First introduced in 2011 by Shao and colleagues,[57] PN with segmental artery clamping has gained acceptance in simple and complex renal masses with equivalent oncologic outcomes. A review of 5 studies looking at selective/super-selective versus on clamp PN concluded that late functional outcomes (absolute eGFR and % change eGFR) were similar between the 2 groups. There were no further differences in transfusion rate, hospital stay or positive surgical margin rates. The Selective/Super-Selective (SS) group did experience a higher blood loss, which was statistically significant as compared with on

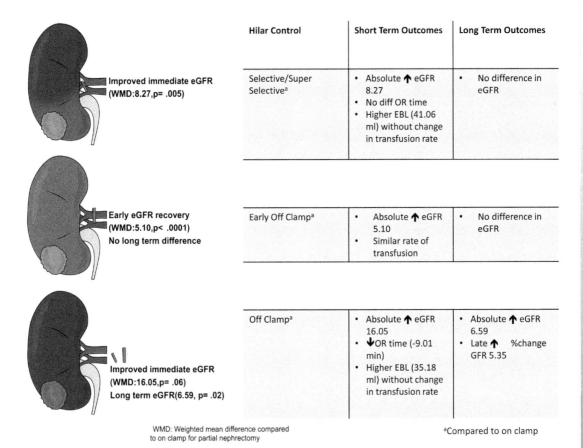

	Hilar Control	Short Term Outcomes	Long Term Outcomes
Improved immediate eGFR (WMD:8.27,p= .005)	Selective/Super Selective[a]	• Absolute ↑ eGFR 8.27 • No diff OR time • Higher EBL (41.06 ml) without change in transfusion rate	• No difference in eGFR
Early eGFR recovery (WMD:5.10,p< .0001) No long term difference	Early Off Clamp[a]	• Absolute ↑ eGFR 5.10 • Similar rate of transfusion	• No difference in eGFR
Improved immediate eGFR (WMD:16.05,p= .06) Long term eGFR(6.59, p= .02)	Off Clamp[a]	• Absolute ↑ eGFR 16.05 • ↓OR time (-9.01 min) • Higher EBL (35.18 ml) without change in transfusion rate	• Absolute ↑ eGFR 6.59 • Late ↑ %change GFR 5.35

WMD: Weighted mean difference compared to on clamp for partial nephrectomy

[a]Compared to on clamp

Fig. 1. Surgical approaches in hilar control: selective/super-selective clamping versus early off clamp versus off clamp and evaluation of short- and long-term outcomes.

clamp group, but no differences in the transfusion rates were seen.[58–62]

In terms of conversion, a single study evaluating differences in conversion rate found no overall differences between the techniques. Postoperative and intraoperative complications were similar among the groups.[58]

The selective/SS clamping did offer improved renal function outcomes immediately after surgery in terms of absolute eGFR (WMD: 8.27, $P = .005$) and % change in eGFR (WMD 8.12, $P = .0003$). However, there were no differences in eGFR or % change eGFR in the late renal functional outcomes.[50,58,59,63]

In addition to the selective and off clamp techniques, the concept of early unclamping (EU) has been developed to further minimize ischemia.[64] EU involves unclamping of the renal hilum before renorrhaphy. Studies evaluating the on clamp versus the early off techniques found no differences in surgical margins, blood loss, length of stay, and operative time. Both groups experienced similar rates of complications and conversion to open. There was a slight improvement in eGFR

with EU (WMD 5.10, $P<.00001$) in the immediate postoperative recovery; however, this benefit was not seen in the long-term follow-up.[50,64–66]

The segmental classification of renal vasculature was first described in 1954 by Graves,[67] which is considered the reference for anatomic description. A classic understanding of renal vasculature involves anterior and posterior renal vessels with segmental branching.[67] To minimize renal ischemia of the healthy tissue in PN, surgeons have taken advantage of selective clamping. Although theoretically sound, cadaveric and near infrared studies evaluating tumor vasculature have shown significant variation in tumor anatomy.[35,68] Studies evaluating renal anatomy, found that almost 53% of the kidneys did not follow the model proposed by Grave. In addition, 43% of the tumors had more than one blood vessel supplying the tumor, most commonly seen in the upper pole and/or in the junction between the anterior and the posterior areas of the kidney.[69] These anatomic variants can explain the differences in blood loss seen among selective and on clamp PNs. Secondarily, it may also partially explain the lack of long-term preservation of kidney function due to the variant anatomy and the likelihood of ischemic damage far beyond the tumor and into the surrounding parenchyma.

Renorrhaphy Techniques

Renorrhaphy techniques have evolved over the past several years, which is largely a reflection of the evolving surgical techniques, new emerging technology, and improved understanding of the complexity of renal tumors undergoing PN. Early PN approaches, primarily performed laparoscopically, focused on ensuring hemostasis and closure of the urinary collecting system with the goal of reducing postoperative complications.[9] Nowadays, surrounding tissue involvement at the time of renorrhaphy is considered an essential determinant of nephron-sparing surgery, and thus a representation of renal function after PN.[70]

Robot-assisted surgery provides key advantages for renorrhaphy during PN, especially in the cases of complex tumors with intraparenchymal components, or hilar renal masses.[14,71] With robot-assisted PN, renorrhaphy typically includes a double-layer technique with medullary suture often performed with a sliding clip fashion.[72,73]

To reduce renorrhaphy time, investigators have reported the use of self-retained barbed suture either for medullary repair, cortical repair, or both. Studies evaluating barbed versus nonbarbed suture found a significant advantage in terms of operating time (mean difference 8 minutes), WIT (6.7 minutes), and blood loss (46.31 mL) in favor of barbed suture. There were no differences in postoperative complications, transfusions and urinary leakages.[74–77]

When evaluating single-layer (SLR) (renorrhaphy without collecting system [CS]) closure versus double-layer closure (CS followed by cortical renorrhaphy), there was a decrease in total operating time (mean difference 11.13 minutes), WIT (3.39 minutes) favoring the single-layer technique. In addition, no differences in blood loss, postoperative complication and urinary leak were observed in the studies comparing the two.[70] In theory, SLR offers preservation of renal volume by fewer suture lines, less parenchymal and segmental artery strangulation.[11] Volumetric analysis post SLR versus double-layer closure shows a decrease of average of 8 cm^3 of renal tissue with SLR.[78] Despite the volumetric differences, studies show no differences with regard to renal function when comparing CS only versus double-layer techniques.[72] A dreaded complication after PN is renal artery pseudoaneurysms (RAP). Reported RAP rate following PN occurs 1% and 1.96% for open

and minimally invasive procedures, respectively.[79] Although one study has suggested renal sinus or CS exposure during PN to be associated with a higher incidence of renal artery pseudoaneurysm, study looking at SLR did not support this.[72]

Among studies evaluating running versus interrupted sutures (most common suture used 2/0 or 3/0 polyglactin), the authors found that the running technique decreases the operating time (mean difference 17.12 minutes), WIT (mean difference 8.73 minutes), and the risk of postoperative complication (odds ratio 0.54) and transfusions (0.3).[80–82]

With the evolution in the renorrhaphy techniques in PN, the use of surgical bolsters to fill the renal defect after the inner layer renorrhaphy has been declining. Overall, the use of hemostatic agents are largely based on surgeon preference, and no formal comparative retrospective or prospective studies have been performed to compare the two within robotic PN literature.

Robotic Laparoscopic Single Site Partial Nephrectomy

Robotic Laparoscopic Single Site Surgery (R-LESS) has emerged as an alternative to the conventional approach with aim to minimize the morbidity as well as to improve the surgical cosmesis.[83] Previously encountered barriers to R-LESS PN included the steep learning curve, as well as the external clashing and robotic arm triangulation. The stated limitations further reduced the maneuverability and the ability to complete complex tasks required in PNs.[84] The recent advent of the da Vinci SP (Intuitive Surgical), an SP robotic platform, has improved the system's feasibility and safety, further allowing wide array of surgical procedures to be completed including a PN.[85]

As in conventional multiport robot-assisted PN, the patient is placed in a semi-lateral position. In contrast to the multiport PN, a single 3.5 cm umbilical incision is made and a GelPOINT advanced access platform (Applied Medical, Rancho Santa Margarita, CA) is inserted after placing a dedicated 25 mm multichannel robotic port and assistant ports. Within the GelPOINT platform, 10 mm and 12 mm ports are included and used as assistant ports. The 12 mm port is used to apply the laparoscopic bulldogs when necessary. The SP system allows for the use of a third arm without placement of an additional trocar. This can be useful to elevate the liver when exposing the hilum and the upper pole of the right kidney.[86]

An additional benefit of the da Vinci SP, as compared with the previous single site platform for the da Vinci Xi System (Xi SSP), is the ability to perform PN on the upper pole tumors, previously not feasible with the Xi SSP system due to system/articulating arm constraints. Another drawback of the XiSSP is the lack of articulating scissors, which limits mobility and dexterity at the time of the tumor resection.[85] These limitations have largely been resolved by the SP system, which not only provides articulation of the instruments, but an additional elbow joint which allows intracorporeal triangulation and articulation with all the instruments.[87]

Kaouk and colleagues[84] reported their successful initial clinical experience in performing R-LESS for small renal mass in their 2019 study with a total of 5 patients who underwent a transperitoneal PN with a mean RENAL score of 5, and tumor size varying from 1.5 cm to 4.6 cm. Authors reported an average WIT 15 to 30 minutes with mean hospital stay 2 days. As this was simply a feasibility study, the authors neither performed a comparative analysis to the multiport system, nor compared the long-term outcomes.[84]

Similarly, a study by Na and colleagues[86] evaluated 14 patients who underwent PNs with either XiSSP (5 patients) or with the SP surgical system (9 patients). The investigators reported 1 conversion to multiport PN within the XiSSP group due to the limited tumor resection and the inability to resect the tumor adequately. They also reported 1 conversion to open in the SP group to a multiport surgery due to tumor fracture. All 14 patients had negative surgical margins.

Since the early 2000s, LESS procedures have been increasingly studied due to their ability to offer improved cosmetic outcomes, less pain, and shortened postoperative recovery time.[84] With the introduction of the da Vinci SP system, many of the previously encountered barriers to dissemination of LESS have been addressed. Despite the steep learning curve, the authors of this review expect the procedure to gain significant traction among robotic surgeons and to improve both the total operating room time and WIT. SP PN offers the ability to perform not only transperitoneal, but also retroperitoneal approach with improved robotic dexterity. As previously reported, retroperitoneal approach allows for decreased gastrointestinal related complications by staying out of the peritoneum and has been shown to decrease estimated blood loss and operating time. Furthermore, it provides access to posterior and lateral renal masses, which otherwise be more difficult with transperitoneal approach.[88]

In summary, surgical techniques for robot-assisted PN are driven by the aims of simplifying the most challenging surgical steps, maximizing functional and oncologic outcomes, and consistently pushing the envelope on possibilities. Over the past several years, we have seen an emergence in not only innovation in surgical technique, and robotic platforms, but integration of a variety of imaging techniques. We believe with developing robotic expertise, practicing urologist will continue to push the envelope in nephron preservation and complication-free recovery.

SUPPORT/FINANCIAL DISCLOSURES AND CONFLICT OF INTEREST

Authors have no conflict relevant to this article.

REFERENCES

1. American Cancer Society. Global Cancer Facts & Figures. 4th Edition. Atlanta: American Cancer Society; 2020.
2. Chow WH, Devesa SS, Warren JL, et al. Rising incidence of renal cell cancer in the United States. JAMA 1999;281(17):1628–31.
3. Basatac C, Akpinar H. Robot-assisted partial nephrectomy with segmental renal artery clamping: a single center experience. Urol J 2019;16(5):469–74.
4. Cooperberg MR, Mallin K, Ritchey J, et al. Decreasing size at diagnosis of stage 1 renal cell carcinoma: analysis from the National Cancer Data Base, 1993 to 2004. J Urol 2008;179(6):2131–5.
5. Chow WH, Dong LM, Devesa SS. Epidemiology and risk factors for kidney cancer. Nat Rev Urol 2010; 7(5):245–57.
6. Campbell S, Uzzo RG, Allaf ME, et al. Renal mass and localized renal cancer: AUA Guideline. J Urol 2017;198:520–9.
7. Ljungberg BCN, Hanbury DC. EAU guidelines on renal cell carcinoma: the 2010 update. Eur Urol 2010;58:398–406.
8. Greco F, Autorino R, Altieri V, et al. Ischemia techniques in nephron-sparing surgery: a systematic review and meta-analysis of surgical, oncological, and functional outcomes. Eur Urol 2019;75(3):477–91.
9. Porpiglia FBR, Amparore D, Fiori C. Nephron-sparing suture of renal parenchyma after partial nephrectomy: which technique to go for?Some best practices. Eur Urol Focus 2017;5(4):600–3.
10. Daugherty M, Bratslavsky G. Surgical techniques in the management of small renal masses. Urol Clin North Am 2017;44(2):233–42.
11. Thompson RH, Lane BR, Lohse CM, et al. Renal function after partial nephrectomy: effect of warm ischemia relative to quantity and quality of preserved kidney. Urology 2012;79(2):356–60.
12. Zabell JR, Wu J, Suk-Ouichai C, et al. Renal ischemia and functional outcomes following partial

nephrectomy. Urol Clin North Am 2017;44(2): 243–55.

13. Aguilar Palacios D, Li J, Mahmood F, et al. Partial nephrectomy for patients with severe chronic kidney disease: is it worthwhile? J Urol 2020;204(3): 434–41.

14. Arora S, Rogers C. Partial nephrectomy in central renal tumors. J Endourol 2018;32(S1):S63–7.

15. Marconi L, Challacombe B. Robotic partial nephrectomy for posterior renal tumours: retro or transperitoneal approach? Eur Urol Focus 2018;4(5):632–5.

16. Marszalek M, Carini M, Chlosta P, et al. Positive surgical margins after nephron-sparing surgery. Eur Urol 2012;61(4):757–63.

17. Sutherland SE, Resnick MI, Maclennan GT, et al. Does the size of the surgical margin in partial nephrectomy for renal cell cancer really matter? J Urol 2002;167(1):61–4.

18. Yossepowitch O, Thompson RH, Leibovich BC, et al. Positive surgical margins at partial nephrectomy: predictors and oncological outcomes. J Urol 2008; 179(6):2158–63.

19. Shah PH, Moreira DM, Okhunov Z, et al. Positive surgical margins increase risk of recurrence after partial nephrectomy for high risk renal tumors. J Urol 2016;196(2):327–34.

20. Shah PH, Moreira DM, Patel VR, et al. Partial nephrectomy is associated with higher risk of relapse compared with radical nephrectomy for clinical stage T1 Renal Cell Carcinoma Pathologically Up Staged to T3a. J Urol 2017;198(2):289–96.

21. Porpiglia F, Checcucci E, Amparore D, et al. Three-dimensional augmented reality robot-assisted partial nephrectomy in case of complex tumours (PADUA ≥10): a new intraoperative tool overcoming the ultrasound guidance. Eur Urol 2020;78(2): 229–38.

22. Qin B, Hu H, Lu Y, et al. Intraoperative ultrasonography in laparoscopic partial nephrectomy for intrarenal tumors. PLoS One. 2018;13(4):e0195911.

23. Assimos DG, Boyce H, Woodruff RD, et al. Intraoperative renal ultrasonography: a useful adjunct to partial nephrectomy. J Urol 1991;146(5):1218–20.

24. Alenezi AN, Karim O. Role of intra-operative contrast-enhanced ultrasound (CEUS) in robotic-assisted nephron-sparing surgery. J Robot Surg 2015;9(1):1–10.

25. Alenezi A, Motiwala A, Eves S, et al. Robotic assisted laparoscopic partial nephrectomy using contrast-enhanced ultrasound scan to map renal blood flow. Int J Med Robot 2017;13(1):e1738.

26. Hekman MCH, Rijpkema M, Langenhuijsen JF, et al. Intraoperative imaging techniques to support complete tumor resection in partial nephrectomy. Eur Urol Focus 2018;4(6):960–8.

27. Rogers CG, Laungani R, Bhandari A, et al. Maximizing console surgeon independence during robot-assisted renal surgery by using the Fourth Arm and TilePro. J Endourol 2009;23(1):115–21.

28. Hoda MR, Popken G. Surgical outcomes of fluorescence-guided laparoscopic partial nephrectomy using 5-aminolevulinic acid-induced protoporphyrin IX. J Surg Res 2009;154(2):220–5.

29. Mitsui Y, Shiina H, Arichi N, et al. Indocyanine green (ICG)-based fluorescence navigation system for discrimination of kidney cancer from normal parenchyma: application during partial nephrectomy. Int Urol Nephrol 2012;44(3):753–9.

30. Tobis S, Knopf J, Silvers C, et al. Near infrared fluorescence imaging with robotic assisted laparoscopic partial nephrectomy: initial clinical experience for renal cortical tumors. J Urol 2011; 186(1):47–52.

31. Tobis S, Knopf JK, Silvers CR, et al. Near infrared fluorescence imaging after intravenous indocyanine green: initial clinical experience with open partial nephrectomy for renal cortical tumors. Urology 2012; 79(4):958–64.

32. Tobis S, Knopf JK, Silvers C, et al. Robot-assisted and laparoscopic partial nephrectomy with near infrared fluorescence imaging. J Endourol 2012; 26(7):797–802.

33. Krane LS, Manny TB, Hemal AK. Is near infrared fluorescence imaging using indocyanine green dye useful in robotic partial nephrectomy: a prospective comparative study of 94 patients. Urology 2012; 80(1):110–6.

34. Manny TB, Krane LS, Hemal AK. Indocyanine green cannot predict malignancy in partial nephrectomy: histopathologic correlation with fluorescence pattern in 100 patients. J Endourol 2013;27(7):918–21.

35. Bjurlin MA, Gan M, McClintock TR, et al. Near-infrared fluorescence imaging: emerging applications in robotic upper urinary tract surgery. Eur Urol 2014;65(4):793–801.

36. Kaczmarek BF, Sukumar S, Petros F, et al. Robotic ultrasound probe for tumor identification in robotic partial nephrectomy: Initial series and outcomes. Int J Urol 2013;20(2):172–6.

37. Rao AR, Gray R, Mayer E, et al. Occlusion angiography using intraoperative contrast-enhanced ultrasound scan (CEUS): a novel technique demonstrating segmental renal blood supply to assist zero-ischaemia robot-assisted partial nephrectomy. Eur Urol 2013;63(5):913–9.

38. Le O, Wood C, Vikram R, et al. Feasibility of contrast-enhanced intraoperative ultrasound for detection and characterization of renal mass undergoing open partial nephrectomy. J Ultrasound Med 2017; 36(8):1547–53.

39. Zhang S, Yang G, Tang L, et al. Application of a functional3-dimensional perfusion model in laparoscopic partial nephrectomy with precise segmental renal artery clamping. Urology 2019;125:98–103.

40. Veccia A, Antonelli A, Hampton LJ, et al. Near-infrared fluorescence imaging with indocyanine green in robot-assisted partial nephrectomy: pooled analysis of comparative studies. Eur Urol Focus 2020;6(3):505–12.

41. Hekman MCH, Rijpkema M, Aarntzen EH, et al. Positron emission tomography/computed tomography with. Eur Urol 2018;74(3):257–60.

42. Hekman MC, Rijpkema M, Muselaers CH, et al. Tumor-targeted dual-modality imaging to improve intraoperative visualization of clear cell renal cell carcinoma: a first in man study. Theranostics. 2018;8(8):2161–70.

43. Porpiglia F, Bertolo R, Checcucci E, et al. Development and validation of 3D printed virtual models for robot-assisted radical prostatectomy and partial nephrectomy: urologists' and patients' perception. World J Urol 2018;36(2):201–7.

44. Hughes-Hallett A, Mayer EK, Marcus HJ, et al. Augmented reality partial nephrectomy: examining the current status and future perspectives. Urology 2014;83(2):266–73.

45. Simpfendörfer T, Gasch C, Hatiboglu G, et al. Intraoperative computed tomography imaging for navigated laparoscopic renal surgery: first clinical experience. J Endourol 2016;30(10):1105–11.

46. Chen Y, Li H, Wu D, et al. Surgical planning and manual image fusion based on 3D model facilitate laparoscopic partial nephrectomy for intrarenal tumors. World J Urol 2014;32(6):1493–9.

47. Thompson RH, Lane BR, Lohse CM, et al. Every minute counts when the renal hilum is clamped during partial nephrectomy. Eur Urol 2010;58(3):340–5.

48. Cacciamani GE, Medina LG, Gill T, et al. Impact of surgical factors on robotic partial nephrectomy outcomes: comprehensive systematic review and meta-analysis. J Urol 2018;200(2):258–74.

49. Agrawal S, Sedlacek H, Kim SP. Comparative effectiveness of surgical treatments for small renal masses. Urol Clin North Am 2017;44(2):257–67.

50. Cacciamani GE, Medina LG, Gill TS, et al. Impact of renal hilar control on outcomes of robotic partial nephrectomy: systematic review and cumulative meta-analysis. Eur Urol Focus 2019;5(4):619–35.

51. White WM, Goel RK, Haber GP, et al. Robotic partial nephrectomy without renal hilar occlusion. BJU Int 2010;105(11):1580–4.

52. Kaczmarek BF, Tanagho YS, Hillyer SP, et al. Off-clamp robot-assisted partial nephrectomy preserves renal function: a multi-institutional propensity score analysis. Eur Urol 2013;64(6):988–93.

53. Satkunasivam R, Tsai S, Syan S, et al. Robotic unclamped "minimal-margin" partial nephrectomy: ongoing refinement of the anatomic zero-ischemia concept. Eur Urol 2015;68(4):705–12.

54. Ficarra V, Novara G, Secco S, et al. Preoperative aspects and dimensions used for an anatomical (PADUA) classification of renal tumours in patients who are candidates for nephron-sparing surgery. Eur Urol 2009;56(5):786–93.

55. Kutikov A, Uzzo RG. The R.E.N.A.L. nephrometry score: a comprehensive standardized system for quantitating renal tumor size, location and depth. J Urol 2009;182(3):844–53.

56. Simone G, Papalia R, Guaglianone S, et al. 'Zero ischaemia', sutureless laparoscopic partial nephrectomy for renal tumours with a low nephrometry score. BJU Int 2012;110(1):124–30.

57. Shao P, QC, Yin C, et al. Laparoscopic partial nephrectomy with segmental renal artery clamping: technique and clinical outcomes. Eur Urol. 2011 May;59(5):849–55. https://doi.org/10.1016/j.eururo.2010.11.037. Epub 2010 Dec 7. PMID: 21146917.

58. Desai MM, de Castro Abreu AL, Leslie S, et al. Robotic partialnephrectomy with superselective versus main artery clamping: a retrospective comparison. Eur Urol 2014;66:713–9.

59. Shin TY, Lim SK, Komninos C, et al. Clinical values of selective-clamp technique in robotic partial nephrectomy. World J Urol 2015;33:763–9.

60. Borofsky MS, Gill IS, Hemal AK, et al. Near-infrared fluorescence imaging to facilitate super-selective arterial clamping during zero-ischaemia robotic partial nephrectomy. BJU Int 2013;111:604–10.

61. Harke N, Schoen G, Schiefelbein F, et al. Selective clamping under the usage of near-infrared fluorescence imaging with indo-cyanine green in robot-assisted partial nephrectomy: a single-surgeon matched-pair study. World J Urol 2014;32:1259–65.

62. Zhang C, Guo F, Jing T, et al. The margin strategy in laparoscopic partial nephrectomy with selective renal artery clamping: Anatomical basis, surgical technique and comparative outcomes. Asian J Surg 2020;43(2):417–22.

63. Bjurlin MA, Renson A, Fantus RJ. Impact of trauma center designation and interfacility transfer on renal trauma outcomes: evidence for universal management. Eur Urol Focus 2019;5(6):1135–42.

64. Baumert H, Ballaro A, Shah N, et al. Reducing warm ischaemia time during laparoscopic partial nephrectomy: a prospective comparison of two renal closure techniques. Eur Urol 2007;52(4):1164–9.

65. Stonier T, Rai BP, Trimboli M, et al. Early vs standard unclamping technique in minimal access partial nephrectomy: a meta-analysis of observational cohort studies and the Lister cohort. J Robot Surg 2017;11(4):389–98.

66. Peyronnet B, Baumert H, Mathieu R, et al. Early unclamping technique during robot-assisted laparoscopic partial nephrectomy can minimise warm ischaemia without increasing morbidity. BJU Int 2014;114(5):741–7.

67. Graves FT. The anatomy of the intrarenal arteries in health and disease. Br J Surg 1956;43(182):605–16.
68. Macchi V, Picardi E, Inferrera A, et al. Anatomic and Radiologic Study of Renal Avascular Plane (Brödel's Line) and Its Potential Relevance on Percutaneous and Surgical Approaches to the Kidney. J Endourol 2018;32(2):154–9.
69. Borojeni S, Borojeni A, Panayotopoulos P, et al. Study of renal and kidney tumor vascularization using data from preoperative three-dimensional arteriography prior to partial nephrectomy. Eur Urol Focus 2020;6(1):112–21.
70. Bertolo R, Campi R, Mir MC, et al. Systematic review and pooled analysis of the impact of renorrhaphy techniques on renal functional outcome after partial nephrectomy. Eur Urol Oncol 2019;2(5):572–5.
71. Rogers CG, Metwalli A, Blatt AM, et al. Robotic partial nephrectomy for renal hilar tumors: a multi-institutional analysis. J Urol 2008;180(6):2353–6 [discussion: 2356].
72. Williams RD, Snowden C, Frank R, et al. Has sliding-clip renorrhaphy eliminated the need for collecting system repair during robot-assisted partial nephrectomy? J Endourol 2017;31(3):289–94.
73. Kaouk JH, Khalifeh A, Hillyer S, et al. Robot-assisted laparoscopic partial nephrectomy: step-by-step contemporary technique and surgical outcomes at a single high-volume institution. Eur Urol 2012;62(3):553–61.
74. Seideman C, Park S, Best SL, et al. Self-retaining barbed suture for parenchymal repair during minimally invasive partial nephrectomy. J Endourol 2011;25(8):1245–7 [discussion: 1247–8].
75. Ramanathan R, Leveillee RJ. A review of methods for hemostasis and renorrhaphy after laparoscopic and robot-assisted laparoscopic partial nephrectomy. Curr Urol Rep 2010;11(3):208–20.
76. Liu W, Chen M, Zu X, et al. The use of self-retaining barbed suture preserves superior renal function during laparoscopic partial nephrectomy: a PADUA score matched comparison. J Laparoendosc Adv Surg Tech A 2015;25(2):130–4.
77. Shang JW, Ma X, Zhang X, et al. Comparison of two different renorrhaphy techniques in retroperitoneal laparoscopic partial nephrectomy for complex tumor. Chin Med J (Engl) 2013;126(24):4629–32.
78. Bahler CD, Dube HT, Flynn KJ, et al. Feasibility of omitting cortical renorrhaphy during robot-assisted partial nephrectomy: a matched analysis. J Endourol 2015;29(5):548–55.
79. Omae K, Kondo T, Takagi T, et al. Renal sinus exposure as an independent factor predicting asymptomatic unruptured pseudoaneurysm formation detected in the early postoperative period after minimally invasive partial nephrectomy. Int J Urol 2015;22(4):356–61.
80. Kim KS, Choi SW, Kim JH, et al. Running-clip renorrhaphy reducing warm ischemic time during laparoscopic partial nephrectomy. J Laparoendosc Adv Surg Tech A 2015;25(1):50–4.
81. Kaygisiz O, Çelen S, Vuruşkan BA, et al. Comparison of two different suture techniques in laparoscopic partial nephrectomy. Int Braz J Urol 2017;43(5):863–70.
82. Canales BK, Lynch AC, Fernandes E, et al. Novel technique of knotless hemostatic renal parenchymal suture repair during laparoscopic partial nephrectomy. Urology 2007;70(2):358–9.
83. Nelson RJ, Chavali JSS, Yerram N, et al. Current status of robotic single-port surgery. Urol Ann 2017;9(3):217–22.
84. Kaouk J, Aminsharifi A, Sawczyn G, et al. Single-port robotic urological surgery using Purpose-built Single-port Surgical System: Single-institutional experience with the first 100 cases. Urology 2020;140:77–84.
85. Fang AM, Saidian A, Magi-Galluzzi C, et al. Single-port robotic partial and radical nephrectomies for renal cortical tumors: initial clinical experience. J Robot Surg 2020;14(5):773–80.
86. Na JC, Lee HH, Yoon YE, et al. True single-site partial nephrectomy using the SP surgical system: feasibility, comparison with the Xi single-site platform, and step-by-step procedure guide. J Endourol 2020;34(2):169–74.
87. Bertolo R, Garisto J, Gettman M, et al. Novel system for robotic single-port surgery: feasibility and state of the art in urology. Eur Urol Focus 2018;4(5):669–73.
88. Mittakanti HR, Heulitt G, Li HF, et al. Transperitoneal vs. retroperitoneal robotic partial nephrectomy: a matched-paired analysis. World J Urol 2020;38(5):1093–9.

Robotic Ureteral Reconstruction

Alice Drain, MD, MS[a], Min Suk Jun, DO, MS[b], Lee C. Zhao, MD, MS[a],*

KEYWORDS

- Robot • Ureteral stricture • Ureteral reimplant • Ureteroureterostomy • Buccal mucosa
- Appendiceal flap • Ileal ureter • Retrocaval ureter

KEY POINTS

- Ureteral strictures should be approached with an algorithmic model with decision of reconstructive technique determined by location, length, and grade.
- Preoperative evaluation after ureteral rest with antegrade and retrograde ureterogram guides the treatment approach.
- Attention to preservation of ureteral blood supply is crucial; anatomic knowledge of the vasculature is critical, circumferential dissection should be avoided, and an onlay is preferred over interposition.
- Ileal ureter remains a salvage option if more minimally invasive techniques are not feasible.

INTRODUCTION

Increasingly sophisticated robotically assisted laparoscopic technology and techniques have led to significant advances in the minimally invasive treatment of ureteral strictures. Stricture etiologies include radiation, iatrogenic injury, trauma, urolithiasis, and congenitalism. Traditionally, ureteral strictures longer than 2 cm, which are refractory to endoscopic treatment, were treated with ureteroneocystotomy with or without psoas hitch or Boari flap, ureteroureterostomy (UU), ileal substitution, or autotransplantation.[1] Laparoscopic ureteral reconstruction was first described in 1992 by Nezhat and colleagues,[2] who performed a UU, but this procedure was not widely adopted owing to the technical challenges of the procedure, which requires dissection and precise suturing in a tight working space with limited exposure. Techniques for ureteral stricture repair were first adapted to the robot in 2003 when Yohannes and associates[3] performed a ureteral reimplantation with a Boari flap for a distal stricture. Middle and proximal ureteral strictures pose a greater challenge owing to both their location

and etiology. The prevalence of robotic-assisted repair of mid and proximal ureteral strictures has increased greatly over the past decade with some now considering it the standard of care.[4,5] The robot's magnified view, stereoscopic vision, freedom of articulation, and availability of adjunct technology such as Indocyanine green and Firefly infrared laparoscopy are particularly advantageous in ureteral repair.[6,7] This article describes the latest advances in the robotic approach to ureteral stricture management.

DIAGNOSIS

Presenting symptoms of ureteral stricture are consistent with renal colic owing to upper tract obstruction, including flank pain, abdominal pain, nausea, vomiting, and pyelonephritis. A computed tomography scan is commonly performed, revealing hydroureteronephrosis with a distinct transition point along the ureter without another obvious cause for obstruction such as a ureteral calculus. In some cases, the obstruction can be asymptomatic and only incidentally found. Laboratory evaluation may reveal worsening renal

[a] NYU Langone Health Department of Urology, 11th Floor, 222 East 41st Street, New York, NY 10017, USA;
[b] Crane CTS, 575 Sir Francis Drake Blvd, Suite 1, Greenbrae, CA 94904, USA
* Corresponding author.
E-mail address: Lee.zhao@nyulangone.org
Twitter: @AliceDrainMD (A.D.); @DrMinJun (M.S.J.); @lee_c_zhao (L.C.Z.)

Urol Clin N Am 48 (2021) 91–101
https://doi.org/10.1016/j.ucl.2020.09.001

function. When patients present acutely, a urologist will often place a ureteral stent for decompression. Some patients who would otherwise be good candidates for repair are managed with serial ureteral stent exchanges.

ANATOMY

The ureters run bilaterally starting posterior to the renal artery, anteriorly along the psoas muscle, posterior to the gonadal vessels, anterior to the bifurcation of the common iliac artery, and along the medial aspect of the internal iliac artery. The ureter then courses medially and runs with the hypogastric nerves into the endopelvic fascia, crossing anterior to the obturator artery, vein, and nerves. In men, the vas deferens loops medially over the ureter at this point, in females the ovary and more distally the uterine artery run anteriorly. In cases requiring distal ureteral mobilization, careful dissection of the hypogastric nerves at this point may help to preserve bladder function.[8]

The ureters can be divided into upper ureter, extending form the ureteropelvic junction to the upper border of the sacrum, the middle ureter, extending from the upper to the lower border of the sacrum, and the lower ureter, which travels from the pelvis to the bladder. There are important differences in blood supply to these 3 anatomic regions. The upper ureter is supplied by branches arising medially from the renal artery and occasionally the abdominal aorta or gonadal artery, the mid ureter posteriorly by branches off the common iliac arteries, and the distal ureter laterally by the superior vesical artery, a branch off the internal iliac artery. These branches further divide to form a longitudinal anastomotic plexus along the ureter, and it is important when determining the location for ureteral spatulation and graft onlay to be aware of arterial supply and minimize disruption. Clinically when determining approach to stricture repair, we divide the ureter into the proximal and mid ureter and the distal ureter with the distal ureter beginning when the ureter runs over the bifurcation of the common iliac artery at the pelvis, which corresponds roughly with the inferior edge of the sacroiliac joint on imaging. There is a normal anatomic narrowing at the levels of the ureteropelvic junction, iliac vessels, and ureterovesical junction, and this must be distinguished on imaging from stricture in preoperative evaluation.

PREOPERATIVE PLANNING

When there is suspicion for ureteral stricture, we recommend placement of a percutaneous nephrostomy tube. If a patient has previously been managed with an indwelling ureteral stent, the stent can be used as a target on imaging. Alternatively, a urethral catheter can be placed and the bladder instilled with irrigation, inducing hydronephrosis and providing a larger target for percutaneous access. At this point, the stent is removed allowing for a period of ureteral rest for 4 to 6 weeks, similar to the urethral rest described for anterior urethral strictures.[9] This period will allow for the ureteral stricture to fully declare itself.[6] After ureteral rest, a renal scan can be performed to assess function and confirm obstruction. Nephrectomy may be appropriate for kidneys providing less than 20% split function in the setting of recurrent pyelonephritis. After the period of ureteral rest, further imaging to visualize the location, length, and grade of stricture with an antegrade and retrograde ureterogram should be performed (**Fig. 1**). Ureteroscopy may be used to definitively rule out malignancy as the cause of obstruction. At this point, the diagnostic workup is complete, and the patient is counseled on the findings before definitive repair. A urine culture is collected and treated preoperatively as needed. The indwelling nephrostomy tube is a nidus for colonization, and patients are at higher risk of bacteremia, funguria, and sepsis. As such, antibiotic coverage is broadened as per the discretion of the surgeon and local guidelines. Routine bowel preparation is not recommended.

PATIENT POSITIONING

Women are placed in dorsal lithotomy with the ipsilateral side elevated. Men may be positioned in lateral decubitus. The genitalia and nephrostomy tube are included in the sterile field. The patient must be well-secured because Trendelenburg is often used in cases of distal stricture. The endotracheal tube is taped to the low side because the buccal graft is harvested from the top (ipsilateral) side. The mouth is prepped and draped separately if a buccal mucosal graft is needed.

PROCEDURAL APPROACH

i. Port placement (**Fig. 2**)
  - Obtain access at the midline, superior to the umbilicus.
  - Distal stricture: Robotic ports are placed similarly to a robotic cystectomy. The ports are placed sufficiently superiorly to allow for bladder manipulation.
  - Proximal or mid stricture: Robotic ports are placed vertically along the midclavicular line

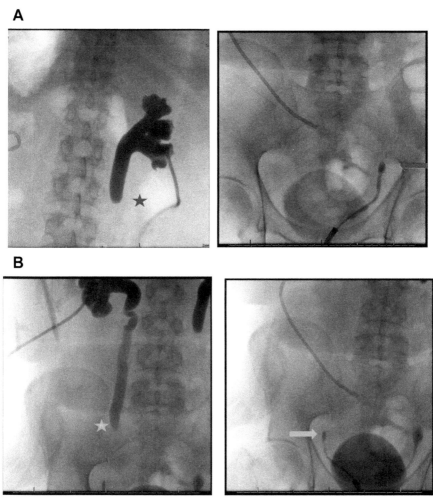

Fig. 1. Antegrade and retrograde pyelograms (*A*). Right ureter: approximately 10 cm stricture. Note moderate hydronephrosis and hydroureter to proximal ureter with abrupt termination (*star*) and narrowing of the distal ureter below pelvic brim (*arrow*). (*B*) Left ureter: approximately 4 to 5 cm stricture. Note severe hydronephrosis, and moderate hydroureter to mid ureter (*star*) with abrupt narrowing of the distal ureter below the pelvic brim (*arrow*). The patient was treated with right ileal ureter and left Boari flap.

starting 2 fingerbreadths below the costal margin to 2 fingerbreadths above the iliac crest. Port placement may be modified as needed based on the presence of adhesions.

ii. Instrumentation
  - Our preference is to use Maryland bipolar forceps, monopolar scissors, and ProGrasp forceps.
  - Camera: 30°

iii. Endoscopy
  - Flexible cystoscopy is performed and a guidewire placed in the ureter.
  - The flexible ureteroscope is advanced over the guidewire to the level of the stricture. TilePro (Intuitive, Sunnyvale, CA) is useful to

enable the console surgeon to see the ureteroscopic view.

iv. Robotic dissection and identification of the stricture
  - The colon is medialized and the ureter is identified. We prefer to avoid circumferential ureterolysis to preserve blood supply. The iliac vessels lie posterior to the ureter, and normal planes are often obliterated in reoperative and irradiated fields. Avoidance of circumferential ureterolysis can minimize injury to these vessels.
  - Maneuvers that can aid in ureteral identification
    a. The Firefly (Intuitive, Sunnyvale, CA) camera can be used because it detects the near-infrared spectrum of the light

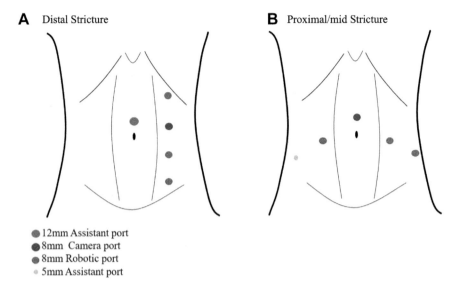

A Distal Stricture

B Proximal/mid Stricture

- 12mm Assistant port
- 8mm Camera port
- 8mm Robotic port
- 5mm Assistant port

Fig. 2. Port placement.

emitted by the ureteroscope, which transmits through tissue more readily than visible light. Note that this will not work if a digital flexible ureteroscope is used because these scopes do not emit light in the near-infrared spectrum.

b. Indocyanine green (ICG) (25 mg ICG in 10 mL water) can be injected intraluminally via nephrostomy or in a retrograde fashion.[6] Of note, once in contact with urothelium, it will be present for the duration of the case, compromising its utility in assessing ureteral vascularity through intravenous (IV) administration.

v. Ureterotomy
- We prefer to make a longitudinal ureterotomy anteriorly to preserve blood supply when the ureteral lumen is patent. This is extended until normal caliber ureter is encountered. If the ureteral lumen is obliterated, the ureter is transected, and the distal and proximal ends are mobilized until the posterior wall can be reestablished in a tension-free manner.
- IV ICG (10 mL × 1 mg/1 mL) may be used to assess ureteral blood supply.[10,11] Within seconds of administration, well-perfused tissue will glow green under the near-infrared camera. If the proximal or distal extent of the ureterotomy is poorly vascularized, consider extending the ureterotomy until well-perfused ureter is encountered.

vi. Ureteral reconstruction
- A detailed discussion of techniques is provided elsewhere in this article.

vii. Stent placement
- A 6 Fr ureteral stent is placed over the wire before completion of the anastomosis.

viii. Evaluation of anastomosis
- Distal stricture: The bladder is instilled with 180 mL of saline to confirm a water-tight anastomosis.
- Proximal or mid stricture: Irrigation through the ureteroscope confirms a water-tight anastomosis. Alternatively, the bladder can be filled and reflux through the ureteral stent can confirm water-tight closure.

ix. Nephrostomy tube removal
- If no longer needed, the assistant should remove the nephrostomy tube while the ureteral stent is grasped to avoid accidental dislocation.

x. Drain placement
- A closed suction drain is placed near the anastomosis. This drain will be removed on postoperative day 1 if output remains low after Foley removal.

DISTAL URETERAL RECONSTRUCTION
Ureteral Reimplantation

Distal ureteral strictures may be managed with ureteral reimplantation. Traditionally, the ureter is circumferentially dissected and a vessel loop is passed to isolate it. The distal ureter is mobilized to facilitate a tension-free anastomosis. The ureter is transected proximal to the stricture. The bladder is then filled with 200 to 300 mL of saline and a cystotomy is made at an appropriate location, usually at the dome. The ureteroneocystotomy anastomosis is then completed with absorbable suture.

In our modification, the ureter is left in situ and a longitudinal ureterotomy is made just proximal to the level of the stricture. This practice ensures maximal blood supply preservation, theoretically decreasing the likelihood of failure. Additionally, avoiding circumferential dissection of the ureter decreases operating time and reduces the risk of injury to the posteriorly located iliac vessels.[12] Lastly, with this approach the native ureteral orifice is maintained, facilitating easy access to the ureter for possible future endoscopic intervention (eg, urolithiasis). The space of Retzius is then developed and the bladder is dropped onto the ureter. The bladder is insufflated with air to avoid fluid extravasation upon making a cystotomy. A cystotomy at a location matching the ureterotomy is made. The anastomosis is completed using 3-0 absorbable barbed suture. Before completion of the anastomosis, a ureteral stent is advanced in retrograde fashion. It is important to ensure adequate mobilization of the bladder to achieve a tension-free anastomosis. If there is any concern regarding this, then the bladder should be thoroughly freed from its anterior attachments. In a retrospective study comparing 10 robotic reimplantations with 24 open repairs, Kozinn and associates[13] found both approaches have durable outcomes, with no recurrence of stricture disease at over 2 years of follow-up.

Psoas Hitch

The psoas hitch is an essential maneuver in the management of distal ureteral stricture. Laparoscopic psoas hitch and Boari flap were first described in 2001.[14,15] The psoas tendon is exposed and an absorbable suture is used to fix the bladder to the psoas tendon to relieve tension at the anastomosis. The suture should be passed longitudinally along the psoas tendon to avoid the genitofemoral nerve. Alternatively, the bladder can be fixed to the side wall peritoneum to similar effect. As in the nontransecting reimplantation described above, the ureter can be left in situ and reimplantation performed in a nontransecting manner.

In the largest prospective series of robotic psoas hitch, all 12 patients who underwent treatment with distal ureteral reimplantation with psoas hitch had successful outcomes with no obstruction on postoperative MAG-3 scan or IV urography.[16]

Boari Flap

When psoas hitch provides inadequate bladder reach to the ureterotomy, a Boari flap is the next adjunctive maneuver that can be used to provide 3 to 15 cm of mobility with success rates reported from 95% to 100%.[17] With the space of Retzius fully developed, a pedicle of bladder is dissected from the anterior bladder wall. The apex is approximately 3 cm proximal to the bladder neck, and the incision is extended toward the dome to create a trapezoidal flap of tissue with the pedicle base wider than the apex. The flap is fixed to the psoas, tubularized, and anastomosed to the ureter.[13,18] In the largest series of robotic ureteral reimplantation with a Boari flap, all 11 patients had durable repair of their distal stricture at 15 months of follow-up.[19]

Distal Ureteroureterostomy

In this technique, the ureter is circumferentially mobilized and the diseased ureter excised. The remaining healthy ends of the ureter are spatulated 1 to 2 cm and reanastomosed using absorbable suture to approximate the mucosal edges. Particular care is taken to avoid manipulation of the tissue or application of monopolar cautery to preserve the periureteric blood supply. As in the previously described repairs, a stent is exchanged over the guidewire after completion of the posterior anastomosis. Traditionally, UU is used for mid and proximal stricture (discussed elsewhere in this article) owing to concern for higher failure rates associated with the tenuous vasculature of the distal ureter. However, there are small series reporting success with this approach distally.[20] Unlike ureteral reimplantation or a Boari flap, this approach preserves the natural integrity of the bladder and ureteral antireflux mechanism. The risk of disruption of blood supply from circumferential ureteral dissection must be balanced with the benefits of this technique. It is best suited to relatively short (<3 cm), unifocal stenosis in nonirradiated fields. Paick and colleagues[21] reported successful open UU in 9 patients. This technique was adapted to the robot by Lee and colleagues[4,22] who reported the first robotic assisted UU in 2010, and expanded on their case series in 2013. Of the 12 patients in the series, only 1 stricture recurred at medium-term follow-up. The largest published series reports successful distal UU in 21 patients.[23]

Middle and Proximal Ureteral Reconstruction

Ureteroureterostomy

UU has traditionally been performed for short strictures (<3 cm) proximal to the crossing of the iliac vessels.[24,25] The stricture is excised and the ureteral ends are mobilized until a tension free anastomosis is possible. Opposite sides of the proximal and distal ureteral ends are spatulated and the anastomosis is completed with absorbable suture over a ureteral stent. It is prudent to re-retroperitonealize the repair to decrease the risk of fistulization. Lee and colleagues advocate for concomitant downward nephropexy in which the proximal ureter and kidney are fully dissected and mobilized caudad. In doing so they estimate 3 to 4 cm of mobilization is possible.

Appendiceal flap

The appendiceal flap ureteroplasty has many advantages, including relative ease of appendiceal mobilization, defined blood supply, negligible absorption of urine over the small surface area, ability to replace totally obliterated ureteral segments, and lack of donor site morbidity compared with a buccal mucosa graft (BMG) ureteroplasty. For this reason, it should be considered when the appendiceal anatomy is favorable. The technique was first described in 1912 by Melnikoff[26] using end-to-end anastomosis, but use was infrequently reported until recently.[27,28] In 2009, Reggio and colleagues[29] reported a successful laparoscopic appendiceal onlay flap ureteroplasty of a nonobliterative right ureteral stricture. Through the use of the onlay technique, not only is the ureteral blood supply minimally disrupted, but the appendiceal flap carries with it its own blood supply and may theoretically be a superior option in cases of impaired vascularity, such as radiation-induced strictures.

Port placement is similar to the previously described setup. Of note, a 12-mm port will need to be placed to accommodate a laparoscopic stapler, which will be used to harvest the appendiceal flap. Once harvested, the 2 ends of the appendix are opened and the lumen is cleared with suction and irrigation. The appendix is opened longitudinally along its antimesenteric border in the case of onlay. The mesentery of the appendix is carefully mobilized to facilitate a tension-free anastomosis (**Fig. 3**). IV ICG can be useful during this maneuver because it will highlight the main vascular trunk of the mesoappendix, which is to be avoided (**Fig. 4**). A ventral ureterotomy is made and anastomosis is performed similarly to that previously described for buccal grafts. If the appendix is not appropriate for ureteroplasty, the mesentery is divided with the stapler and appendectomy completed.

Outcome data for minimally invasive appendiceal graft techniques are favorable. In 2015, a case series of 6 patients from Reggio and colleagues[30] reported no recurrences at 16 months of follow-up. All strictures were right sided with an average length of 2.5 cm. Case reports have shown that this procedure translates well into

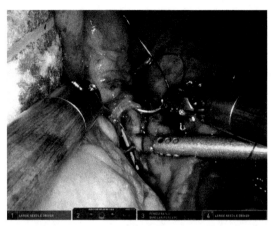

Fig. 3. Proximal right ureteral stricture. The lateral edge anastomosis of an appendiceal onlay is nearing completion. The opened appendiceal flap is seen underneath the suction tip while the needle is seen entering the distal apex of the opened right ureter.

robotic technique, with Yarlagadda and colleagues[31] reporting the use of tubularized appendiceal interposition for a 5 cm obliterative right ureteral stricture with no recurrence at 10 months. More complex repairs are also possible; Gn and colleagues[32] described a panureteral appendiceal ureteroplasty for an iatrogenic avulsion, requiring simultaneous downward nephropexy, psoas hitch, and calycostomy.

Oral mucosa graft onlay

Buccal mucosa graft (BMG) is particularly well-suited for urinary reconstruction owing to a panvascular lamina propria, epithelium adapted to a wet environment, well-tolerated donor site morbidity, and good take even in irradiated and

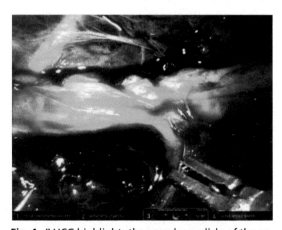

Fig. 4. IV ICG highlights the vascular pedicle of the appendiceal flap with near infrared laparoscopy, confirming viability of the mobilized flap at its new location.

reoperative fields.[33,34] BMG ureteroplasty was first reported by Naude in 1999.[35] Although it has been increasingly prominent in urethroplasty over the past 2 decades, it was not frequently used in ureteroplasty over this period.[36] In 2015, Zhao and colleagues[37] reported their experience with robotic BMG ureteroplasty with a follow-up multi-institutional study. In that study, 19 patients with average stricture length of 4 cm treated with BMG ureteroplasty showed 90% success at a median follow-up of 26 months.

After initial robotic access and exposure of the ureter is obtained, an anterior ureterotomy is extended the length of the stricture. We prefer a ventral onlay because this allows one to preserve the posterior blood supply and avoid circumferential dissection, as mentioned elsewhere in this article. In cases of short obliterative strictures, the obliterated section is excised and the ventral portion of the 2 ureteral ends are spatulated. A posterior ureteral plate is established through the anastomosis of the dorsal ureteral ends with absorbable barbed suture (**Fig. 5**). IV ICG may be used to confirm adequate blood supply to the ureter. Once adequate blood supply is confirmed, stay sutures are placed to mark the apices. The stricture length is measured to determine the necessary graft size and the BMG harvest is performed. If adjunctive maneuvers, such as downward nephropexy, do not result in a tension-free anastomosis, one should consider an ileal ureter.

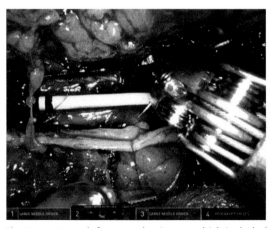

Fig. 5. An 11-cm left ureteral stricture, which included a 3-cm segment of complete obliteration owing to a cryoablation injury for a lower pole renal mass. An augmented anastomotic ventral onlay buccal mucosal graft ureteroplasty with downward nephropexy was performed. The posterior wall has been reestablished in an interrupted fashion. Seen in the picture is the anastomosis of the medial edge of an 8 cm buccal graft.

A mouth retractor with a tongue blade is positioned and 2 to 3 holding sutures are placed on the lip for retraction. A headlamp is useful for visualization. Stenson's duct is identified and marked. Lidocaine (1%) with 1:100,000 epinephrine is used for hydrodissection and to minimize bleeding. A buccal graft 1 cm wide by the length of the ureteral stricture is harvested. The graft is defatted and passed to the robotic surgeon with a suture to facilitate graft handling. The buccal defect can be left open or closed at the surgeon's preference. The BMG is oriented over the ureterotomy with mucosal surface facing the ureteral lumen, and the edges are anastomosed with barbed absorbable suture. A flap of omentum or perinephric fat is then fixed over the graft to provide a vascular source on which to take.

Retrocaval ureter

Retrocaval ureter is a congenital abnormality in which the right ureter runs posterior to the inferior vena cava. A few options for patients with symptomatic ureteral obstruction are reported. Traditionally, these choices have been UU or pyelopyelostomy. Robotic-assisted UU for retrocaval ureter was first described in 2006 in the pediatric population and further developed in 2011 by LeRoy and colleagues.[38,39] In the latter approach, the normal ureter is transected leaving the retrocaval segment of the ureter in situ. The normal ureter is then transposed anterior to the vena cava and a UU is performed, taking care to minimize distal ureteral dissection to avoid stricture recurrence.[40] Although there is a theoretic risk that the retained retrocaval ureter may undergo malignant transformation, the rarity of this condition precludes any evidence-based conclusion. Simforoosh and colleagues[41] reported 6 cases in which the retrocaval ureter was left in situ without complication.

Ileal ureter

Ileal ureteral substitution is an important fallback technique, and all patients should be counseled on the possibility of requiring one if the previously mentioned approaches are insufficient. Ileal ureter may be contraindicated in patients with inflammatory bowel disease, bladder outlet obstruction, neurogenic bladder, and short gut.[42] Potential complications include bowel obstruction, fistula, bowel leak, and long-term metabolic complications, including metabolic acidosis, vitamin B_{12} malabsorption, and increased risk of nephrolithiasis and cholelithiasis owing to bile acid malabsorption.[43]

The first ileal ureter was described in 1959[44] and further refined in the 1990s by Yang and Monti and colleagues for longer strictures.[45,46] Robotic ileal ureter was first described in 2008 by Wagner and colleagues[47] and has since been modified further to be performed entirely intracorporeally.[48] In 2016, Chopra and colleagues[49] reported a 3-case series of robotic ileal ureter in which 1 patient suffered a volvulus resulting in loss of ileal ureter on postoperative day 4. The remaining 2 cases were successful. Most recently, Ubrig and colleagues[50] reported a 7-patient series of robotic intracorporeal ileal ureter of which 5 patients underwent simultaneous psoas hitch. The mean length of transposed ileum was 20.4 cm. All patients were symptom free at the 3-month follow-up.[50]

After the ureter is isolated and the patent ends of the ureter exposed (or bladder and renal pelvis), an appropriate length of ileum 20 cm proximal to the ileocecal valve is harvested with a laparoscopic stapler. Bowel continuity is restored in standard fashion. Proximally, the bowel may be anastomosed to the ureter, renal pelvis, or lower pole calyx, depending on stricture severity. One must ensure adequate spatulation to accommodate anastomosis to the end of the bowel. Alternatively, a side-to-side anastomosis may be more appropriate; this should be judged on a case-by-case basis. Distally, the end of the ureter is anastomosed to the bladder or spatulated distal ureteral stump. For bilateral ureteral stricture, a longer segment of ileum may be harvested and the ureteral anastomoses performed on both ends. The most dependent portion of the bowel segment is allowed to lay on the bladder in a U configuration. An approximately 5-cm enterotomy is made on the antimesenteric side, and a matching cystotomy is made at the dome of the bladder. An anastomosis between the two is completed with absorbable barbed suture. IV ICG is useful to confirm adequate perfusion at the level of the anastomoses. A ureteral stent is placed in usual fashion over a wire before complete closure. The bladder is irrigated to confirm a water-tight anastomosis.

Autotransplantation

Robotic-assisted kidney autotransplantation is reserved as a salvage procedure. It was first described in 1962 by Hardy[51] as an open procedure. In 2000, Fabrizio and colleagues[52] reported the first laparoscopic renal autotransplant, which consisted of a laparoscopic donor nephrectomy, extraction of the kidney through a midline incision, and standard transplantation through a Gibson incision. Completely intracorporeal robotic-assisted kidney autotransplantation was first reported in 2014 and has since been replicated at several institutions.[53–56] It remains a technically demanding but feasible procedure when all other options have been exhausted.

POSTOPERATIVE MANAGEMENT
Distal Reconstruction

If a drain is placed intraoperatively, it will be removed before discharge unless output is high. Because a cystotomy has been performed, patients are discharged from the hospital with a Foley catheter. A cystogram is performed at 1 to 2 weeks postoperatively, and the Foley is removed if there is no evidence of leak. The stent is removed at the 4-week postoperative visit.

Proximal and Mid Reconstruction

The Foley catheter is removed on postoperative day 1. The drain is removed after Foley removal the same day if output remains low. The stent is removed in the clinic 4 weeks later.

Ileal Ureter

If an ileovesical anastomosis was performed, a cystogram is obtained 2 weeks postoperatively, and the Foley catheter is removed if there is no evidence of leakage. The ureteral stent is removed 4 weeks postoperatively.

Postoperative Imaging

Although we have not found retrograde pyelogram necessary at the time of stent removal, this is an option based on practice preference We obtain a renal ultrasound examination 6 to 12 weeks after stent removal followed by a diuretic renal scan at 6 months. If ultrasound findings or patient symptoms are concerning for ureteral obstruction, the renogram may be obtained sooner.

Nephrostomy Management

A nephrostomy tube is kept or removed at the end of surgery on a case-by-case basis. For example, if the patient has a history of recurrent obstruction and sepsis, it may be prudent to keep the nephrostomy, which will remain through stent removal. The patient will then be instructed to place the nephrostomy to drainage if renal colic or pyelonephritis ensues. The nephrostomy tube is generally removed 1 week after stent removal if the patient remains symptom free.

MANAGEMENT

We use an algorithmic approach for the treatment of ureteral stricture. For distal ureteral strictures, we prefer a nontransecting ureteral reimplantation, performing a psoas hitch and then a Boari flap as

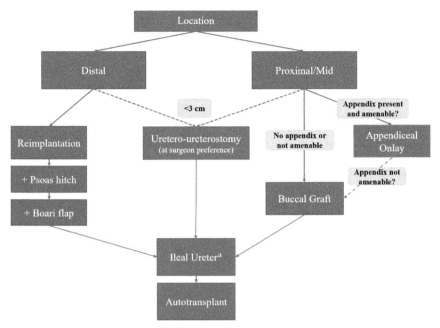

Fig. 6. Treatment decision tree. [a]Consider if prior radiation or multiple surgeries.

needed for added length. For middle to proximal right-sided ureteral strictures, if the appendix is available, we prefer to use it as a ventral onlay. For obliterated lumens, we prefer an augmented anastomotic approach. If one cannot perform an appendiceal flap reconstruction, we will perform buccal graft ureteroplasty. If a buccal graft is impractical, we will perform ileal ureteral substitution. The need for autotransplantation is rare and reserved for salvage cases. For multifocal unilateral or bilateral strictures, one may combine techniques. For example, one may perform a nontransecting ureteral reimplantation and a ventral buccal onlay at the same time (**Fig. 6**).

SUMMARY

The last 2 decades have seen the rapid adaption of time-tested techniques of ureteroplasty to the robotic-assisted laparoscopic approach. With that, morbidity continues to improve as techniques become less invasive. This article has sought to describe those techniques with an algorithm to guide their application. Although more advancements will undoubtedly be made, it is important to adhere to fundamental reconstructive principles and to have a contingency procedure, such as ileal ureteral substitution, should the need arise. Ureteral stricture management with serial ureteral stent exchanges is an all too common history encountered in reconstructive urology. The current armamentarium of ureteroplasty techniques now provides a safe, effective, and tolerable means of surgical cure.

CLINICS CARE POINTS

- One should strive to minimally disrupt the ureteral blood supply by avoiding circumferential dissection and transection. Onlay is preferred to interposition.
- An algorithmic approach ensures that the most effective and least invasive method of ureteral reconstruction is undertaken.
- The surgeon should be prepared at the time of surgery to perform an ileal ureter in the event if less invasive techniques are not feasible.

DISCLOSURE

L.C. Zhao is a consultant for Intuitive Surgical. M.S. Jun and A. Drain do not have any conflicts of interest to declare.

REFERENCES

1. Babbar P, Yerram N, Sun A, et al. Robot-assisted ureteral reconstruction – current status and future direction. Urol Ann 2018;10:7–14.
2. Nezhat C, Nezhat F, Green B. Laparoscopic treatment of obstructed ureter due to endometriosis by resection and ureteroureterostomy: a case report. J Urol 1992;148:865–8.

3. Yohannes P, Chiou RK, Pelinkovic D. Rapid communication: pure robot-assisted laparoscopic ureteral reimplantation for ureteral stricture disease: a case report. J Endourol 2003;17(10):891–3.

4. Lee Z, Llukani E, Reilly CE, et al. Single surgeon experience with robot-assisted ureteroureterostomy for pathologies at the proximal, middle, and distal ureter in adults. J Endourol 2013;27:994–9.

5. Tracey AT, Eun DD, Stifelman MD, et al. Robotic-assisted laparoscopic repair of ureteral injury: an evidence-based review of techniques and outcomes. Minerva Urol Nefrol 2018;70(3):231–41.

6. Lee Z, Moore B, Giusto L, et al. Use of indocyanine green during robot-assisted ureteral reconstructions. Eur Urol 2015;67:291–8.

7. Arora S, Campbell L, Tourojman M, et al. Robotic buccal mucosal Graft ureteroplasty for complex ureteral stricture. Urology 2017;110:257–8.

8. Casale P, Patel RP, Kolon TF. Nerve sparing robotic extravesical ureteral reimplantation. J Urol 2008; 179:1987–90.

9. Terlecki RP, Steele MC, Valadez C, et al. Urethral rest: role and rationale in preparation for anterior urethroplasty. Urology 2011;77:1477–81.

10. Bjurlin MA, Gan M, McClintock TR, et al. Near-infrared fluorescence imaging: emerging applications in robotic upper urinary tract surgery. Eur Urol 2014;65:793–801.

11. van Manen L, Handgraaf HJM, Diana M, et al. A practical guide for the use of indocyanine green and methylene blue in fluorescence-guided abdominal surgery. J Surg Oncol 2018;118(2):283–300.

12. Slawin J, Patel NH, Lee Z, et al. Ureteral Reimplantation via Robotic Nontransecting Side-to-Side Anastomosis for Distal Ureteral Stricture. J Endourol 2020 Aug;34(8):836–9. https://doi.org/10.1089/end. 2019.0877. Epub 2020 May 5. PMID: 32233674.

13. Kozinn SI, Canes D, Sorcini A, et al. Robotic versus open distal ureteral reconstruction and reimplantation for benign stricture disease. J Endourol 2012; 26(2):147–51.

14. Ahn M, Loughlin KR. Psoas hitch ureteral reimplantation in adults—analysis of a modified technique and timing of repair. Urology 2001;58:184–7.

15. Fugita OE, Dinlenc C, Kavoussi L. The laparoscopic Boari flap. Urology 2001;166(1):51–3.

16. Patil NN, Mottrie A, Sundaram B, et al. Robotic-assisted laparoscopic ureteral reimplantation with psoas hitch: a multi-institutional, multinational evaluation. Urology 2008;72(1):47–50.

17. Nakada SY, Best SL. Management of upper urinary tract obstruction. In: Wein AJ, Kavoussi LR, Partin AW, et al, editors. Campbell-Walsh urology. 11th edition. Philadelphia: Elsevier; 2016. p. 1135.

18. Schimpf MO, Wagner JR. Robot-assisted laparoscopic Boari flap ureteral reimplantation. J Endourol 2008;22(12):2691–4.

19. Stolzenburg JU, Rai BP, Do M, et al. Robot-assisted technique for Boari flap ureteric reimplantation: replicating the techniques of open surgery in robotics. BJU Int 2016;118:482–4.

20. Asghar AM, Lee RA, Yang KK, et al. Robot-assisted distal ureteral reconstruction for benign pathology: current state. Investig Clin Urol 2020;61(Suppl 1): S23–32.

21. Paick JS, Hong SK, Park MS, et al. Management of postoperatively detected iatrogenic lower ureteral injury: should ureteroureterostomy really be abandoned? Urology 2006;67(2):237–41.

22. Lee DI, Schwab CW, Harris A. Robot-assisted ureteroureterostomy in the adult: initial clinical series. Urology 2010;75:570–3.

23. Buffi NM, Lughezzani G, Hurle R, et al. Robot-assisted surgery for benign ureteral strictures: experience and outcomes from four tertiary care institutions. Eur Urol 2017;71:945–51.

24. Andrade HS, Kaouk JH, Zargar H, et al. Robotic ureteroureterostomy for treatment of a proximal ureteric stricture. Int Braz J Urol 2016;42:1041–2.

25. Raheem AA, Alatawi A, Kim DK, et al. Feasibility of robot-assisted segmental ureterectomy and ureteroureterostomy in patient with high medical comorbidity. Int Braz J Urol 2017;43:779–80.

26. Melnikoff AE. Sur le replacement de l'uretere par anse isolee de l'intestine grele. Rev Clin Urol 1912;1:601–3.

27. Richter F, Stock JA, Hanna MK. The appendix as right ureteral substitute in children. J Urol 2000; 163:1908–12.

28. Juma S, Nickel JC. Appendix interposition of the ureter. J Urol 1990;144:130–1.

29. Reggio E, Richstone L, Okeke Z, et al. Laparoscopic ureteroplasty using on-lay appendix graft. Urology 2009;73(4):928.

30. Duty BD, Kreshover JE, Richstone L, et al. Review of appendiceal onlay flap in the management of complex ureteric strictures in six patients: appendiceal onlay flap in management of ureteric strictures. BJU Int 2015;115:282–7.

31. Yarlagadda VK, Nix JW, Benson DG, et al. Feasibility of intracorporeal robotic-assisted laparoscopic appendiceal interposition for ureteral stricture disease: a case report. Urology 2017;109:201–5.

32. Gn M, Lee Z, Strauss D, et al. Robotic appendiceal interposition with right lower pole calycostomy, downward nephropexy, and psoas hitch for the management of an iatrogenic near-complete ureteral avulsion. Urology 2018;113:e9–10.

33. Somerville JJ, Naude JH. Segmental ureteric replacement: an animal study using a free non-pedicled graft. Urol Res 1984;12(2):115–9.

34. Naude JH. Buccal mucosal grafts in the treatment of ureteric lesions. BJU Int 2001;83:751–4.

35. Naude JH. Buccal mucosal grafts in the treatment of ureteric lesions. BJU Int 1999;83(7):751–4.

36. Wessells H, Angermeier KW, Elliott S, et al. Male urethral stricture: American Urological Association guideline. J Urol 2017;197:182–90.

37. Zhao LC, Yamaguchi Y, Bryk DJ, et al. Robot-assisted ureteral reconstruction using buccal mucosa. Urology 2015;86:634–8.

38. Gundeti MS, Duffy PG, Mushtaq I. Robotic-assisted laparoscopic correction of pediatric retrocaval ureter. J Laparoendosc Adv Surg Tech 2006;16:422–4.

39. LeRoy TJ, Thiel DD, Igel TC. Robot-assisted laparoscopic reconstruction of retrocaval ureter: description and video of technique. J Laparoendosc Adv Surg Tech 2011;21(4):349–51.

40. Liu E, Sun X, Guo H, et al. Retroperitoneoscopic ureteroplasty for retrocaval ureter: report of nine cases and literature review. Scand J Urol 2016;50:319–22.

41. Simforoosh N, Nouri-Mahdavi K, Tabibi A. Laparoscopic pyelopyelostomy for retrocaval ureter without excision of the retrocaval segment: first report of 6 cases. J Urol 2006;175:2166–9.

42. Mattos RM, Smith JJ 3rd. Ileal Ureter. Urol Clin North Am 1997;24(4):813–25.

43. Martini A, Villari D, Nicita G. Long-term complications arising from bowel interposition in the urinary tract. Int J Surg 2017;44:278–80.

44. Goodwin WF, Winter CC, Turner RD. Replacement of the ureter by small intestine: clinical application and results of the 'ileal ureter'. J Urol 1959;81:406–18.

45. Yang H. Yang needle tunneling technique in creating anti-reflux and continent mechanisms. J Urol 1993;150:830–46.

46. Monti PR, Lara RC, Dutra MA, et al. New techniques for construction of efferent conduits based on the Mitrofanoff principle. Urology 1997;49:112–5.

47. Wagner JR, Schimpf MO, Cohen JL. Robot-assisted laparoscopic ileal ureter. JSLS 2008;12(3):306–9.

48. Brandao LF, Autorino R, Zargar H, et al. Robotic ileal ureter: a completely intracorporeal technique. Urology 2014;83:951–4.

49. Chopra S, Metcalfe C, Satkunasivam R, et al. Initial series of four-arm robotic completely intracorporeal ileal ureter. J Endourol 2016;30:395–9.

50. Ubrig B, Janusonis J, Paulics L, et al. Functional outcomes of completely intracorporeal robotic ileal ureteric replacement. Urology 2018;114:193–7.

51. Hardy JD. High ureteral injuries. Management by autotransplantation of the kidney. JAMA 1963;184:97–101.

52. Fabrizio MD, Kavoussi LR, Jackman S, et al. Laparoscopic nephrectomy for autotransplantation. Urology 2000;55:145.

53. Gordon ZN, Angell J, Abaza R. Completely intracorporal robotic renal autotransplantation. J Urol 2014;192:1516–22.

54. Lee JY, Alzahrani T, Ordon M. Intra-corporeal robotic renal autotransplantation. Can Urol Assoc J 2015;9:E748–9.

55. Decaestecker K, Van Parys B, Van Besien J, et al. Robot-assisted kidney autotransplantation: a minimally invasive way to salvage kidneys. Eur Urol Focus 2018;4(2):198–205.

56. Doumerc N, Beauval JB, Roumiguie M, et al. Total intracorporeal robotic auto-transplantation: a new minimally invasive approach to preserve the kidney after major ureteral injuries. Int J Surg Case Rep 2018;49:176–9.

Robotic Lower Urinary Tract Reconstruction

Sunchin Kim, MD[a], Jill C. Buckley, MD[b],*

KEYWORDS

- Robotic lower urinary tract reconstruction • Bladder neck contracture • Proximal urethral stricture
- Genitourinary fistula • Rectourethral fistula

KEY POINTS

- Robotic reconstruction for the lower urinary tract is novel and currently rare but is promising as a new technique to approach complicated repairs.
- Bladder neck contractures and vesicourethral anastomotic strictures have been successfully repaired robotically with good patency rates and improved rates of urinary incontinence versus traditional approaches.
- Robotic-assisted surgery versus traditional approaches enable better visualization and greater control of anastomotic sutures during proximal and posterior urethral stricture repair.
- Although reports and case series are promising more studies, and higher-level evidence are needed to conclusively support robotic reconstruction of the lower urinary tract.

INTRODUCTION

Reconstruction of the urinary tract was first described in 1851 with a ureterosigmoidostomy,[1] followed by the ileal conduit described by Bricker in the 1950s as the primary form of urinary diversion from the lower urinary tract (LUT).[2] Over the last several decades, there has been development of numerous novel techniques to facilitate the reconstruction of the LUT instead of urinary diversion. The advent of laparoscopy and subsequent robotic techniques have allowed even further innovation to allow complex LUT issues to be managed as orthotopically as possible with the addition of numerous benefits offered by laparoscopic techniques. Reconstructive urologists have increasingly adopted the robotic platform to address a wide variety of upper and LUT pathologies.

The LUT anatomy includes the bladder, bladder neck, prostate, urinary sphincter, and the urethra. Not all disease processes in this anatomic region require laparoscopic surgery to repair. This article instead focuses on the anatomy and disease processes in the LUT that are appropriate for robotic repair, including bladder neck contractures (BNCs), proximal urethral strictures, and genitourinary fistulas. Given the rare occurrence of these pathologies and the relatively new robotic techniques that have been described, most of the data presented are case series and reports that speak to the technical feasibility of the robotic approach rather than comparative effectiveness with traditional open techniques.

BLADDER NECK CONTRACTURES AND VESICOURETHRAL ANASTOMOTIC STRICTURES

BNCs and vesicourethral anastomotic strictures (VUAS) are well-known complications that occur after prostate procedures for both benign and malignant conditions. These 2 complications are discussed together given their similar locations and general approaches to successful reconstruction. Although the precise pathophysiology of BNC remains unclear, scar hypertrophy is considered to

[a] Department of Urology, University of California San Diego, San Diego, CA, USA; [b] Department of Urology, University of California San Diego, 200 West Arbor Drive, San Diego, CA 92103, USA
* Corresponding author.
E-mail address: jcbuckley@health.ucsd.edu

Urol Clin N Am 48 (2021) 103–112
https://doi.org/10.1016/j.ucl.2020.09.006

be the basis for recurrence due to a prolonged inflammatory phase and/or ischemia.[3] BNC has a reported incidence after transurethral resection of prostate between 0% and 9.6%,[4,5] although rates have varied between different techniques used to treat benign conditions such as outlet obstruction. After a radical prostatectomy, VUAS rates have historically been reported to be as high 16%[6-8]; however, the advent of robotic surgery and improved visualization enables better mucosal apposition and watertight anastomosis, and rates have decreased to 2.2%.[9]

Initial treatment of BNC is highly variable, ranging from a simple dilation to endoscopic procedures using cold knife, electrocautery, lasers, and loop resection. These procedures can also be augmented with the addition of a steroid or a cytotoxic agent such as mitomycin C. Treatment success has ranged from 58% to 89% after these techniques.[10-12] However, when conservative or endoscopic treatment fails, a more invasive option is considered. Open reconstruction of BNC has historically been performed in patients with highly recalcitrant BNC. Because of the rare nature of these procedures, most published series are limited by a small sample size and may vary significantly in techniques, ranging from abdominoperineal, perineal, and transpubic approaches.[13-15] Although the reported patency rates have been as high as 93.3%, dissection through the external urinary sphincter is associated with significant risk for urinary incontinence.[16]

Robotic reconstruction of BNC is becoming a more widely adopted technique that has been described as advantageous in regard to lower estimated blood loss, reduced postoperative pain, shorter hospitalization, and improved continence rates, as the dissection is above the level of the sphincter, and avoids the morbidity of a pubectomy described in open procedures. There is also the potential advantage of improved durability in placing a future artificial urinary sphincter due to the lack of prior perineal dissection.

Procedural Approach

The surgical principles for a successful anastomosis for urethral strictures are applicable to BNC repairs. A tension-free, watertight, mucosa to mucosa apposition, well-vascularized, and catheterized anastomosis using resorbable sutures is crucial.

The patient is placed in a steep Trendelenburg position, and the abdomen is entered using a similar approach to robotic prostatectomy. Port placement includes a supraumbilical midline camera port, a robotic port and assistant port on the right side, and 2 robotic ports on the left side (**Fig. 1**A).

Patients with a history of outlet deobstruction procedure

Patients who have had a transurethral procedure of the prostate or a simple prostatectomy can be approached anteriorly by developing the space of Retzius and dropping the bladder off the anterior surface of the abdominal wall. This dissection is carried inferiorly underneath the pubic symphysis to the junction between the prostate and bladder neck. Given most patients have undergone several transurethral procedures prior for recurrent BNC, there may be a dense desmoplastic reaction that may require careful dissection to separate the bladder and prostate from the anterior pelvis (**Fig. 1**B). After dissection of the desmoplastic reaction off of the bladder neck junction (**Fig. 1**C), a flexible cystoscope is passed retrograde through the urethra to identify the location and extent of BNC. Firefly technology can be used to help delineate the location of the contracture (**Fig. 1**D).

The bladder is then opened anteriorly just proximal to the bladder neck and continued distally to determine the proximal extent of the contracture (**Fig. 1**E). Using sharp dissection and electrocautery, the scar tissue is completely excised. The mucosal edges are then brought together to create a posterior plate using interrupted 4-0 Vicryl sutures (**Fig. 1**F). A Y-V plasty is then performed (**Fig. 1**G). The long arm of the Y is a longitudinal incision of the bladder neck scar on the anterior aspect. An inverted V incision is made on the anterior aspect of the bladder neck. A 16-Fr Foley catheter is brought through as the final catheter. The apex of the V bladder flap is then advanced to the distal aspect of the anterior longitudinal incision through the scar, which is then closed with a running V-loc suture. After anastomosis, a leak test is performed by flushing the catheter with saline (**Fig. 1**H).

Patients with a history of prostatectomy

The procedure is approached similarly to described earlier, although the dissection is usually more difficult due to the more distal location and severe adherence to the pubic symphysis. The bladder neck is approached anteriorly by developing the space of Retzius and dropping the bladder off the anterior surface of the abdominal wall. This dissection is carried inferiorly underneath the pubic symphysis to the area of the vesicourethral anastomosis, which is notably very distal. A flexible cystoscope is then passed through the urethra to identify the location and

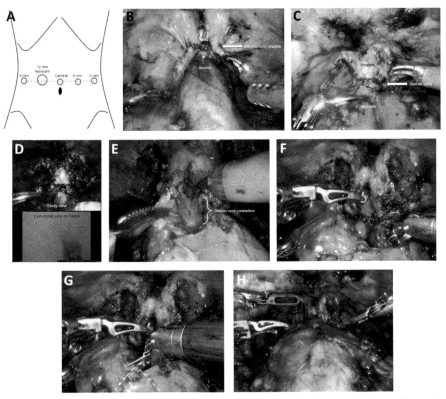

Fig. 1. (*A*) Robotic port placement for bladder neck reconstruction. (*B*) Desmoplastic reaction from prior transurethral procedures for bladder neck contractures. (*C*) Bladder neck junction after dissection of desmoplastic reaction. (*D*) Determination of location of bladder neck contracture using Firefly technology and TilePro. (*E*) Longitudinal incision from bladder through bladder neck contracture. (*F*) After excision of bladder neck contracture, the posterior plate is brought together with interrupted sutures. (*G*) A Y-V plasty performed to bring the anterior bladder wall distal to excised bladder neck contracture and into prostatic urethra. (*H*) A leak test with saline is performed to ensure watertight anastomosis.

extent of the anastomotic stricture. The bladder neck is completely freed from the pubic symphysis as well as 1 cm distal to where the scar tissue ends. The bladder is opened anteriorly just cephalad to VUAS and carried through the contracture. Using sharp dissection, the scar tissue is completely excised posteriorly and anteriorly. Healthy posterior bladder mucosa and urethra is mobilized to allow for a tension-free anastomosis. The anastomosis is performed similarly to a radical prostatectomy with running V-loc sutures. For a mild VUAS, a Y-V plasty approach may be used, although this would be the exception. The advantage to this approach is that it avoids the dissection of the posterior bladder neck and the potential of a rectal injury. If the repair seems tenuous for radiated VUAS, the authors strongly recommend placing an anterior omental flap to cover the anastomosis.

A suprapubic tube can be placed to maximize drainage, along with a pelvic drain. A Foley catheter is left in place for about 3 weeks depending on the degree of reconstruction. A voiding cystourethrogram or retrograde urethrogram can be performed at the time of catheter removal to ensure no leakage.

Outcomes

There are small case series that show the feasibility of a robotic approach to reconstructing the bladder neck. Kirshenbaum and colleagues[17] showed that 12 patients who have undergone robotic bladder neck reconstruction were assessed with a cystoscopy postoperatively with an average follow-up of 98 days. Eight of 11 patients had a wide-open, patent bladder neck, whereas 3 of 11 were deemed to have failure, with less than 17 Fr urethral strictures identified. One patient who did not have a cystoscopy had a uroflow rate of 24 mL/s with postvoid residual volume of 12 cc. Nine of 11 patients were continent. Overall, the success rate as defined by being able to pass a 17-Fr cystoscope or uroflow rate greater than

15 mL/s was 75%, with an incontinence rate of 18%.

Granieri and colleagues[18] showed the robotic reconstruction of BNC in 7 patients using Y-V plasty, which showed all cases successful with no evidence of recurrence after a median follow-up of 8 months. Two of 7 patients had persistent urinary incontinence. Musch and colleagues[19] showed a Y-V plasty performed on 12 patients, which was successful in 83.3% of patients after a follow-up of 23.3 months. One of 12 patients had documented stress urinary incontinence.

Overall, the success rate of a robotic reconstruction ranges from 75% to 100%, although the definition of success can vary. The ability to maintain a patent urethral channel, based on this small case series, is high. The rate of incontinence ranges from 8% to 28%, and this is a significant improvement from previous incontinence rates from open procedures that can range from 85% to 93%.[20]

Summary

BCNs/VUAS can be a very difficult issue to manage both from the patient and surgeon perspective. The recalcitrant nature of contractures through endoscopic approaches has necessitated novel techniques that attempt to reduce morbidity and complications. The robotic approach of bladder neck reconstruction is a viable surgical option for recalcitrant contractures, with good patency and minimal exacerbation of urinary incontinence. The robotic-assisted technique offers many advantages over the open technique for BNC/VUAS reconstruction: improved access to the deep and narrow retropubic space, fine and precise dissection and suturing, significant magnification, and improved ergonomics to perform the surgery. There is a growing body of literature to support the role of robotic-assisted reconstructive surgery for recurrent BNC/VUAS.

Clinics Care Points

- BNCs are a devastating complication of commonly performed procedures such as a prostatectomy or transurethral resection of the prostate and can be recalcitrant to endoscopic attempts to keep them open.
- Delineation of the contracture with a cystoscope intraoperatively is crucial to excising the scar tissue and performing a confident repair with mucosa to mucosa apposition.
- The surgical principles of a urethral anastomosis should be applied to BNC/VUAS repair: tension-free, watertight, well-vascularized,

mucosa to mucosa apposition, and catheterized anastomosis.

PROXIMAL URETHRAL STRICTURE

The management of urethral stricture disease has varied considerably depending on location, length, and severity of the stricture. It can develop anywhere along the length of the male or female urethra and has been attributed to multiple causes including injury, infection, and iatrogenic instrumentation. The urethroplasty has long been considered as the gold standard for repair of urethral stricture,[21] and most of the anterior urethral strictures can be managed with an open technique with a transecting, nontransecting, onlay, or augmentation urethroplasty.

Proximal bulbar and posterior urethral injuries represent a different challenge in reconstructive urology. It is most commonly associated with pelvic fractures,[22] although it can also be found with radiation treatment. There exists a wide variety of techniques available for posterior injury management, a common principle being the excision of scar tissue and a spatulated end-to-end anastomosis of healthy mucosa.[23] However, given the anatomic complexity of these injuries, the exposure and visualization can be much more challenging than more distal urethral strictures. The location of the posterior urethral stricture can be difficult to access, as we are limited laterally by aspects of the pubic rami and by the pubic symphysis anteriorly. This has necessitated the development of ancillary maneuvers such as corporeal body separation, inferior pubectomy, and retrocrural urethral rerouting to bridge the gap between the prostatic urethral apex and bulbar urethra.[24] This long and narrow channel can also make it very difficult to place the proximal urethral sutures, and this can result in inadequate mucosal apposition. The robotic platform has been used extensively in urology to improve visualization, access to deep and narrow spaces, precise suturing, and ergonomics, and proximal urethral strictures is no exception.

Procedural Approach

The surgical principles of a urethral anastomosis are described earlier in the article. There are 2 described approaches to urethroplasty for proximal strictures. Depending on the location and distal extent of the stricture, a transabdominal versus perineal approach can be taken. A transabdominal approach can be considered when the urethral stricture is proximal to the membranous urethra, and the steps are described earlier in the article. The focus of this portion of the article will be the robotic perineal approach.

The steps of the procedure are similar to an open urethroplasty procedure, with highlighted improvement in visualization of proximal urethral mucosa and placement of reliable sutures due to the articulation of the needle driver arms in a relatively tight space. The patient is placed in a high lithotomy position and perineal dissection performed in standard urethroplasty fashion until the area of urethral stricture is encountered. The preferred urethroplasty approach is then performed, whether it is a primary anastomosis or a nontransecting technique. The robot is then brought in for suturing, angled in such a way that the camera arm is positioned facing toward the perineal incision. A total of 3 floating robotic arms are used, with 2 working arms using needle drivers and the middle arm using for the 0-degree camera lens (**Fig. 2**A).

For an excision and primary anastomosis, a spatulation is made dorsally on the proximal end and ventrally on the distal end. The distal end of the urethra is then tucked away from the field of view (**Fig. 2**B). A total of 12 full-thickness absorbable monofilament sutures are placed in a clockwise fashion circumferentially initially on the proximal urethra (**Fig. 2**C). Once these sutures are placed, the distal throw can be performed either open or with the robotic arms. It is important

for the bedside assistant to keep the sutures organized and straightened throughout the case to avoid tangling issues. For a nontransecting urethroplasty, a dorsal longitudinal incision is made through the urethral stricture. A total of 7 sutures are placed starting with the middle stitch to bring the 2 apexes of the incision together. Three sutures are then placed on each side of the middle stitch and closed in a Heineke-Mikulicz fashion. It may be preferable to tie down each stitch, as they are thrown to help reduce future clash with the sutures and the robotic arms.

The Foley catheter is then placed before closure of the final suture and is standard care for urethroplasty. The catheter is left in place from 10 to 21 days. A cystoscopy and voiding cystourethrogram (VCUG) are performed postoperatively to rule out extravasation or anastomotic leak before catheter removal.

Outcomes

Use of the robotic approach for a proximal urethroplasty is rare. A case series[25] describes 10 patients with an average stricture length of 2.2 cm who underwent a robotic urethral reconstruction. The set-up time for the robotic portion of the case was 15 minutes and 30 to 45 minutes for suture placement. All patients had a VCUG before catheter removal, which showed no evidence of extravasation and had a 3- and 12-month

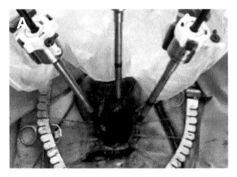
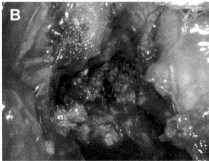
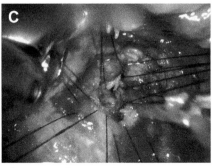

Fig. 2. (*A*) Robotic arm placement for repair of proximal urethral strictures. (*B*) Visualization of proximal urethra after excision of urethral stricture. (*C*) Placement of 12 proximal stitches.

cystoscopy follow-up. All patients were patent as demonstrated by the ability to easily pass a 17-Fr flexible cystoscope.

Summary

Proximal urethral strictures can be challenging to access, and its repair requires a deep perineal dissection for adequate visualization and suture placement. The robotic perineal approach can provide improved visualization and ergonomics needed for reliable suture placement to overcome the anatomic challenges inherent to this location. Operative times and outcomes are comparable to the standard open approach with improved surgeon comfort/ergonomics. Although proximal urethral strictures can be successfully managed with an open approach, the utility of robot-assisted surgery and all of its technical advantages can enhance the ability to perform the surgery.

Clinics Care Points

- Proximal urethral strictures can be difficult to access with the anatomic restraints afforded by the pubic rami and symphysis.
- The robotic perineal approach allows improved visualization with the magnified view to better visualize the proximal mucosa and greater control of the anastomosis with articulating arms of the needle driver in a deep, tight space.

LOWER URINARY TRACT FISTULA

LUT fistulas encompass a wide range of conditions that include vesicovaginal, rectourethral, colovesical, and other enterovesical fistulas. The cause of these fistulas vary significantly, but the overall impact they have on social life, mental and physical well-being, and sexual function can be debilitating. Robotic-assisted dissection and repair of urologic fistulas is a useful and highly successful approach that has significant benefit to the patient and the surgeon preforming the surgery.

Rectourethral Fistula

Rectourethral fistulas (RUF) represent a challenging problem; however, the incidence is fortunately rare. Most of the RUF are now a result of ablative therapy, mostly commonly radiation therapy for prostate cancer. Other less common causes are surgically induced RUF, medical conditions such as inflammatory bowel disease, diverticulitis, and perirectal abscesses,[26,27] and other pelvic cancer therapies. Patients with these fistulas encounter many debilitating symptoms including irritative voiding, recurrent cystitis, fecaluria, urine leakage per rectum, and significant pain (pelvic, perineal, and lower extremity).[28]

Both conservative and surgical approaches have been described in its management. It is rare for ablative fistula to resolve with simply urinary diversion, although this is often the first step preformed. In radiated patients it is found that hyperbaric oxygen therapy is a very useful tool to help alleviate many of the symptomatic complaints the patient experiences, in addition to overall improved healing if an operative approach is pursued.[29] All patients who have been radiated to have hyperbaric oxygen therapy before any surgical intervention if possible are encouraged.

There are numerous surgical techniques described such as the York-Mason,[30] anterior rectal wall advancement,[31] anterior transanal mucosal advancement flap,[32] and the Latzko technique.[33] Among these techniques is also a multitude of vascular interposition tissue flaps used, including the omentum, gracilis muscle, and peritoneum. Accepted success rates of the different surgical approaches by high-volume centers vary between 75% and 100%.[34] When done open, urologist tends to favor the perineal approach, as it allows for the range of various surgical techniques needed to close the fistula including an interposition muscle flap. The robotic approach to fistula repairs is still in the early phase of data collection and publication but offers some real advantages. The ability to access deep narrow spaces with precise dissection and suturing with increased magnification and comfort is a significant advantage over open fistula repair and closure.

Vesicovaginal Fistula

Vesicovaginal fistulas (VVF), a communication between the bladder and vagina, are a result of pelvic surgery, radiation, or gynecologic malignancies. They can also occur from obstructed labor or instrumental vaginal delivery in developing countries.[35] It results in a continuous involuntary loss of urine through the vagina that is socially distressing. A careful history, physical examination, and cystoscopy is essential to establish the size, number, and location of the fistula. A biopsy of the site is performed when malignancy is suspected.

VVFs can be managed conservatively with prolonged catheterization or even with a minimally invasive approach with a fibrin sealant and collagen as a plug after electrocoagulation[36]; however, only the small fistulas are likely to spontaneously close. There are 2 typical approaches to the repair, either transvaginal or transabdominal. The approach depends on characteristics of the fistula, along with surgeon preference. The authors focus on the transabdominal extravesical approach. Indications for transabdominal approach include involvement of the ureteral orifice, small capacity bladders requiring augmentation, vaginal stenosis, high VVF, redo VVF, involvement of the cervix or uterus, and ureterovaginal fistulas.[37]

Colovesical Fistula

Colovesical fistula is a communication between bowel and the bladder (**Fig. 3**A, B). Unlike VVFs or RUFs, colovesical fistulas are more likely due to colorectal conditions rather than from iatrogenic injury, most commonly due to diverticular disease or colon cancer.[37] The symptoms of CVFs are similar to RUFs, presenting with pneumaturia, fecaluria, and recurrent cystitis, and diagnosed with a combination of cystoscopy, computed tomography, or MRI. Given that the cause is typically a colorectal process, a colonoscopy or sigmoidoscopy is indicated, and a biopsy may be taken for suspected malignancy.[38]

Management for colovesical fistula is largely done by colorectal surgery, as the primary disease is managed first with a diversion or excision of affected bowel segment with primary anastomosis. A urologist is called on to help for more complex repair of the bladder for large openings or for augmentation of a small bladder. The importance of managing or removing the original bowel cause cannot be overemphasized for a success and permanent fistula closure.

Procedural Approach

Overall principles of a fistula repair remain unchanged with a robotic approach. It requires adequate exposure of the fistula, separation of the bladder or urethra from the vagina, colon, or rectum, trimming of the devascularized edges, a tension-free closure of the respective fistulous connections, interposition of a vascularized tissue, and adequate postoperative drainage. The repair approach for rectourethral, vesicovaginal, or colovesical fistula is similar and described later.

The patient is positioned in a dorsal lithotomy position, and the procedure is started first with cystoscopy. The C-arm fluoroscopy should also be available, should the fistula be difficult to visualize (**Fig. 3**C). Once the fistula is identified by

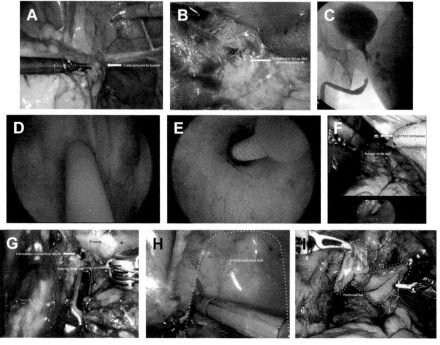

Fig. 3. (A) Colovesical fistula, with densely adherent colon to bladder. (B) Fistulous site seen after dissection of colon off of bladder, with saline irrigation confirming lumen of bladder. (C) Retrograde urethrogram with extravasation of contrast into rectum. (D) Cannulation of fistula from the urethral side with catheter. (E) Cannulation of fistula from rectal side. (F) Visualization of location of fistula with light from rectoscope. (G) Separation of rectal wall from prostatic urethra, confirmed with catheter visualization. (H) Peritoneal flap creation. (I) The flap is inverted and brought down into the deep pelvis to cover the urinary repair by securing it over and at least 1 cm distal to the prostatic urethral closure.

cystoscopy (**Fig. 3**D), it is cannulated with a wire and 5-Fr open-ended ureteral catheter and externalized through the vagina or anus (**Fig. 3**E). Should identification of the fistula be questionable or difficult to cannulate, contrast can be injected into an opening with a ureteral catheter and confirmed with fluoroscopy showing contrast or with methylene blue to directly visualize the fistula. Bilateral ureteral stents may also be placed at this time to be able to identify any potential injuries to the ureters that may occur in this case.

Once the fistula has been identified, the robot is then docked with the patient in low lithotomy Trendelenburg position. Ports are placed in similar fashion to a radical prostatectomy (see **Fig. 1**A). The posterior bladder is first mobilized. A flexible cystoscope is then placed through the urethra to assist with visualization of the level of the fistula, using the light visualized with near-infrared frequency technology. Light from a rectoscope can also be helpful to visualize the fistula (**Fig. 3**F). It is helpful to place a vaginal or rectal retractor to get some separation of the planes between the 2 fistulous sites. Once the dissection down to the fistula is performed with adequate exposure (**Fig. 3**G) the 2 systems are separated and dropped away from each other (ie, prostate from the rectum or the rectum from the bladder). The urethral or bladder wound is closed in a tension-free manner with interrupted absorbable sutures. The additional organ system (ie the vaginal, colon or rectal wound) is closed or resected and dropped away from the urinary tract closure. Ideally there are no overlapping suture lines.

Critical to a successful closure is the development of an interposition rotational flap placed between the 2 fistulous sites, including the peritoneum, gracilis muscle, and omentum. Robotically, the authors prefer to harvest a peritoneal inverted U flap (**Fig. 3**H). When possible, a 4-cm base width flap is harvested for adequate blood supply and the length measured to reach at least 1 cm distal to the fistula repair. The flap is then inverted into the inferior pelvis (**Fig. 3**I), creating an additional layer between the fistula repairs. For RUF, the gracilis muscle can be harvested and rotated from a perineal approach. Once the urinary side of the RUF is closed, the perineal dissection is performed with harvest of the gracilis muscle described earlier. The gracilis flap is placed between the rectal and the urethral closure.

A catheter is then left indwelling for about 2 to 4 weeks depending on the cause of the fistula. A retrograde urethrogram and/or voiding cystourethrogram can be performed after this period to check for patency and ensure no leakage of the repair.

Gracilis muscle harvest

The patient is placed in a lithotomy position with the thigh placed in minimal flexion, abduction, and external rotation at the hip. The muscle is marked on the inner thigh from the pubic tubercle to the medial condyle of the tibia. The skin is then incised, and after dividing through the subcutaneous fat and muscular fascia, the gracilis muscle is identified. The tendinous insertion near the tibia is divided and the muscle is separated. Small vessels supplying the muscle distally are then divided, while preserving the most proximal vascular supply. The vascular pedicle and nerve are identified 8 to 10 cm below the ischiopubic rami[27] and preserved. The muscle is then rotated 180° and tunneled beneath the subcutaneous tissue for interposition between the rectum and urethra.

Outcomes

Rectourethral fistula

The robotic approach to RUF is rare.[39–41] These are case reports with 1 or 2 patients, and more data are needed. One case report discusses a patient with a fistula secondary to a prostatectomy who had failed previous open repair. After the described robotic approach with a gracilis flap, a cystoscopy was performed 40 days postoperatively, showing no evidence of fistula recurrence. Another case report described 2 patients who had cryotherapy and salvage radiation as the cause of their fistula who underwent robotic repair using an omental flap placement. Both had no reported symptoms at 4 and 9 months, and the patency of the repair was confirmed with imaging studies. In the authors' own experience they have repaired several rectourethral fistulae using the robotic approach with no recurrences to date. It is especially valuable for a high bladder/trigone fistula to the rectum that is amenable to pelvic dissection and a peritoneal flap.

Vesicovaginal fistula

Robotic approach to VVF repair is well tolerated and effective. In several robotic VVF repair case series and case reports[42–47] in the posthysterectomy setting for 2- to 4-cm defects, operative times ranged from 110 to 240 minutes, length of stay from 2 to 5 days, and minimal blood loss. All reported successful outcomes defined subjectively as lack of leak symptoms or objectively with an imaging study.

SUMMARY

Fistulas involving the genitourinary tract are a challenging problem with many described methods for repair, although comparative effectiveness data are lacking to define a superior approach. Although there is early evidence for a robotic approach to repair, the technique has shown to be feasible, effective, and successful. A robotic approach to repair will continue to gain a larger presence in fistula repair surgery, as there are many advantages of the robotic approach over open fistula repair.

CLINICS CARE POINTS

- Genitourinary fistulas have a wide range of causes, and malignancy should always be ruled out as a cause.
- Careful preoperative workup and cannulation of the fistulas before the repair are critical to dissection of the correct plane between the fistulous connection.
- Interposition flaps are critical to success fistula closures and should be able to reach 1 to 2 cm beyond the fistula tract closure.

DISCLOSURE

The authors have nothing to disclose.

REFERENCES

1. Basic DT, Hadzi-Djokic J, Ignjatovic I. The history of urinary diversion. Acta Chir Iugosl 2007;54(4):9–17.
2. Bricker EM. Bladder substitution after pelvic evisceration. 1950. J Urol 2002;167(2 Pt 2):1140–6.
3. Zhang L, Liu S, Wu K, et al. Management of highly recurrent bladder neck contractures via transurethral resection combined with intra- and postoperative triamcinolone acetonide injections. World J Urol 2020. https://doi.org/10.1007/s00345-020-03224-w.
4. Cindolo L, Marchioni M, Emiliani E, et al. Bladder neck contracture after surgery for benign prostatic obstruction. Minerva Urol Nefrol 2017;69(2):133–43.
5. Primiceri G, Castellan P, Marchioni M, et al. Bladder Neck Contracture After Endoscopic Surgery for Benign Prostatic Obstruction: Incidence, Treatment, and Outcomes. Curr Urol Rep 2017;18(10):79.
6. Tomschi W, Suster G, Höltl W. Bladder neck strictures after radical retropubic prostatectomy: still an unsolved problem. Br J Urol 1998;81(6):823–6.
7. Surya BV, Provet J, Johanson KE, et al. Anastomotic strictures following radical prostatectomy: risk factors and management. J Urol 1990;143(4):755–8.
8. Dalkin BL. Endoscopic evaluation and treatment of anastomotic strictures after radical retropubic prostatectomy. J Urol 1996;155(1):206–8.
9. Breyer BN, Davis CB, Cowan JE, et al. Incidence of bladder neck contracture after robot-assisted laparoscopic and open radical prostatectomy. BJU Int 2010;106(11):1734–8.
10. Vanni AJ, Zinman LN, Buckley JC. Radial urethrotomy and intralesional mitomycin C for the management of recurrent bladder neck contractures. J Urol 2011;186(1):156–60.
11. Redshaw JD, Broghammer JA, Smith TG 3rd, et al. Intralesional injection of mitomycin C at transurethral incision of bladder neck contracture may offer limited benefit: TURNS Study Group. J Urol 2015;193(2):587–92.
12. Cotta BH, Buckley JC. Endoscopic Treatment of Urethral Stenosis. Urol Clin North Am 2017;44(1):19–25.
13. Schlossberg S, Jordan G, Schellhammer P. Repair of obliterative vesicourethral stricture after radical prostatectomy: a technique for preservation of continence. Urology 1995;45(3):510–3.
14. Theodoros C, Katsifotis C, Stournaras P, et al. Abdomino-perineal repair of recurrent and complex bladder neck-prostatic urethra contractures. Eur Urol 2000;38(6):734–41.
15. Wessells H, Morey AF, McAninch JW. Obliterative vesicourethral strictures following radical prostatectomy for prostate cancer: reconstructive armamentarium. J Urol 1998;160(4):1373–5.
16. Reiss CP, Pfalzgraf D, Kluth LA, et al. Transperineal reanastomosis for the treatment for highly recurrent anastomotic strictures as a last option before urinary diversion. World J Urol 2014;32(5):1185–90.
17. Kirshenbaum EJ, Zhao LC, Myers JB, et al. Patency and Incontinence Rates After Robotic Bladder Neck Reconstruction for Vesicourethral Anastomotic Stenosis and Recalcitrant Bladder Neck Contractures: The Trauma and Urologic Reconstructive Network of Surgeons Experience. Urology 2018;118:227–33.
18. Granieri MA, Weinberg AC, Sun JY, et al. Robotic Y-V Plasty for Recalcitrant Bladder Neck Contracture. Urology 2018;117:163–5.
19. Musch M, Hohenhorst JL, Vogel A, et al. Robot-assisted laparoscopic Y-V plasty in 12 patients with refractory bladder neck contracture. J Robot Surg 2018;12(1):139–45.
20. Pfalzgraf D, Beuke M, Isbarn H, et al. Open retropubic reanastomosis for highly recurrent and complex bladder neck stenosis. J Urol 2011;186(5):1944–7.
21. Mangera A, Chapple C. Management of anterior urethral stricture: an evidence-based approach. Curr Opin Urol 2010;20(6):453–8.
22. Ingram MD, Watson SG, Skippage PL, et al. Urethral injuries after pelvic trauma: evaluation with urethrography. Radiographics 2008;28(6):1631–43.
23. Kulkarni SB, Joshi PM, Hunter C, et al. Complex posterior urethral injury. Arab J Urol 2015;13(1):43–52.
24. Mehmood S, Alsulaiman OA, Al Taweel WM. Outcome of anastomotic posterior urethroplasty with various ancillary maneuvers for post-traumatic urethral injury. Does prior urethral manipulation

affect the outcome of urethroplasty? Urol Ann 2018; 10(2):175–80.

25. Unterberg SH, Patel SH, Fuller TW, et al. Robotic-assisted Proximal Perineal Urethroplasty: Improving Visualization and Ergonomics. Urology 2019;125:230–3.

26. Benoit RM, Naslund MJ, Cohen JK. Complications after radical retropubic prostatectomy in the medicare population. Urology 2000;56(1):116–20.

27. Gupta G, Kumar S, Kekre NS, et al. Surgical management of rectourethral fistula. Urology 2008; 71(2):267–71.

28. Shin PR, Foley E, Steers WD. Surgical management of rectourinary fistulae. J Am Coll Surg 2000;191(5): 547–53.

29. Marguet C, Raj GV, Brashears JH, et al. Rectourethral fistula after combination radiotherapy for prostate cancer. Urology 2007;69(5):898–901.

30. Renschler TD, Middleton RG. 30 years of experience with York-Mason repair of recto-urinary fistulas. J Urol 2003;170(4 Pt 1):1222–5.

31. al-Ali M, Kashmoula D, Saoud IJ. Experience with 30 posttraumatic rectourethral fistulas: presentation of posterior transsphincteric anterior rectal wall advancement. J Urol 1997;158(2):421–4.

32. Vose SN. A technique for the repair of recto-urethral fistula. J Urol 1949;61(4):790–4.

33. Razi A, Yahyazadeh SR, Gilani MA, et al. Transanal repair of rectourethral and rectovaginal fistulas. Urol J 2008;5(2):111–4.

34. Prabha V, Kadeli V. Repair of recto-urethral fistula with urethral augmentation by buccal mucosal graft and gracilis muscle flap interposition - our experience. Cent Eur J Urol 2018;71(1):121–8.

35. Malik MA, Sohail M, Malik MT, et al. Changing trends in the etiology and management of vesicovaginal fistula. Int J Urol 2018;25(1):25–9.

36. Sharma SK, Perry KT, Turk TM. Endoscopic injection of fibrin glue for the treatment of urinary-tract pathology. J Endourol 2005;19(3):419–23.

37. Dorairajan LN, Hemal AK. Lower urinary tract fistula: the minimally invasive approach. Curr Opin Urol 2009;19(6):556–62.

38. Cochetti G, Del Zingaro M, Boni A, et al. Colovesical fistula: review on conservative management, surgical techniques and minimally invasive approaches. G Chir 2018;39(4):195–207.

39. Tseng SI, Huang CW, Huang TY. Robotic-assisted transanal repair of rectourethral fistula. Endoscopy 2019;51(5):E96–7.

40. Sun JY, Granieri MA, Zhao LC. Robotics and urologic reconstructive surgery. Transl Androl Urol 2018;7(4):545–57.

41. Medina LG, Cacciamani GE, Hernandez A, et al. Robotic Management of Rectourethral Fistulas After Focal Treatment for Prostate Cancer. Urology 2018; 118:241.

42. Hemal AK, Kolla SB, Wadhwa P. Robotic reconstruction for recurrent supratrigonal vesicovaginal fistulas. J Urol 2008;180(3):981–5.

43. Schimpf MO, Morgenstern JH, Tulikangas PK, et al. Vesicovaginal fistula repair without intentional cystotomy using the laparoscopic robotic approach: a case report. JSLS 2007;11(3):378–80.

44. Sundaram BM, Kalidasan G, Hemal AK. Robotic repair of vesicovaginal fistula: case series of five patients. Urology 2006;67(5):970–3.

45. Melamud O, Eichel L, Turbow B, et al. Laparoscopic vesicovaginal fistula repair with robotic reconstruction. Urology 2005;65(1):163–6.

46. Nóbrega L, Andrade C, Schmidt R, et al. Robotic Vesicovaginal Fistula Repair. J Minim Invasive Gynecol 2020;27(3):580.

47. Kelly E, Wu MY, MacMillan JB. Robotic-assisted vesicovaginal fistula repair using an extravesical approach without interposition grafting. J Robot Surg 2010;12(1):173 6.

Robotics in Pediatric Urology
Evolution and the Future

Sameer Mittal, MD, MS*, Arun Srinivasan, MD

KEYWORDS

- Minimally invasive surgery • Pediatric robotic surgery • Pediatric urologic reconstruction
- Ureteropelvic junction obstruction • Vesicoureteral reflux • Bladder augmentation

KEY POINTS

- Robotic-assisted surgery in children is increasing in utilization for common reconstructive procedures such as pyeloplasty and ureteral reimplantation.
- Similar to open surgery, careful attention to surgical technique and outcomes allows robotic-assisted surgery to be a safe and effective alternative treatment option.
- Further complex reconstructions are being reported with encouraging preliminary results.

 Video content accompanies this article at http://www.urologic.theclinics.com.

INTRODUCTION

Pediatric urologists were early adopters of laparoscopy and subsequently robotic-assisted (RA) surgery. The first reported pediatric urologic surgery performed robotically was performed in 2002 by Dr Craig Peters at Boston Children's Hospital.[1] As is discussed, robot utilization in pediatric urology has been ubiquitous with most major academic institutions offering access to this technology. As surgeon comfort, access, and indications for robotic surgery in children expand, utilization will likely continue to increase. Here we review the current state of robotic surgery in pediatric urology, including utilization and general and case-specific technical considerations.

UTILIZATION AND LEARNING CURVE OF ROBOTIC-ASSISTED SURGERY IN PEDIATRIC UROLOGY

Between 2000 and 2010, the number of pediatric urology cases published increased gradually with rapid increases seen after 2010.[2,3] The most common cases performed robotically are pyeloplasty and ureteral reimplantation which combined account for 80% of RA procedures performed?[4] Recent studies have shown that from 2003 to 2015, the overall number of pyeloplasty cases and open pyeloplasty cases has declined 7% and 10% annually, respectively, while RA pyeloplasty increased by 29% annually, accounting for 40% of pyeloplasties in 2015.[5] Currently at our own institution, the Children's Hospital of Philadelphia, more than 75% of pyeloplasties and reimplants are performed robotically.

As in other surgical procedures, adoption of new technology is dependent on many factors and a major component is its reproducibility and the associated learning curve. Within pediatric urology, Tasian and colleagues[6] initially reported attempts to understand the learning curve in performing robotic pyeloplasty and showed that via multivariate linear regression, fellow trainees were projected to achieve the median operative time of the attending surgeon after 37 cases. Other studies have shown similar findings of in the

Division of Urology, Children's Hospital of Philadelphia, Perelman School of Medicine, University of Pennsylvania, 3401 Civic Center Boulevard, Philadelphia, PA 19104, USA
* Corresponding author.
E-mail address: mittals3@chop.edu

Urol Clin N Am 48 (2021) 113–125
https://doi.org/10.1016/j.ucl.2020.09.008
0094-0143/21/© 2020 Elsevier Inc. All rights reserved.

relatively quick learning curve of this common procedure,[7,8] but studies have been limited in investigating the other types of cases. As RA surgical experience and comfort increases in urologic residencies nationwide, we are likely to see decreased learning curves in pediatric urology trainees with further increased utilization.

IMPORTANT PRINCIPLES IN PEDIATRIC ROBOT-ASSISTED SURGERY

Anesthesia considerations for robotic surgery are very similar compared with other minimal invasive approaches that involve pneumoperitoneum. Efforts to minimize insufflation pressure (<10 mm Hg) and reduce flow-rate are necessary in children as the ratio to peritoneal surface is larger relative to body weight, the systemic absorption of carbon dioxide may be higher. In addition, increased intraperitoneal pressure can lead to increased peak inspiratory pressure and decreased pulmonary compliance as well as decreases cardiac output and renal perfusion and increased renal vascular resistance. Bradyarrhythmias have also been documented during insufflation possibly secondary to vagal stimulation. Immediate reversal of pneumoperitoneum is generally enough to reverse these arrhythmias.

PORTS: CHOICE, PLACEMENT, AND REMOVAL

The most common robotic port size used across the country is 8 mm but for the Si version of the da Vinci, 5 mm is an option. The differences between the 8 mm and 5 mm instrumentation are that the 5 mm lacks a wrist joint and lacks surgical shears as an instrument option. Hence, the hook is the dissecting tool of choice with the 5-mm instruments. More recently, the single-port version of the Xi has been introduced although not specifically approved for pediatric use. Whether a single 25-mm incision is beneficial in children is unclear.

Port Placement

There are a number of techniques for robotic port placement and we will define the basic principles of safe port placement and some strategies to consider in this population. It is important to emphasize that a child's abdomen is very pliable and hence provides little, if any counter resistance when a port is pushed through an incision. This process has to be taken into consideration to ensure safe port placement.

1. Adequate skin incision: in our experience smaller incisions have been the most common

reason excessive force used during port placement.
2. Place port under vision whenever possible. If in doubt, use a visual obturator during port placement. We also prefer to incise the fascia and peritoneum and use blunt obturators for robotic port placement.
3. Laparoscopic literature has not demonstrated any clear difference in outcome between an open technique (Hasson) versus Veress needle for initial access into the peritoneum.[9] Surgeons should pursue the technique he or she is most comfortable with. Our preference is to use the Veress needle but dissect partially through the abdominal fascia before we introduce the needle.
4. It is ideal to have 4 finger breadths between ports, although this not uniformly available during infant cases.
5. Ensure adequate distance from the point of port entry to the surgical field to allow for adequate mobility and safety during instrument exchange.

Literature on incision site aesthetics and patient preferences have trended toward incisions below the umbilicus, preferably at the level of the Pfannenstiel incision, which can be covered easily. The development of "hidden incision endoscopic surgery (HIdES)" has gained some momentum in this regard.[10] Skin incisions are made lower in the abdomen and the camera is placed above the pubic symphysis with trocars triangulating on the organ of interest (**Fig. 1**). Similarly, making skin incisions in the inguinal crease and tunneling the robotic trocars subcutaneously while entering the abdomen in their standard location has also

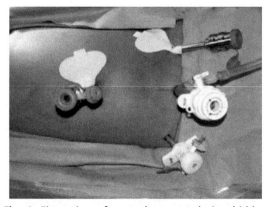

Fig. 1. Figuration of port placement during hidden incision ("HIdES") technique. (*From* Gargollo PC. Hidden incision endoscopic surgery: description of technique, parental satisfaction and applications. J Urol. 2011;185(4):1425-1431.)

been described (**Fig. 2**). Early reports are encouraging but long-term and aesthetic outcomes including patient preferences remain unknown.

Although port site hernia in children is an infrequent complication, we routinely close fascia at port sites, including the 5-mm ports. We perform this, because unlike adults, children have much less abdominal wall muscle mass and subcutaneous tissue, which could allow for port site hernias.

ROBOTIC-ASSISTED RECONSTRUCTION FOR UPPER TRACT PATHOLOGY
Ureteropelvic Junction Obstruction (UPJO)

Indications and technique
RA pyeloplasty remains the most common robotic procedure performed in pediatric urology. The indications for RA pyeloplasty are the same as those for open surgery. Declines in the overall number of pyeloplasty cases performed nationally likely reflect judicious selection of patients being recommended for surgery who exhibit even severe degrees of upper tract dilation.

The steps of RA pyeloplasty are shown in **Box 1**. We give patients a broad-spectrum, intravenous antibiotic based on previous urine culture data or empiric cefazolin. A Foley catheter is placed. After peritoneal insufflation is obtained, ports are placed and the robot is docked. Our practice is to begin the procedure by medially reflecting the bowel, although others have used a transmesenteric window to gain access to the ureteropelvic junction (UPJ). A hitch stitch is used to bring the renal pelvis closer to the abdominal wall to allow for suturing without using a third-arm or assistant port (**Fig. 3**). We use 5 to 0 monocryl for the anastomosis with 1 to 3 interrupted sutures placed at

the most dependent portion of the UPJ followed by continuous suture. The use of interrupted sutures throughout and knotless self-anchoring barbed suture[11] have also been reported. We generally do not place a drain, except in more challenging cases (eg, redo cases or ureterocalicostomy).

Utilization of stents and their method of effective placement is a topic of continued debate in the field. Traditional placement of pigtail stents requires an additional anesthetic for their removal, which contributes to additional morbidity and cost. To mitigate this, groups have popularized the utilization of a ureteral stent secured to the patient via a string placed at the beginning of the procedure and removal within 7 to 10 days or utilization of a percutaneous pyeloureteral stent (Salle stent; Cook Urologic, Spencer, Indiana).[12,13] Furthermore, groups have shown comparable perioperative outcomes in stentless reconstructions in small case series with relatively short follow-up.[14,15] In our practice, stents are placed antegrade while the bladder is filled with a methylene blue/saline mix. This allows for confirmation of appropriate placement in the bladder, via visualization of blue fluid effluxing through the stent, and avoids the potential complication of the stent deploying in the distal ureter.

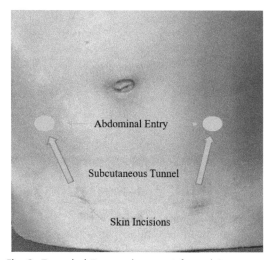

Fig. 2. Tunneled Trocar placement for pelvic surgery. (*Courtesy of* Aseem Shukla MD, Philadelphia, PA.)

> **Box 1**
> **Operative steps for robotic-assisted pyeloplasty**
>
> 1. Position patient in modified flank at the edge of operative table
> 2. Port placement
>   - Camera placed in umbilicus
>   - 5-mm working ports in the midline above umbilicus and ipsilateral to midline 4 fingers below the umbilicus
> 3. Dock robot over kidney
> 4. Medial reflection of colon to expose UPJ
> 5. Mobilization of ureter and renal pelvis
>   - Identification and mobilization of UPJ from possible crossing vessel
> 6. Percutaneous hitch stitch placed to anchor renal pelvis
> 7. Incision of dilated renal pelvis and lateral spatulation of ureter
> 8. Anastomosis of ureter to renal pelvis with continuous monofilament suture
>   - Percutaneous placement of double pigtail stent antegrade across UPJO

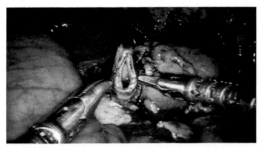

Fig. 3. Demonstration of utility of percutaneous hitch stitch on renal pelvis during pyeloplasty to avoid use of an assistant port and stabilization during reanastomosis.

Outcomes, costs, and complications

Most series show a success rate, defined as improvement of hydronephrosis, resolution of symptoms, and/or improved T1/2 on diuretic renogram of robotic pyeloplasty of greater than 92% to 98%,[16–23] which is equivalent to that of the open experience. Benefits of RA pyeloplasty include decreased narcotic requirements[24] and shorter length of stay. Despite this, RA is associated with increased operating room (OR) time and equipment costs[5] with an absolute difference of $1060 per case. Efforts to identify areas of cost-saving during the procedure have shown areas such as OR turnover, positioning, and increasing overall utilization,[25] as well as efforts to quantify downstream costs such as decreased lost parental wages and lower hospitalization expenses[26] associated with the RA approach. In addition, patient-/family-centered outcomes have shown higher parent satisfaction noted after RA than open surgery.[27] Comparable to the open experience, complications have been reported to occur in 10% of cases and most are Clavien-Dindo 1 to 2 grade complications.[28]

Special considerations: infant robotic pyeloplasty

The first reported case series of patients younger than 1 year undergoing RA pyeloplasty was in 2006 and offered encouraging results.[20] Despite this, the appropriate approach to UPJO in this patient population continues to be debated due to the decreased working space and increased robotic arm collisions. Finkelstein and colleagues[29] proposed the distance between both anterior superior iliac spines and the puboxyphoid distance of 13 cm and 15 cm,[30] respectively, decreased collisions and operative time, although adoption of this metric is unreported. As groups report positive outcomes in this patient population,[29,31] we expect further adoption in approaching this unique group robotically.

Special considerations: bilateral ureteropelvic junction obstruction

In rare instances of bilateral UPJO, the RA approach has been used with simultaneous bilateral repair with good short-term results.[32] Both sides can be repaired if midline port placement is used without the need to place additional ports. We use an iodine impregnated drape over the port sites during repositioning and draping of the patient.

Special considerations: Reobstruction after initial repair

Persistent obstruction occurs in ∼5% of patients and management of these cases can be difficult. Initially, endopyelotomy was shown to be a viable option in small case series with short-term follow-up.[33,34] As the minimally invasive surgery experience was further adopted, reports of laparoscopic salvage pyeloplasty showed promise in adults[35] and that experience has been mirrored in the pediatric population. Multiple groups have shown good success rates with RA redo pyeloplasty.[36–40] It our institutional preference to address these cases with this approach. In cases in which significant renal pelvis reduction was performed at the initial procedure, significant intrarenal pelvis dilation is present, or if the UPJ is unable to be safely mobilized, an RA ureterocalicostomy has proven an effective method to overcome these challenges and relieve the obstruction.[41] [Video 1]

Duplex anomalies: ureteroceles, ureteral ectopia, single-moiety ureteral reflux

Patients presenting with ureteroceles or ureteral ectopia historically presented with febrile urinary tract infections, but contemporarily are identified via antenatal ultrasonography. This shift in presentation has changed the natural history and treatment recommendations for these diseases. Despite this, the goals are the same: relief of obstruction, reduction in infection and preservation of renal function. The RA platform has allowed for decreased morbidity when correcting these anomalies.

Robot-assisted ureteroureterostomy (Video 2)

The ipsilateral ureteroureterostomy is a common procedure to address this pathology. Laparoscopic ureteroureterostomy initially gained momentum in the late 2000s.[42] This was quickly replaced with the RA approach as access to the technology increased[43,44] and it offers superior visualization and more delicate handling of the ureters. The procedure is completed by performing an end-to-side anastomosis between the donor and recipient ureters.[45] [Fig. 4] At our institution, a ureteral stent is placed in the recipient ureter with no

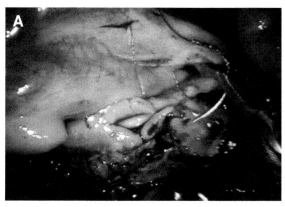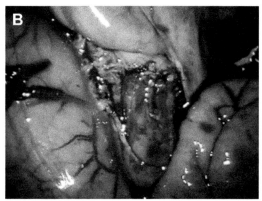

Fig. 4. (*A*) Example of upper-to-lower pole ureteroureterostomy reanastomosis. (*B*) Final end-to-side anastomosis after ureteroureterostomy.

stent across the anastomosis and is removed ~6 weeks after the procedure. One group has reported good short-term outcomes after external ureteral stent removal on postoperative day 1,[46] which may offset further costs associated with subsequent indwelling ureteral stent removal. The overall success rate in resolving the obstruction is greater than 90% with rare complications noted. Further surgical management of the infected residual donor ureteral stump may be required in up to 12% of cases.[47] During the initial procedure, we aim to excise this ureteral stump as far distally as possible, generally to the area where the ureters cross close the ureterovesical junction. This procedure is used most often at our institution to address these cases.

Robot-assisted heminephroureterectomy with partial ureterectomy

In the hopes of leaving the unaffected renal moiety undisturbed, many advocate for heminephrectomy and partial ureterectomy in cases of obstructed duplex systems. This approach allows for removal of the poorly functioning unit that is, associated with recurrent infections and/or symptomatology. In the open approach, during excision of the upper pole, the associated ureter is mobilized from a posterior to superior position along the renal vessels, which allows for its complete removal. Unfortunately, this technique as well as complete kidney mobilization is associated with a 5% incidence of vascular injury or vasospasm affecting the functional moiety. This risk is decreased via a minimally invasive approach by allowing for decreased manipulation of the entire kidney and an in situ dissection.[48] Comparison between the open and robotic approach have shown similar complication rates, success, need for additional interventions but with decreased length of stay.[49]

Minimally invasive techniques have been reported by using a variety of approaches including both intraperitoneal[50,51] and retroperitoneal approaches.[52] Regardless, the robotic approach with its increase magnification will allow for accurate distinction between the upper and lower pole moieties and further preservation of the unaffected moiety vasculature. In addition, using advanced imaging with near infrared fluorescence and indocyanine green (ICG) to perform intraoperative selective arterial mapping[53] theoretically may further decrease the risk of injury to the vasculature. The RA approach has also allowed for reconstruction/closure of the renal capsule after excision, which has been shown to decrease the formation of postoperative fluid collections from 42% to 11% when performed.[50]

ROBOTIC-ASSISTED RECONSTRUCTION FOR LOWER TRACT PATHOLOGY
Vesicoureteral Reflux

Ureteral reimplantation is performed for vesicoureteral reflux with recurrent febrile urinary tract infections with or without evidence of renal scarring. Open ureteral reimplantation, either via an intravesical or extravesical approach, is considered the gold standard for this procedure and the robotic approach is being perfected to achieve the same standards.

Patient selection and optimization

Children with recurrent febrile urinary tract infections despite continuous antibiotic prophylaxis in the setting of vesicoureteral reflux are ideal candidates for this procedure. Other indications, although controversial, are patients with renal scarring, worsening reflux, or unresolved high-grade reflux particularly in girls. Pre-procedure evaluation and optimization should include treatment directed toward bladder and bowel dysfunction. We recommend all children who are toilet trained have a uroflowmetry and estimation of post void residual to objectively evaluate bladder function. Bladder habits should be quizzed in terms of frequency of voiding, continence issues, and adequacy of hydration. Stooling frequency and consistency should be optimized before surgery. If problems with bladder and bowel dysfunction persist despite treatment, consideration should be given for neurologic evaluation of the spine and/or additional medical/behavioral therapy.

Technique

RA ureteral reimplantation can be done both intravesically or extravesically, with the latter more commonly used. The surgical technique in both mimics the open approach. The intravesical replicates a Cohen cross-trigonal reimplantation, whereas the extravesical replicates the Lich-Gregoir technique.

Patient positioning

Patients younger than 2 years are positioned supine on the operating table, whereas older children are positioned in dorsal lithotomy with stirrups. In addition, we have found that the robot can be brought in the midline stopping at the patient's feet or alternatively side docked. We have found no difference between these 2 approaches. The patient is secured to the operating table with silk tape across their chest with extreme care to avoid compromising ventilation, especially in smaller children. As the patient is in steep Trendelenburg position, we place a heavy gel bolster secured to the operating table above their head to prevent intraoperative sliding in a cranial direction (**Fig. 5**). We place a soft thick cushion over the patient's face and the endotracheal tube to protect both from the robotic arms. Special attention is paid to appropriate padding of pressure points and neutral positioning of the joints.

Intravesical technique

The anterior abdominal wall from the xiphoid to pubis including external genitalia is included in the sterile field. Cystoscopy is performed and the bladder is distended with fluid. Under direct visual guidance of cystoscopy, port placement sites are selected and "box stitches" are placed. These are full-thickness sutures from the fascia through the bladder and back out through the fascia. These sutures allow for traction anchoring the bladder to the abdominal wall during port placement and to allow for easy closure at the conclusion of the procedure. Pneumovesicum is achieved after draining

the bladder. Similar to a Cohen cross-trigonal reimplantation, feeding tubes are used to intubate the ureters and secured. Using this tube for traction, periureteral dissection is performed to mobilize the ureter(s) further into the bladder. A mucosal tunnel is then created with a natural shallow angle to the old hiatus across the trigone. The ureter is then passed through the tunnel and the neo-orifice is created with interrupted monofilament suture. Dissected mucosa over the old orifice is closed. Continuous drainage via Foley catheter is used for 3 to 5 days, at which point a cystogram is performed before trial of void.

Extravesical technique

After draping the patient, a Foley is placed. A camera port in the inferior border of the umbilicus, 2 working arm ports on either side at the mid clavicular line are placed and either hook or endoshears in the working arm and a Maryland dissector are used. In girls, the dissection is started between the fallopian tube and broad ligament on one side and the bladder on the other. In boys, the peritoneum is opened on the ureter distal to the vas which is visualized and protected throughout the procedure. Proximal dissection of the ureter in the retroperitoneum is performed to gain adequate length at avoid tension during tunneling. Dissection distal to the ureterovesical junction is then performed. Avoiding the use of traction sutures, directly handling, crushing or the use of cautery on the ureter during dissection to avoid injury or compromising vascularity is important.

A traction suture is placed near the posterior dome of the bladder to aid visualization of the ureterovesical junction and to aid detrussorotomy. The detrussorotomy should be performed to allow for a tunnel length approximately 4 times the diameter of the ureter and in a trajectory to avoid kinking as it enters the bladder. The indwelling urethral

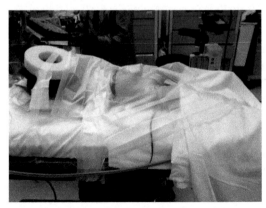

Fig. 5. Patient positioned for robotic-assisted reimplantation.

catheter is used to fill the bladder about one-third full with sterile water/saline. Using cautery and blunt dissection, the detrussorotomy is then created down to the mucosal layer. Filling the bladder allows for early identification of the mucosal layer, which bulges out like a blue dome and allows for efficient dissection. If the mucosal layer is breeched, we recommend simple closure to avoid subsequent leak. The detrussorotomy is extended distally in a Y-shaped configuration around the ureterovesical junction on either side with sparing use of cautery in this area. The bladder is then deflated and the ureter is placed in this tunnel and the detrusor closed behind it in an interrupted fashion. The Foley is left overnight and removed the following day.

Outcomes and success in a modern cohort

The robotic approach to ureteral reimplantation has been controversial as institutions with varying degrees of experience reported varying initial success rates. Understanding factors such as the technique used and surgeon experience as well as patient-specific factors including the age of the child, if the child is toilet trained or not, presence and treatment of bowel-bladder dysfunction, baseline bladder dynamics, the grade of reflux, and gender of child all play an important role in success. Furthermore, there is significant controversy in how we define success. If the goal of surgery is to reduce the risk of urinary tract infections, should that be the primary end point rather than radiologic success? **Table 1** provides the results from studies evaluating the efficacy of RA ureteral reimplantation for primary vesicoureteral reflux. We believe these encouraging results show this approach leading to greater than 90% success rate.

Pediatric urologists have modified the diagnostic patterns and treatment recommendations of this disease notably over the past 2 decades. This has led to a significant decline in the number of patients undergoing surgery.[54,55] When critically evaluating the patients with vesicoureteral reflux undergoing surgery, historical cohorts are different by age at surgery, grades of reflux and other confounders like the presence of bowel-bladder dysfunction. Studies comparing the 2 approaches in a modern cohort with a controlled research design are lacking.

Grimsby and colleagues[56] also reported a multi-institutional experience that provides a cautionary tale when implementing a novel surgical technique and the importance of recognizing areas for improvement and sharing experiences. We acknowledge that the technique for reimplantation at our institution has evolved and improved over time. To this point, Boysen and colleagues[57] reported on a multi-institutional effort that demonstrated how institutions vary in technique, success and benefit from this type of collaboration, which continues to develop and expand.

Complications

Table 1 shows that complications after robotic ureteral extravesical ureteral reimplantation are few and infrequent. Transient urinary retention has been reported and in our experience, is self-limited and resolves spontaneously. There is a general belief that this occurs more common in bilateral procedures, but Kawal and colleagues[58] showed that this did not appear to be a risk factor. Ureteral injury and ureteral obstruction are other possible complications reported in about 1.0% to 2.5% of patients. Careful use of cautery during the ureteral dissection, discontinued use of traction sutures on the ureters and avoiding traction injuries to the ureter are critical to decrease the likelihood of these complications. In addition, avoiding pressure on the ureter during detrusorrhaphy is essential. Transient hydronephrosis has also been reported after ureteral reimplantation in about 30% of patients and typically resolves within 1 year,[59] which is similar to open surgery.[60]

ADVANCED ROBOTIC-ASSISTED PROCEDURES

As pediatric robotic surgeons gained more experience with the procedures discussed previously, centers began to apply these techniques to more complex operations such as augmentation cystoplasty and appendicovesicostomy creation. The first robotic case was reported in 2008 by Dr Mohan Gundeti and colleagues[61] and provided the framework to approaching this operation in the pediatric population. The open approach continues to be the most common technique to for these cases, but as experience is further published and disseminated, the authors feel adoption will continue to increase.

Robot-Assisted Augmentation Cystoplasty and Mitrofanoff Appendicovesicostomy

Indications for this surgery include diseases that leads to impaired bladder function with reduced capacity and decreased compliance. Commonly, patients with diseases such as spina bifida, neurogenic bladder, posterior urethral valves, and prune belly syndrome may benefit from these reconstructions. In addition to the contraindications noted in open surgery, such as history of inflammatory bowel diseases, inability to perform catheterization and poor access to care, the minimally

Table 1
Results from studies evaluating efficacy of robotic-assisted ureteral reimplantation

Study	Technique	Patients, n/Ureters, n	Median Age, y	Bowel-Bladder Dysfunction: Yes/No, %	Complications, %	Success, %
Marchini et al,[74] 2011	RALUR-IV and EV OR-IV and EV	RALUR-IV – 19 RALUR-EV – 20 OR-IV – 22 OR-EV - 7	RALUR IV-9.9 RALUR EV – 8.6 OR-IV -8.8 OR – EV -6.0	No	RALUR IV- 5 (retention = 1, leak = 4) RALUR EV – 4 (retention = 2, ureteral leak = 2)	RALUR IV-92.2 RALUR EV – 100 OR – IV -93.2 OR – EV – 94.2
Casale,[75] 2008	RALUR-EV	41(82)	3.2	Addressed preoperatively but numbers not included	0	97.6
Smith et al,[76] 2011	RALUR-EV OR IV	RALUR-EV -25(33) OR-IV – 25(46)	RALUR IV- 5.8 OR IV – 4.2	Addressed preoperatively but numbers not included	RALUR EV – 3 (urinary retention) OR IV – 1 (bladder leak)	RALUR EV- 97 OR IV - 100
Kasturi et al, 2012[77]	RALUR-EV	150 (300)	3.55	Addressed preoperatively but numbers not included	0	99.3
Chalmers et al,[78] 2012	RALUR-EV	17(23)	6.23	No	0	90.9
Schomburg et al,[79] 2014	RALUR-EV OR EV	RALUR 21 OR 20	RALUR 6.2 OR4.3	No	RALUR 2 OR 7	RALUR 100 OR 95
Akhavan et al,[80] 2014	RALUR-EV	50(78)	6.2	No	6: ileus = 2, obstruction = 2, ureteral injury = 1, perinephric fluid = 1	92.3

Boysen et al,[57] 2018 – Multi-institutional	RALUR-EV	143 (199)	6.6	Yes: 45, of those 35.4% dysfunction resolved completely before surgery	12: obstruction = 2, urine leak = 3, port site hernia = 1, catheter and drain complications = 2, transient urinary retention = 4	93.8–1 had redo surgery
Grimsby et al,[56] 2015 – Multi-institutional	RALUR-EV	61(93)	6.7	Addressed preoperatively, included in a multivariate analysis but numbers and outcomes not provided	6: obstruction = 3, urine leak = 2, readmission = 1	72–4 had redo surgery

Abbreviations: EV, extravesical; IV, intravesical; OR, open ureteral reimplant; RALUR-EV, robot-assisted laparoscopic extravesical ureteral reimplantation.
Data from Refs.[56,57,74–80]

invasive approach may be hampered in patients with history of multiple prior abdominal surgeries or severe spinal abnormalities that may affect appropriate positioning. Many of these patients have a history of ventriculo-peritoneal shunt placement, which may benefit from isolation by using an Endopouch bag (Ethicon Endo-Surgery, Cincinnati, OH)[62] during surgery, although our practice does not commonly use this approach.

Technique and outcomes

The steps of the procedure have been reported in great detail in previous publications.[63,64] Differing slightly from these techniques, it has been our preference to perform the bowel mobilization by using a conventional laparoscopic approach. Reports have shown success with RA intracorporeal hand-sewn bowel anastomosis,[65] but we prefer to perform the bowel reanastomosis by using surgical stapling devices.

Interim studies have shown RA procedures had longer operative time (623 vs 287 mins; $P<.01$) and a decreased length of stay compared with open surgery, but comparable increases in measured bladder capacity, narcotic use, and complication rates.[66] We believe these initial results are optimistic and encourage further implantation of these procedures.

Additional Procedures in Pediatric Urology

A number of additional complex procedures have been performed robotically, including bladder neck repair,[67] bladder diverticulectomy,[68] and excision of prostatic utricles.[69] Unlike the adult experience, RA technology being applied to pediatric urologic oncology is just beginning to be reported both in cases of renal tumors[70,71] as well as retroperitoneal lymph node dissections[72] with good initial results. Further adoption of these techniques is likely to continue as these cases are managed at high-volume centers and in collaboration with adult urologic oncologists.

THE FUTURE IN PEDIATRIC UROLOGY

As discussed previously and likely in many of the articles reported herein, in an era of rising health care expenditures, aside from outcomes, procedural costs will continue to play a role in deciding appropriate treatment of disease. With the development and approval of competing robotic platforms,[73] the authors hope that industry will consider application of their technologies on pediatric patients and their procedures. This competition will hopefully decrease cost as well as provide further diversity and specificity in instrumentation that may be further tailored to pediatric

urology. RA procedures within pediatric urology will continue to play a major part of the care provided and training opportunities for our next generation of trainees. Pediatric urologists, in conjunction with their adult counterparts, will continue to champion this technology in hopes of providing good results with less morbidity in this population.

DISCLOSURE

The author has nothing to disclose.

SUPPLEMENTARY DATA

Supplementary data related to this article can be found online at https://doi.org/10.1016/j.ucl.2020.09.008.

REFERENCES

1. Peters CA. Robotically assisted surgery in pediatric urology. Urol Clin North Am 2004;31(4):743–52.
2. Cundy TP, Shetty K, Clark J, et al. The first decade of robotic surgery in children. J Pediatr Surg 2013; 48(4):858–65.
3. Mahida JB, Cooper JN, Herz D, et al. Utilization and costs associated with robotic surgery in children. J Surg Res 2015;199(1):169–76.
4. Cundy TP, Harley SJD, Marcus HJ, Hughes-Hallett A, Khurana S. Global trends in paediatric robot-assisted urological surgery: a bibliometric and Progressive Scholarly Acceptance analysis. J Robot Surg 2018;12(1):109–15.
5. Varda BK, Wang Y, Chung BI, et al. Has the robot caught up? National trends in utilization, perioperative outcomes, and cost for open, laparoscopic, and robotic pediatric pyeloplasty in the United States from 2003 to 2015. J Pediatr Urol 2018; 14(4):336 e331–8.
6. Tasian GE, Wiebe DJ, Casale P. Learning curve of robotic assisted pyeloplasty for pediatric urology fellows. J Urol 2013;190(4 Suppl):1622–6.
7. Dothan D, Raisin G, Jaber J, Kocherov S, Chertin B. Learning curve of robotic-assisted laparoscopic pyeloplasty (RALP) in children: how to reach a level of excellence? J Robot Surg 2020.
8. Junejo NN, Alotaibi A, Alshahrani SM, et al. The learning curve for robotic-assisted pyeloplasty in children: Our initial experience from a single center. Urol Ann 2020;12(1):19–24.
9. Vilos GA, Ternamian A, Dempster J, Laberge PY, Clinical Practice Gynaecology C. Laparoscopic entry: a review of techniques, technologies, and complications. J Obstet Gynaecol Can 2007;29(5): 433–47.

10. Gargollo PC. Hidden incision endoscopic surgery: description of technique, parental satisfaction and applications. J Urol 2011;185(4):1425–31.

11. Yilmaz O, Tanriverdi HI, Cayirli H, et al. Successful outcomes in laparoscopic pyeloplasty using knotless self-anchoring barbed suture in children. J Pediatr Urol 2019;15(6):660 e661–5.

12. Braga LH, Lorenzo AJ, Farhat WA, Bagli DJ, Khoury AE, Pippi Salle JL. Outcome analysis and cost comparison between externalized pyeloureteral and standard stents in 470 consecutive open pyeloplasties. J Urol 2008;180(4 Suppl):1693–8. discussion1698-1699.

13. Chu DI, Shrivastava D, Van Batavia JP, et al. Outcomes of externalized pyeloureteral versus internal ureteral stent in pediatric robotic-assisted laparoscopic pyeloplasty. J Pediatr Urol 2018;14(5):450 e451–6.

14. Silva MV, Levy AC, Finkelstein JB, Van Batavia JP, Casale P. Is peri-operative urethral catheter drainage enough? The case for stentless pediatric robotic pyeloplasty. J Pediatr Urol 2015;11(4). 175 e171-175.

15. Rodriguez AR, Rich MA, Swana HS. Stentless pediatric robotic pyeloplasty. Ther Adv Urol 2012;4(2): 57–60.

16. Yee DS, Shanberg AM, Duel BP, Rodriguez E, Eichel L, Rajpoot D. Initial comparison of robotic-assisted laparoscopic versus open pyeloplasty in children. Urology 2006;67(3):599–602.

17. Tasian GE, Casale P. The robotic-assisted laparoscopic pyeloplasty: gateway to advanced reconstruction. Urol Clin North Am 2015;42(1):89–97.

18. Salo M, Sjoberg Altemani T, Anderberg M. Pyeloplasty in children: perioperative results and long-term outcomes of robotic-assisted laparoscopic surgery compared to open surgery. Pediatr Surg Int 2016;32(6):599–607.

19. Lee RS, Retik AB, Borer JG, Peters CA. Pediatric robot assisted laparoscopic dismembered pyeloplasty: comparison with a cohort of open surgery. J Urol 2006;175(2):683–7. discussion 687.

20. Kutikov A, Nguyen M, Guzzo T, Canter D, Casale P. Robot assisted pyeloplasty in the infant-lessons learned. J Urol 2006;176(5):2237–9. discussion 2239-2240.

21. Chang SJ, Hsu CK, Hsieh CH, Yang SS. Comparing the efficacy and safety between robotic-assisted versus open pyeloplasty in children: a systemic review and meta-analysis. World J Urol 2015;33(11): 1855–65.

22. Atug F, Woods M, Burgess SV, Castle EP, Thomas R. Robotic assisted laparoscopic pyeloplasty in children. J Urol 2005;174(4 Pt 1):1440–2.

23. Braga LH, Pace K, DeMaria J, Lorenzo AJ. Systematic review and meta-analysis of robotic-assisted versus conventional laparoscopic pyeloplasty for patients with ureteropelvic junction obstruction: effect on operative time, length of hospital stay, postoperative complications, and success rate. Eur Urol 2009;56(5):848–57.

24. Lee Z, Schulte M, DeFoor WR, et al. A Non-Narcotic Pathway for the Management of Postoperative Pain Following Pediatric Robotic Pyeloplasty. J Endourol 2017;31(3):255–8.

25. Bodar YJL, Srinivasan AK, Shah AS, Kawal T, Shukla AR. Time-Driven activity-based costing identifies opportunities for process efficiency and cost optimization for robot-assisted laparoscopic pyeloplasty. J Pediatr Urol 2020.

26. Behan JW, Kim SS, Dorey F, et al. Human capital gains associated with robotic assisted laparoscopic pyeloplasty in children compared to open pyeloplasty. J Urol 2011;186(4 Suppl):1663–7.

27. Freilich DA, Penna FJ, Nelson CP, Retik AB, Nguyen HT. Parental satisfaction after open versus robot assisted laparoscopic pyeloplasty: results from modified Glasgow Children's Benefit Inventory Survey. J Urol 2010;183(2):704–8.

28. Autorino R, Eden C, El-Ghoneimi A, et al. Robot-assisted and laparoscopic repair of ureteropelvic junction obstruction: a systematic review and meta-analysis. Eur Urol 2014;65(2):430–52.

29. Finkelstein JB, Levy AC, Silva MV, Murray L, Delaney C, Casale P. How to decide which infant can have robotic surgery? Just do the math. J Pediatr Urol 2015;11(4):170 e171-174.

30. Chan YY, Durbin-Johnson B, Sturm RM, Kurzrock EA. Outcomes after pediatric open, laparoscopic, and robotic pyeloplasty at academic institutions. J Pediatr Urol 2017;13(1):49 e41–6.

31. Kawal T, Srinivasan AK, Shrivastava D, et al. Pediatric robotic-assisted laparoscopic pyeloplasty: Does age matter? J Pediatr Urol 2018;14(6):540 e541–6.

32. Bora GS, Bendapudi D, Mavuduru RS, et al. Robot-assisted bilateral simultaneous pyeloplasty: safe and feasible. J Robot Surg 2017;11(2):145 9.

33. Faerber GJ, Ritchey ML, Bloom DA. Percutaneous endopyelotomy in infants and young children after failed open pyeloplasty. J Urol 1995;154(4):1495–7.

34. Capolicchio G, Homsy YL, Houle AM, Brzezinski A, Stein L, Elhilali MM. Long-term results of percutaneous endopyelotomy in the treatment of children with failed open pyeloplasty. J Urol 1997;158(4): 1534–7.

35. Shapiro EY, Cho JS, Srinivasan A, et al. Long-term follow-up for salvage laparoscopic pyeloplasty after failed open pyeloplasty. Urology 2009;73(1):115–8.

36. Braga LH, Lorenzo AJ, Skeldon S, et al. Failed pyeloplasty in children: comparative analysis of retrograde endopyelotomy versus redo pyeloplasty. J Urol 2007;178(6):2571–5. discussion 2575.

37. Helmy TE, Sarhan OM, Hafez AT, Elsherbiny MT, Dawaba ME, Ghali AM. Surgical management of

failed pyeloplasty in children: single-center experience. J Pediatr Urol 2009;5(2):87–9.

38. Romao RL, Koyle MA, Pippi Salle JL, et al. Failed pyeloplasty in children: revisiting the unknown. Urology 2013;82(5):1145–7.

39. Abdrabuh AM, Salih EM, Aboelnasr M, Galal H, El-Emam A, El-Zayat T. Endopyelotomy versus redo pyeloplasty for management of failed pyeloplasty in children: A single center experience. J Pediatr Surg 2018;53(11):2250–5.

40. Jacobson DL, Shannon R, Johnson EK, et al. Robot-Assisted Laparoscopic Reoperative Repair for Failed Pyeloplasty in Children: An Updated Series. J Urol 2019;201(5):1005–11.

41. Casale P, Mucksavage P, Resnick M, Kim SS. Robotic ureterocalicostomy in the pediatric population. J Urol 2008;180(6):2643–8.

42. Gonzalez R, Piaggio L. Initial experience with laparoscopic ipsilateral ureteroureterostomy in infants and children for duplication anomalies of the urinary tract. J Urol 2007;177(6):2315–8.

43. Passerotti CC, Diamond DA, Borer JG, Eisner BH, Barrisford G, Nguyen HT. Robot-assisted laparoscopic ureteroureterostomy: description of technique. J Endourol 2008;22(4):581–4. discussion 585.

44. Smith KM, Shrivastava D, Ravish IR, Nerli RB, Shukla AR. Robot-assisted laparoscopic ureteroureterostomy for proximal ureteral obstructions in children. J Pediatr Urol 2009;5(6):475–9.

45. Leavitt DA, Rambachan A, Haberman K, DeMarco R, Shukla AR. Robot-assisted laparoscopic ipsilateral ureteroureterostomy for ectopic ureters in children: description of technique. J Endourol 2012;26(10):1279–83.

46. Biles MJ, Finkelstein JB, Silva MV, Lambert SM, Casale P. Innovation in Robotics and Pediatric Urology: Robotic Ureteroureterostomy for Duplex Systems with Ureteral Ectopia. J Endourol 2016; 30(10):1041–8.

47. Lee YS, Hah YS, Kim MJ, et al. Factors associated with complications of the ureteral stump after proximal ureteroureterostomy. J Urol 2012;188(5): 1890–4.

48. Jayram G, Roberts J, Hernandez A, et al. Outcomes and fate of the remnant moiety following laparoscopic heminephrectomy for duplex kidney: a multicenter review. J Pediatr Urol 2011;7(3):272–5.

49. Varda BK, Rajender A, Yu RN, Lee RS. A contemporary single-institution retrospective cohort study comparing perioperative outcomes between robotic and open partial nephrectomy for poorly functioning renal moieties in children with duplex collecting systems. J Pediatr Urol 2018;14(6):549 e541–8.

50. Mason MD, Anthony Herndon CD, Smith-Harrison LI, Peters CA, Corbett ST. Robotic-assisted partial nephrectomy in duplicated collecting systems in the pediatric population: techniques and outcomes. J Pediatr Urol 2014;10(2):374–9.

51. Lee RS, Sethi AS, Passerotti CC, et al. Robot assisted laparoscopic partial nephrectomy: a viable and safe option in children. J Urol 2009;181(2):823–8. discussion 828-829.

52. Olsen LH, Jorgensen TM. Robotically assisted retroperitoneoscopic heminephrectomy in children: initial clinical results. J Pediatr Urol 2005;1(2):101–4.

53. Herz D, DaJusta D, Ching C, McLeod D. Segmental arterial mapping during pediatric robot-assisted laparoscopic heminephrectomy: A descriptive series. J Pediatr Urol 2016;12(4):266 e261–266.

54. Kurtz MP, Leow JJ, Varda BK, et al. The Decline of the Open Ureteral Reimplant in the United States: National Data From 2003 to 2013. Urology 2017; 100:193–7.

55. Bowen DK, Faasse MA, Liu DB, Gong EM, Lindgren BW, Johnson EK. Use of Pediatric Open, Laparoscopic and Robot-Assisted Laparoscopic Ureteral Reimplantation in the United States: 2000 to 2012. J Urol 2016;196(1):207–12.

56. Grimsby GM, Dwyer ME, Jacobs MA, et al. Multi-institutional review of outcomes of robot-assisted laparoscopic extravesical ureteral reimplantation. J Urol 2015;193(5 Suppl):1791–5.

57. Boysen WR, Akhavan A, Ko J, et al. Prospective multicenter study on robot-assisted laparoscopic extravesical ureteral reimplantation (RALUR-EV): Outcomes and complications. J Pediatr Urol 2018; 14(3):262 e261–6.

58. Kawal T, Srinivasan AK, Chang J, Long C, Chu D, Shukla AR. Robotic-assisted laparoscopic ureteral re-implant (RALUR): Can post-operative urinary retention be predicted? J Pediatr Urol 2018;14(4): 323 e321–5.

59. Kim EJ, Song SH, Sheth K, et al. Does de novo hydronephrosis after pediatric robot-assisted laparoscopic ureteral re-implantation behave similarly to open re-implantation? J Pediatr Urol 2019;15(6): 604.e601–6.

60. Rosman BM, Passerotti CC, Kohn D, Recabal P, Retik AB, Nguyen HT. Hydronephrosis following ureteral reimplantation: when is it concerning? J Pediatr Urol 2012;8(5):481–7.

61. Gundeti MS, Eng MK, Reynolds WS, Zagaja GP. Pediatric robotic-assisted laparoscopic augmentation ileocystoplasty and Mitrofanoff appendicovesicostomy: complete intracorporeal–initial case report. Urology 2008;72(5):1144–7. discussion 1147.

62. Marchetti P, Razmaria A, Zagaja GP, Gundeti MS. Management of the ventriculo-peritoneal shunt in pediatric patients during robot-assisted laparoscopic urologic procedures. J Endourol 2011; 25(2):225–9.

63. Cohen AJ, Pariser JJ, Anderson BB, Pearce SM, Gundeti MS. The robotic appendicovesicostomy

and bladder augmentation: the next frontier in robotics, are we there? Urol Clin North Am 2015; 42(1):121–30.

64. Gundeti MS, Acharya SS, Zagaja GP, Shalhav AL. Paediatric robotic-assisted laparoscopic augmentation ileocystoplasty and Mitrofanoff appendicovesicostomy (RALIMA): feasibility of and initial experience with the University of Chicago technique. BJU Int 2011;107(6):962–9.

65. Gundeti MS, Wiltz AL, Zagaja GP, Shalhav AL. Robot-assisted laparoscopic intracorporeal hand-sewn bowel anastomosis during pediatric bladder reconstructive surgery. J Endourol 2010;24(8): 1325–8.

66. Murthy P, Cohn JA, Selig RB, Gundeti MS. Robot-assisted Laparoscopic Augmentation Ileocystoplasty and Mitrofanoff Appendicovesicostomy in Children: Updated Interim Results. Eur Urol 2015;68(6): 1069–75.

67. Gargollo PC, White LA. Robotic-Assisted Bladder Neck Procedures for Incontinence in Pediatric Patients. Front Pediatr 2019;7:172.

68. Christman MS, Casale P. Robot-assisted bladder diverticulectomy in the pediatric population. J Endourol 2012;26(10):1296–300.

69. Goruppi I, Avolio L, Romano P, Raffaele A, Pelizzo G. Robotic-assisted surgery for excision of an enlarged prostatic utricle. Int J Surg Case Rep 2015;10:94–6.

70. Varda BK, Cho P, Wagner AA, Lee RS. Collaborating with our adult colleagues: A case series of robotic surgery for suspicious and cancerous lesions in children and young adults performed in a free-standing children's hospital. J Pediatr Urol 2018;14(2):182 e181–8.

71. Meignan P, Ballouhey Q, Lejeune J, et al. Robotic-assisted laparoscopic surgery for pediatric tumors: a bicenter experience. J Robot Surg 2018;12(3): 501–8.

72. Cost NG, Geller JI, DeFoor WR Jr, Wagner LM, Noh PH. A robotic-assisted laparoscopic approach for pediatric renal cell carcinoma allows for both nephron-sparing surgery and extended lymph node dissection. J Pediatr Surg 2012;47(10): 1946–50.

73. Sheth KR, Koh CJ. The Future of Robotic Surgery in Pediatric Urology: Upcoming Technology and Evolution Within the Field. Front Pediatr 2019;7:259.

74. Marchini GS, Hong YK, Minnillo BJ, et al. Robotic assisted laparoscopic ureteral reimplantation in children: case matched comparative study with open surgical approach. J Urol 2011;185(5):1870–5.

75. Casale P, Patel RP, Kolon TF. Nerve sparing robotic extravesical ureteral reimplantation. J Urol 2008; 179(5):1987–9. discussion 1990.

76. Smith RP, Oliver JL, Peters CA. Pediatric robotic extravesical ureteral reimplantation: comparison with open surgery. J Urol 2011;185(5):1876–81.

77. Kasturi S, Sehgal SS, Christman MS, Lambert SM, Casale P. Prospective long-term analysis of nerve-sparing extravesical robotic-assisted laparoscopic ureteral reimplantation. Urology 2012;79(3):680–3.

78. Chalmers D, Herbst K, Kim C. Robotic-assisted laparoscopic extravesical ureteral reimplantation: an initial experience. J Pediatr Urol 2012;8(3): 268–71.

79. Schomburg JL, Haberman K, Willihnganz-Lawson KH, Shukla AR. Robot-assisted laparoscopic ureteral reimplantation: a single surgeon comparison to open surgery. J Pediatr Urol 2014; 10(5):875–9.

80. Akhavan A, Avery D, Lendvay TS. Robot-assisted extravesical ureteral reimplantation: outcomes and conclusions from 78 ureters. J Pediatr Urol 2014; 10(5):864–8.

Robotic Surgery for Male Infertility

Annie Darves-Bornoz, MD, Evan Panken, BS, Robert E. Brannigan, MD, Joshua A. Halpern, MD, MS*

KEYWORDS

• Robotic surgical procedures • Infertility • Male • Vasovasostomy • Varicocele

KEY POINTS

• Robotic-assisted approaches to male infertility microsurgery have potential practical benefits including reduction of tremor, 3-dimensional visualization, and decreased need for skilled surgical assistance.
• Several small, retrospective studies have described robotic-assisted vasectomy reversal with comparable clinical outcomes to the traditional microsurgical approach.
• Few studies have described application of the robot to varicocelectomy, testicular sperm extraction, and spermatic cord denervation.
• The use of robotic-assistance for male infertility procedures is evolving, and adoption has been limited. Rigorous studies are needed to evaluate outcomes and cost-effectiveness.

INTRODUCTION

Up to 15% of couples have infertility, with approximately 50% of cases involving a male factor.[1,2] A substantial proportion of men with subfertility have surgically treatable and even reversible etiologies, such as a varicocele or vasal obstruction. The introduction of the operating microscope revolutionized the field of male infertility, dramatically improving visualization of small, complex anatomic structures. The technical precision afforded has improved operative outcomes across the board. For decades, microsurgery has been considered the gold standard for many male infertility procedures.

As robotic-assisted laparoscopic surgery was widely adopted in urology, male infertility surgeons began to explore potential applications of the robotic platform to microsurgical operations. On the one hand, most male infertility procedures are extra-abdominal and extra-corporeal, rendering them less amenable to the benefits of the robotic approach that are best recognized with intraperitoneal and pelvic surgery. On the other hand, many of the theoretic and practical advantages offered by the robotic approach are highly transferrable to surgery for male infertility:

High quality, 3-dimensional visualization is essential for any microsurgical procedure.

Improved surgeon ergonomics are always desirable, particularly given the surgeon morbidity associated with microsurgery.[3]

Filtering of physiologic tremor can improve precision during technically demanding microsurgical operations.

The robotic arm may obviate the need for a skilled surgical assistant that is often required in microsurgical cases (**Table 1**).

This article reviews the application of robotic surgery to each of the 4 primary male infertility procedures: vasectomy reversal, varicocelectomy, testicular sperm extraction, and spermatic cord denervation. For each, a brief historic perspective is presented alongside the data, limited in most cases, examining its use.

Department of Urology, Northwestern University Feinberg School of Medicine, Chicago, IL, USA
* Corresponding author. Department of Urology, Northwestern University Feinberg School of Medicine, 676 North St. Clair Street, Arkes 2300, Chicago, IL 60611.
E-mail address: joshua.halpern@northwestern.edu

Urol Clin N Am 48 (2021) 127–135
https://doi.org/10.1016/j.ucl.2020.09.009
0094-0143/21/Published by Elsevier Inc.

Table 1
Theoretic advantages of the robotic approach for male infertility surgery

Advantage	Description
3-dimensional visualization	High-quality, 3-dimensional visualization is comparable and possibly superior to conventional microscopy in certain anatomic areas.
Ergonomics	Improved surgeon comfort and ergonomics may reduce morbidity associated with conventional microsurgery.
Tremor reduction	Filtering of physiologic tremor can improve precision during technically demanding microsurgical operations.
Minimal assistance	Fourth robotic arm may obviate the need for a skilled surgical assistant, often required for complex microsurgical cases.

ROBOTIC-ASSISTED MICROSURGICAL VASECTOMY REVERSAL

Vasectomy is a commonly used method of contraception with over 500,000 vasectomies performed annually in the United States.[4] It is estimated that up to 6% of these men will eventually pursue vasectomy reversal.[5] In most men, vasectomy reversal is technically feasible; however, long-term success rates with respect to pregnancy and live birth are variable.[6]

From a technical perspective, the vasal anastomosis is the critical operative step. The vasal lumen is exceedingly small, with an average diameter of approximately 1.0 mm.[7] The key surgical principles are the achievement of a tension-free, water-tight, vasal anastomosis, and taking great care to avoid iatrogenic obstruction with placement of a cross-luminal suture. Early vasectomy reversals were performed without magnification; however the introduction of the operating microscope greatly improved both patency and pregnancy rates, and thus microsurgical vasectomy reversal became the standard of care.[8,9] The technique and microsurgical skills require dedicated training experience and often a skilled microsurgical assistant. Robot-assisted microsurgical approaches offer advantages to overcome some of the challenges associated with pure microsurgery for this challenging procedure. As such, vasectomy reversal was the first application of robotic microsurgery to male infertility.

Initial descriptions of robotic vasal surgery were small feasibility studies in ex vivo models.[10–12] In 2003, Schoor and colleagues[10] performed en bloc resection of the spermatic cord and testis in euthanized rats, following which they sharply divided the bilateral vasa and performed a robotic-assisted single-layer vasal anastomosis using 10-0 nylon suture. The authors noted that both surgeons found the robotic instruments sufficiently delicate for manipulation of the vasal tissue and suture material. Other benefits described in this initial report were "complete elimination of tremor, and enhanced comfort." Soon thereafter, Kuang and colleagues[11] compared vasovasostomy (VV) outcomes of a single surgeon using the robotic versus microsurgical approaches in an ex vivo human model consisting of fresh vasal specimens from radical cystectomy patients. Although operative time was longer using the robotic approach, there was no difference in the number of needle passes, surgeon fatigue, or anastomotic patency between the 2 approaches. The authors also noted that surgeon tremor was substantially reduced with the robotic approach.

The first comparative study of robotic vasal surgery in rats was published by Schiff and colleagues in 2004.[13] The authors performed vasectomy in 24 rats, returning 2 weeks later to perform robotic versus microsurgical VV or vasoepididymostomy (VE). Robotic VV was significantly faster than the conventional microsurgical procedure (68.5 vs 102.5 minutes, $P=.002$), whereas there was no significant difference for VE (90.3 vs 107.3 minutes, $P = .29$). Similar anastomotic patency rates were seen between the two groups for both VV (robotic 100% vs conventional 90%, $P=.23$) and VE (robotic 100% vs conventional 90%, $P=.16$). Although the study was not designed to assess the surgeon learning curve, the authors noted that experienced microsurgeons were able to adapt their skills to the robotic approach during a short, 6-hour training period before the study, during which they performed robotic-assisted suture placement and knot tying on a practice card.

It was not until almost a decade later that the first retrospective studies of robotic vasectomy reversal in people were published. Parekattil and colleagues reported the largest study to date, comparing 110 robotic and 45 conventional microsurgical cases performed by a single fellowship-trained microsurgeon.[14] Median obstructive interval was similar between the 2 groups (7 vs 6.5 years, respectively; $P=.3$), and 2-layer anastomotic technique was used in both approaches. Median operative time was shorter for the robotic VV compared with the microsurgical VV (97 vs 120 minutes, $P < .001$), although the authors excluded time required for setup of either the robot or the microscope. Patency (defined as sperm concentration >1 million/mL) was higher in the robotic group compared with the microsurgical group (96% vs 80%, $P=.02$), although there was no difference in pregnancy rates (65% vs 55%, P-value not reported). Kavoussi reported results from a smaller, retrospective study of 25 men who underwent robotic VV compared with 27 men who underwent conventional microsurgical VV.[15] The author found that there was no difference in operative time, anastomotic patency, or total motile sperm counts between the 2 groups.

Early adopters of the robotic approach also reported their experience with the robotic learning curve. As mentioned previously, Schiff and colleagues[16] found the robotic approach to be easily adoptable with 6 hours of laboratory-based practice, although the authors did not report any subsequent results in human studies. Parekattil and colleagues[17] noted that the initial 10 robotic cases had substantially higher operative times (range 150–180 minutes), needle bending, and suture breakage, all of which improved thereafter. Most recently, Kavoussi and colleagues reported a single-surgeon learning curve experience with robotic vasectomy reversal. The authors divided the surgeon's initial 100 cases into quartiles, finding that while high patency was achieved early in the learning curve, approximately 75 cases were required to achieve optimal operative and anastomotic time.[18] Santomauro and colleagues[19] examined trainee experience with the robotic approach, reporting on 20 patients in whom an experienced staff surgeon performed unilateral vasal reconstruction and a trainee performed the contralateral anastomosis. Mean anastomotic time was lower for staff surgeons compared with trainees, but the difference was not significant (37.6 vs 54 minutes, $P=.13$); however, the study was likely underpowered. In aggregate, these findings

suggest that the learning curve for the robotic approach is short, at least for the well-trained microsurgeon. A summary of studies examining robotic-assisted vasal reconstruction is presented in **Table 2**.

From a technical perspective, there is no significant difference between the robotic and microsurgical approach for vasectomy reversal (**Fig. 1**). In either circumstance, conventional open identification, mobilization, and exteriorization of the vas deferens are performed, followed by vasal transection and examination of vasal fluid. The technical aspects of robotic vasal anastomosis are comparable to the microsurgical procedure. Small differences in technique have been described, but all utilize 9-0 and 10-0 suture to perform either single- or 2-layer anastomoses using conventional microsurgical principles.[14,15,20,21]

Procedures involving high or intra-abdominal vasal obstruction may be uniquely suited to the robotic approach, as the conventional microsurgical approach has limited access to the high-inguinal and intra-abdominal vas deferens. Najari and colleagues initially described robot-assisted intra-abdominal mobilization of the vas deferens for a patient with iatrogenic bilateral vasal obstruction secondary to a prior bilateral hernia repair. Abdominal mobilization allowed for a tension-free anastomosis that was externalized and performed microscopically. At 12-month follow-up, the patient had return of sperm to the ejaculate with normal concentration.[22] Trost and colleagues[23] subsequently described a purely intracorporeal robotic vasectomy reversal with an intra-abdominal vasal anastomosis in the setting of bilateral obstruction secondary to prior inguinal hernia repair with mesh. The authors demonstrated technical success with semen analysis at 8-week follow-up demonstrating normal sperm concentration.

At present, there is little consensus among reproductive urologists regarding the role for robotic vasectomy reversal.[24] Although the few retrospective studies demonstrate encouraging results with relatively short learning curves and high patency rates, there are no randomized trials comparing the 2 approaches. And despite the theoretical and subjective advantages of potentially decreased surgeon tremor and increased comfort, these metrics have not been rigorously studied.

ROBOTIC-ASSISTED MICROSURGICAL VARICOCELECTOMY

Varicoceles are found in up to 15% of all men[25] and in up to 35% of men presenting with

Table 2
Summary of animal and human studies examining robotic-assisted vasal reconstruction

Author	Year	Subjects	N	Study Characteristics	Significant Findings
Schoor, R[10]	2003	Rats	8	Ex vivo, combination of experienced and inexperienced microsurgeons performing vasal anastomosis	• Elimination of tremor • Enhanced surgeon comfort • Improved visual acuity • Robotic instruments sufficiently delicate for manipulation of vasal tissue and suture material
Kuang, W[11]	2004	Humans	10	Ex vivo, fresh vasa from radical cystectomy specimens, 5 RAVV vs 5 MAVV	• Mean operating time higher for RAVV • # of adverse haptic events higher for RAVV • Similar # of needle passes • No tremor in RAVV, minimal to moderate in MAVV • Equivalent vasal patency
Fleming, C[12]	2004	Humans	1	Case report of RAVV in a human subject	• Demonstrated feasibility in vivo
Schiff, J[16]	2004	Rats	24	In-vivo, randomized trial, 11 RAVV vs 10 MAVV and 12 RAVE vs 10 MAVE	• Shorter operative time for RAVV • Equivalent anastomotic patency • Fewer sperm granulomas with RAVV vs MAVV
Kuang, W[21]	2005	Rabbits	4	In vivo, 4 RAVV vs 4 MAVV	• Longer operative time for RAVV • Similar # of needle passes • No tremor for RAVV, minimal to moderate in MAVV
Santomauro, M[19]	2012	Humans	20	In vivo, case series of MAVV with either single (n = 17) or double (n = 3) anastomosis	• Mean operative time 187 min • Among 13 men with follow-up, 12 (92.3%) patent • Mean sperm concentration 14 million/mL, motility of 26.4%
Parekattil, S[14]	2012	Humans	155	Retrospective, case series	• Higher patency with RAVV (96%) vs MAVV (80%), P=.02 • No difference in total motile sperm count or pregnancy at 1-y
Trost, L[23]	2014	Humans	1	Case report of intracorporeal robotic vasovasostomy for bilateral vasal obstruction secondary to inguinal mesh	• Total operative time was 278 min. • No intraoperative or postoperative complications
Kavoussi, P[15]	2015	Humans	52	Retrospective, cohort study of RAVR (N = 25) vs MAVR (N = 27)	• No difference in operative time, though RAVR had longer anastomotic time (74 vs 63 min) • Equivalent patency • No difference in total motile sperm count operative time: no difference

(continued on next page)

Table 2 (continued)				
Author	**Year**	**Subjects**	**N**	**Study Characteristics**	**Significant Findings**
Marshall, M[20]	2017	Humans	79	Case series of RAVV with single-layer layer anastomosis	• Mean operative time was 192 min • Among men with follow-up (N = 42), 37 (88%) patent

Data from Refs.[10–12,14–16,19–21,23]

infertility.[26] In a proportion of these men, the varicocele may contribute to the impairment of semen parameters. Hypothesized pathophysiologic mechanisms include increased oxidative stress, testicular hypoperfusion, and alteration of the countercurrent heat exchange that is necessary for maintenance of optimal scrotal temperature resultant from the variocele.[27] Studies have shown improvements in semen parameters, pregnancy rate, and live birth rate following varicocele repair, and as such, the diagnosis and treatment of varicoceles have become crucial in the management of male infertility.[28–30]

Varicocele ligation can be performed by a retroperitoneal (high ligation via open incision or laparoscopic), inguinal, or subinguinal, approach. Some evidence suggests that the microsurgical subinguinal approach is associated with lower risks of recurrence and lower rates of postoperative complications including hydrocele and testicular atrophy, compared with other approaches.[31] Thus, rather than translating the laparoscopic approach to a robotic modification, initial reports of robotic-assisted varicocelectomy used the goldstandard subinguinal approach, leveraging the advantages of the robotic platform including excellent visualization and potential reduction of hand tremor in an extracorporeal fashion.[32] Additionally, the fourth robotic arm allows for Doppler mapping of the testicular arteries, minimizing the need for a surgical assistant (**Fig. 2**). Beyond these differences, the basic principles of robotic-

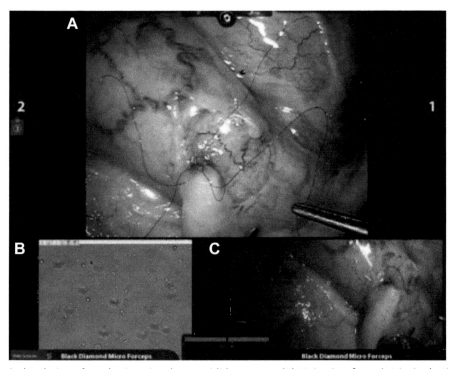

Fig. 1. Surgical technique for robotic assisted vasoepididymostomy.(*A*) Main view from da Vinci robotic platform. (*B*) Live image of andrology optical microscope. (*C*) View from the right side for enhanced magnification. (*From* Gudeloglu A., Brahmbhatt JV., Parekattil SJ. Robot-Assisted Microsurgery in Male Infertility and Andrology. Urologic Clinics of North America. 2014;41(4) 559–566; with permission.)

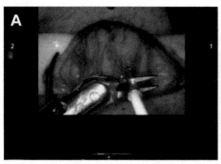
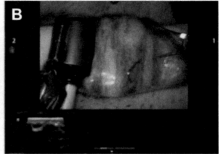

Fig. 2. Surgical technique for robotic assisted varicocelectomy. (*A*) Main view from da Vinci robotic platform of spermatic cord with audio micro-Doppler. (*B*) Video micro-Doppler. (*From* Gudeloglu A., Brahmbhatt JV., Parekattil SJ. Robot-Assisted Microsurgery in Male Infertility and Andrology. Urologic Clinics of North America. 2014;41(4) 559–566; with permission.)

assisted varicocelectomy are essentially unchanged from the conventional microsurgical approach.

Shu and colleagues reported the first series of robotic-assisted subinguinal varicocelectomy in 8 patients, demonstrating no difference in operative time compared with the conventional microsurgical approach, although the authors did not report outcomes such as postoperative complications, recurrence, or changes in semen parameters.[32] Parekattil and colleagues reported outcomes of robotic-assisted varicocelectomy in 154 patients with median follow-up of 22 months. Two patients (1.3%) had recurrences during follow-up; 1 patient (0.6%) developed a postoperative hydrocele, and 2 patients (1.3%) suffered postoperative hematomas.[33]

Most recently, McCullough and colleagues reported a single-surgeon experience in 140 consecutive men who underwent robotic-assisted varicocelectomy for subfertility. Mean operative time for robotic-assisted versus conventional microsurgical approach was 57 plus or minus 16 versus 49 plus or minus 13 minutes per side (no *P*-value provided). However, the authors also noted that mean robotic dock time for bilateral robotic-assisted approach was 39 plus or minus 9 minutes, a substantial addition to operative time that was not included in the operative time for each side. Median follow-up was not reported, but recurrence or failure rate was 9.7%, substantially higher than reported in the literature for the conventional approach. Other observed complications included hematoma (2.7%) and hydrocele (0.8%), with no incidence of testicular loss.[34] Postoperative improvements were noted in serum testosterone (median 145 ng/dL; *P*<.01) and sperm concentration (3.0 million/mL), although pregnancy and birth outcomes were not reported.

These studies are limited by their retrospective nature, single-institution experience, and lack of comparison groups. However, the reported outcomes are roughly comparable to historical data from the conventional microsurgical approach, although the higher recurrence rate reported by McCullough and colleagues does raise some concern. At this time, more rigorous studies are needed to meaningfully compare the robotic approach with the conventional subinguinal microsurgical approach. The authors' anecdotal observation is that the adoption of robot-assisted approaches for varicocele repair is currently limited.

ROBOT-ASSISTED MICRODENERVATION OF THE SPERMATIC CORD

Chronic groin or scrotal content pain (CGSCP) is a common condition, estimated to represent 2.5% of all urology clinic visits.[35] Defined as intermittent or constant pain or discomfort lasting more than 3 months in the groin, scrotum, testis, or epididymis, CGSCP can be frustrating for the patient and provider, as there is no universally accepted treatment algorithm.[36] Although some patients will have an attributable cause such as varicocele, infection, trauma, inflammation, or history of inguinal surgery, up to 50% of cases remain idiopathic.[37] In men refractory to medical management with nonsteroidal anti-inflammatory drugs, antibiotics, and neurotransmitter inhibitors, surgical options may be considered including microdenervation of the spermatic cord (MDSC), epididymectomy, and orchiectomy. Initially described by Levine and colleagues,[38] MDSC offers high success rates with a testis-sparing approach, rendering this an attractive surgical option for these men.

Similar to varicocelectomy, the robotic approach to MDSC is virtually identical to the conventional microsurgical procedure with the exception of robotic in lieu of microsurgical instrumentation. Parekettil and colleagues were first to describe robotic MDSC. In their initial series of 24 cases, they reported a mean operative time of 41 minutes (range 19–80 minutes). Complete resolution of pain was seen in 18 (75%) patients, with an additional 4 (17%) reporting greater than 50% improvement in pain and 2 patients having no benefit. No control group was described.[39] The authors noted that advantages of the robotic approach were elimination of surgeon tremor and decreased dependence on a surgical assistant because of the availability of the fourth robotic arm.

Most recently, the same group reported outcomes of robot-assisted MDSC in a large, single-institutional series of 772 patients with chronic orchalgia.[40] Median patient age was 41 years, and median postoperative follow-up was 24 months. Complete resolution of pain was observed in 426 (49%) cases, improvement in pain in 292 cases (34%), and persistent pain in 142 cases (17%). Complications included hydrocele (2.7%), wound infection (1.5%), and testicular artery injury (0.2%). Overall, these success rates are slightly lower than those with the conventional microsurgical approach, but postoperative complication rates are similar.[41]

ROBOT-ASSISTED MICRODISSECTION TESTICULAR SPERM EXTRACTION

Nonobstructive azoospermia (NOA) affects approximately 10% of men presenting with infertility.[42] As was the case for the aforementioned procedures, the operating microscope revolutionized treatment for NOA with the initial description of the microTESE (microdissection testicular sperm extraction) procedure in 1998 by Schlegel.[43] Under high-power magnification, individual seminiferous tubules more likely to harbor sperm are identified and selectively harvested for further processing, resulting in higher success rates than conventional TESE.[44]

The theoretic advantages of the robotic platform for microTESE are few. Parekattil and colleagues reported the only series of robot-assisted microTESE, which they suggested could facilitate simultaneous visualization of the operative field and the andrology laboratory microscope, thereby allowing the surgeon to continue operating while assessing the testicular tissue, resulting in improved operative workflow and efficiency. The authors also reported easier testicular tissue dissection and tissue handling, along with improved surgeon ergonomics, compared with conventional microTESE, although no objective data or comparisons were performed.[33] In their

small series of 12 procedures, no complications were observed, and the authors found that robot-assisted microTESE was safe and effective. Patient characteristics, operative time, and sperm retrieval rates were not reported.

Certainly, additional studies are needed to assess the robotic approach to microTESE and determine its value added. The ability of the robotic platform to integrate video and imaging inputs from other sources does open the possibility for easy adoption of advanced imaging techniques for visualization of seminiferous tubules and sperm, should these become clinically available. For now, the data supporting this approach are limited.

THE FUTURE OF ROBOTIC SURGERY FOR MALE INFERTILITY

Although the robotic platform has been rapidly adopted by other urologic subspecialties, it has not yet taken hold among reproductive urologists. The paucity of data on robot-assisted male infertility surgery and the authors' anecdotal experience suggest that the robotic approach is rarely utilized by most reproductive urologists. Despite the theoretic benefits of robotic surgery, the outcomes to date have not justified its widespread use.

The reasons for low utilization of robotic surgery in this field are likely multifactorial. First, as mentioned previously, the data examining the approach are sparse. For each of the procedures described, the data are limited to case series. Where advantages of the robotic approach are posited (eg, better visualization or surgeon ergonomics), no studies have attempted to measure these outcomes rigorously. The few studies that have shown equivalent outcomes to the conventional microsurgical approaches will, at best, lead toward noninferiority of the robotic platform. However, this is an insufficient impetus for a paradigm shift in surgical approach for male infertility.

Second, traditional microsurgeons have remained skeptical regarding the delicate tissue handling capabilities of the robotic approach. Some have pointed to the lack of haptic feedback and dedicated microsurgical robotic instruments as limitations of the robotic approach, and additional studies are needed to examine the difference in tissue handling across platforms. Additionally, although early studies suggest relatively quick learning with the robotic approach, surgeon experience and comfort with the traditional microscope may limit widespread adaptability of the robot.

Third, costs have also been touted as a substantial drawback of robotic surgery. Initial capital investment for acquisition of a surgical robot can exceed that of an operating microscope by a factor of 10, which does not account for the high disposable costs of the robotic platform that are virtually nonexistent with the operating microscope.[45] Parekattil and colleagues[33] noted that the only path toward financial viability for the robotic model is to dramatically increase case volume. The authors found that the robotic platform almost doubled their operative efficiency, which justified the increased robotic costs. However, operative efficiency is not the only driver of patient volume. Some urologists may not have sufficient case volume (whether because of the nature their practice, size of catchment area, or other factors) to increase operative volume. In such instances, the robotic investment may not be financially viable. Alternatively, some reproductive urologists may operate within a health care system already in possession of a surgical robot, in which case the added use costs would be substantially less.

Beyond these concerns, the more recent arrival of video microsurgery for male infertility, although in its infancy, has the potential to undermine and outpace the potential advantages of robotic surgery in this specialty. Video microsurgery employs a heads-up approach, combining 3-dimensional imaging with 4K video output to provide a laparoscopy-like experience with high magnification and high-quality visualization.[46] This approach maintains the haptic feedback and delicate tissue-handling capabilities of traditional microsurgery while improving surgeon ergonomics and visualization. Like the robotic platform, it has the potential to integrate advanced imaging techniques with simultaneous video input, should these technologies arise. Although video microsurgery does not reduce surgeon tremor or obviate the need for a surgical assistant, it does have the potential to substantially improve on the conventional microsurgical experience. Importantly, the initial capital investment and ongoing disposable costs for video microsurgery are substantially lower than those for robotics.[45]

In order for robotic surgery to take hold and gain widespread adoption, multicenter, randomized trials are needed. The obstacles to performing these trials are many, not the least of which is the small number of centers currently performing this type of surgery. Moreover, other techniques, such as video microsurgery, that offer greater technical advantages have the potential to leapfrog robotic surgery for male infertility. Although the robotic platform offers potential added benefits for male infertility, rigorous clinical trials are needed to

compare outcomes and costs to those of other surgical platforms with validated outcomes. In the meantime, the evidence does not support the postulated incremental technical benefits justifying the substantial barriers to adoption.

DISCLOSURE

The authors have nothing to disclose.

REFERENCES

1. Thonneau P, Marchand S, Tallec A, et al. Incidence and main causes of infertility in a resident population (1,850,000) of three French regions (1988-1989). Hum Reprod 1991;6(6):811–6.
2. Pathak UI, Gabrielsen JS, Lipshultz LI. Cutting-edge evaluation of male infertility. Urol Clin North Am 2020;47(2):129–38.
3. Howarth AL, Hallbeck S, Mahabir RC, et al. Work-related musculoskeletal discomfort and injury in microsurgeons. J Reconstr Microsurg 2019;35(5):322–8.
4. Barone MA, Hutchinson PL, Johnson CH, et al. Vasectomy in the United States, 2002. J Urol 2006;176(1):232–6. discussion 236.
5. Dickey RM, Pastuszak AW, Hakky TS, et al. The evolution of vasectomy reversal. Curr Urol Rep 2015;16(6):40.
6. Belker AM, Thomas AJ, Fuchs EF, et al. Results of 1,469 microsurgical vasectomy reversals by the Vasovasotomy Study Group. J Urol 1991;145(3):505–11.
7. Schmidt SS, Brueschke EE. Anatomical sizes of the human vas deferens after vasectomy.** Presented at the Annual Meeting of the Pacific Coast Fertility Society, Palm Springs, California, October 18, 1975. Fertil Steril 1976;27(3):271–4.
8. Silber SJ. Microscopic vasectomy reversal. Fertil Steril 1977;28(11):1101–02.
9. Belker AM. Urologic microsurgery–current perspectives: I. Vasovasostomy. Urology 1979;14(4):325–9.
10. Schoor RA, Ross L, Niederberger C. Robotic assisted microsurgical vasal reconstruction in a model system. World J Urol 2003;21(1):48–9.
11. Kuang W, Shin PR, Matin S, et al. Initial evaluation of robotic technology for microsurgical vasovasostomy. J Urol 2004;171(1):300–3.
12. Fleming C. Robot-assisted vasovasostomy. Urol Clin North Am 2004;31(4):769–72.
13. Schiff J, Li PS, Goldstein M. Robotic microsurgical vasovasostomy and vasoepididymostomy: a prospective randomized study in a rat model. J Urol 2004;171(4):1720–5.
14. Parekattil SJ, Gudeloglu A, Brahmbhatt J, et al. Robotic assisted versus pure microsurgical vasectomy reversal: technique and prospective database control trial. J Reconstr Microsurg 2012;28(7):435–44.

15. Kavoussi PK. Validation of robot-assisted vasectomy reversal. Asian J Androl 2015;17(2):245–7.

16. Schiff J, Li PS, Goldstein M. Robotic microsurgical vasovasostomy and vasoepididymostomy in rats. Int J Med Robot 2005;1(2):122–6.

17. Parekattil SJ, Gudeoglu A, Brahmbhatt J, et al. Robotic assisted versus pure microsurgical vasectomy reversal: prospective control trial. Fertil Steril 2011; 96(3):S230–1.

18. Kavoussi PK, Harlan C, Kavoussi KM, et al. Robot-assisted microsurgical vasovasostomy: the learning curve for a pure microsurgeon. J Robot Surg 2019; 13(3):501–4.

19. Santomauro MG, Choe CH, L'Esperance JO, et al. Robotic vasovasostomy: description of technique and review of initial results. J Robot Surg 2012; 6(3):217–21.

20. Marshall MT, Doudt AD, Berger JH, et al. Robot-assisted vasovasostomy using a single layer anastomosis. J Robot Surg 2017;11(3):299–303.

21. Kuang W, Shin PR, Oder M, et al. Robotic-assisted vasovasostomy: a two-layer technique in an animal model. Urology 2005;65(4):811–4.

22. Najari BB, Li PS, Mehta A, et al. V1593 robotic-assisted laparoscopic mobilization of the vas deferens for correction of obstructive azoospermia induced by mesh herniorrhaphy. J Urol 2013; 189(4S). https://doi.org/10.1016/j.juro.2013.02.3143.

23. Trost L, Parekattil S, Wang J, et al. Intracorporeal robot-assisted microsurgical vasovasostomy for the treatment of bilateral vasal obstruction occurring following bilateral inguinal hernia repairs with mesh placement. J Urol 2014;191(4):1120–5.

24. Chan P, Parekattil SJ, Goldstein M, et al. Pros and cons of robotic microsurgery as an appropriate approach to male reproductive surgery for vasectomy reversal and varicocele repair. Fertil Steril 2018;110(5):816–23.

25. Clarke BG. Incidence of varicocele in normal men and among men of different ages. JAMA 1966; 198(10):1121.

26. Gorelick JI, Goldstein M. Loss of fertility in men with varicocele. Fertil Steril 1993;59(3):613–6.

27. Clavijo RI, Carrasquillo R, Ramasamy R. Varicoceles: prevalence and pathogenesis in adult men. Fertil Steril 2017;108(3):364–9.

28. Abdel-Meguid TA, Al-Sayyad A, Tayib A, et al. Does varicocele repair improve male infertility? An evidence-based perspective from a randomized, controlled trial. Eur Urol 2011;59(3):455–61.

29. Agarwal A, Deepinder F, Cocuzza M, et al. Efficacy of varicocelectomy in improving semen parameters: new meta-analytical approach. Urology 2007;70(3): 532–8.

30. Schauer I, Madersbacher S, Jost R, et al. The impact of varicocelectomy on sperm parameters: a meta-analysis. J Urol 2012;187(5):1540–7.

31. Al-Kandari AM, Shabaan H, Ibrahim HM, et al. Comparison of outcomes of different varicocelectomy techniques: open inguinal, laparoscopic, and subinguinal microscopic varicocelectomy: a randomized clinical trial. Urology 2007;69(3):417–20.

32. Shu T, Taghechian S, Wang R. Initial experience with robot-assisted varicocelectomy. Asian J Androl 2008;10(1):146–8.

33. Parekattil SJ, Gudeloglu A. Robotic assisted andrological surgery. Asian J Androl 2013;15(1):67–74.

34. McCullough A, Elebyjian L, Ellen J, et al. A retrospective review of single-institution outcomes with robotic-assisted microsurgical varicocelectomy. Asian J Androl 2018;20(2):189–94.

35. Costabile RA, Hahn M, McLeod DG. Chronic orchialgia in the pain prone patient: the clinical perspective. J Urol 1991;146(6):1571–4.

36. Levine LA, Hoeh MP. Evaluation and management of chronic scrotal content pain. Curr Urol Rep 2015; 16(6):36.

37. Davis BE, Noble MJ, Weigel JW, et al. Analysis and management of chronic testicular pain. J Urol 1990; 143(5):936–9.

38. Levine LA. Microsurgical denervation of the spermatic cord. J Sex Med 2008;5(3):526–9.

39. Parekattil SJ, Cohen MS. Robotic surgery in male infertility and chronic orchialgia. Curr Opin Urol 2010;20(1):75–9.

40. Calixte N, Tojuola B, Kartal I, et al. Targeted robotic assisted microsurgical denervation of the spermatic cord for the treatment of chronic orchialgia or groin pain: a single center, large series review. J Urol 2018;199(4):1015–22.

41. Strom KH, Levine LA. Microsurgical denervation of the spermatic cord for chronic orchialgia: long-term results from a single center. J Urol 2008; 180(3):949–53.

42. Wosnitzer M, Goldstein M, Hardy MP. Review of azoospermia. Spermatogenesis 2014;4:e28218.

43. Schlegel PN. Testicular sperm extraction: microdissection improves sperm yield with minimal tissue excision. Hum Reprod 1999;14(1):131–5.

44. Deruyver Y, Vanderschueren D, Van der Aa F. Outcome of microdissection TESE compared with conventional TESE in non-obstructive azoospermia: a systematic review. Andrology 2014;2(1):20–4.

45. Barbash GI, Glied SA. New technology and health care costs–the case of robot-assisted surgery. N Engl J Med 2010;363(8):701–4.

46. Hayden RP, Chen H, Goldstein M, et al. A randomized controlled animal trial: efficacy of a 4K3D video microscope versus an optical operating microscope for urologic microsurgery. Fertil Steril 2019;112(3):e93.

Robotic Surgery Training
Current Trends and Future Directions

Robert S. Wang, MD, Sapan N. Ambani, MD*

KEYWORDS

- Education • Curriculum • Robotics • Training • Simulation

KEY POINTS

- Current robotic surgery training during residency has not yet developed to reflect the increasing role of robotic surgery in the field of urology.
- A comprehensive robotic surgery curriculum should include robotic platform familiarization, preclinical simulation-based training, bedsiding and laparoscopic exposure, clinical exposure with competency-based progression, and nontechnical skills development.
- A variety of published curricula exist, but none has been adopted as the gold standard in the way the Fundamentals of Laparoscopic Surgery (FLS) has been for laparoscopic surgery training.

INTRODUCTION

The use of robotic surgery in urology has grown exponentially in the United States since the first robotic prostatectomy was performed in 2000. From 2003 to 2012, the percentage of radical prostatectomies performed robotically increased from 13.6% to 72.6%.[1] Similar expansions were observed in radical nephrectomies, pyeloplasties, and partial nephrectomies, among others.[1–3] Early efforts in education focused on promoting adoption by practicing urologists. Now that robotic surgery has firmly established itself within the field, proficiency has become an expectation, and attention has shifted toward ensuring that trainees are able to safely and effectively perform robotic surgery by the time they graduate. This article aims to provide an up-to-date overview of the current literature in the area of robotic surgery education, detailing existing resources and curricula available to learners and program directors, as well as upcoming innovations in how to best train the robotic surgeons of tomorrow.

NEEDS ASSESSMENT

Adoption of robotic surgery by urologists has been accompanied by an increasing recognition of the need for structured training. Studies early in the adoption of robotic surgery demonstrated uncertainty of the future role of this technology. In 2006, a survey of 372 residents and 56 program directors revealed limited experience and significant uncertainty about the role of robotics at the time.[4] Approximately 15% believed robotics was a "fad that will fail," 35% felt that it was "here to stay," and 50% were "unsure." Most residents were either unsure (33%) or doubtful (30%) that they would perform robotic surgery in practice. However, 74% of residents and program directors felt that use of robotic surgery would increase in the future. A survey of 56 senior urology residents in Canada from 2007 and 2008 revealed similar proportions of graduates expecting to perform robotic surgery in the future (29%–39%) and who felt that robotic surgery would increase in the future (71%–75%).[5]

A more recent 2019 survey of 59 American urology program directors and 61 chief residents/recent graduates revealed improved but persistent deficiencies in exposure, access to simulation, and comfort performing robotic urologic surgery independently.[6] Chief residents reported a lack of readiness for independent practice in pyeloplasty (60%), radical prostatectomy (61%), cystectomy (79%), and retroperitoneal surgery

Department of Urology, Michigan Medicine, 1500 East Medical Center Drive, TC 3875, Ann Arbor, MI 48109, USA
* Corresponding author.
E-mail address: sapan@med.umich.edu

Urol Clin N Am 48 (2021) 137–146
https://doi.org/10.1016/j.ucl.2020.09.014
0094-0143/21/© 2020 Elsevier Inc. All rights reserved.

(88%). Respondents reported rates of exposure to robotic surgery at 60% and access to a robotic simulator at 54% during residency. Program directors (PDs), on the other hand, reported robot exposure and simulator access at 98% and 88%, respectively. It is unclear whether this discrepancy represented hesitancy of PDs to report program deficiencies, perceived inadequacy of available exposure by trainees, or ongoing expansion of robotic training in the middle of the survey period. Whatever the reason, this survey provides strong evidence that current robotics training in the United States has not yet expanded to reflect the increasing importance of robotic surgery in our field.

PATIENT-SIDE TRAINING

Mastery of robotic surgery requires preparation before performing surgery at the console. Preconsole training involves ensuring the trainee has comfort in 3 areas: understanding the robotic system, bedside assistance, and basic laparoscopic skills. Comfort with each of these areas equips the trainee with the skills to troubleshoot issues when they become the lead surgeon.

Robotic Basics

An understanding of the components of the robotic system is critical for an effective robotic training curriculum, including the console and secondary console if available, remote manipulator arms, visualization support system (the "tower"), and robotic accessories, cables, and connectors. Trainees should be familiar with the various configurable console settings before their first robotic surgical experience. These include adjustable options such as console ergonomics, camera features, motion scaling, digital zoom, energy control, secondary console control, and communication. Robotic surgical systems come with a wide array of instruments, and training should include an awareness of all instruments and their uses. It is also helpful to be familiar with troubleshooting common errors, such as expired instruments or instrument collision.

Bedside Training

Bedside training offers learners 2 educational benefits.[7] As bedside trainees, residents are directly exposed to and interacting with the steps of the surgical procedure, and therefore have the opportunity to learn how the console surgeon conducts the operation. Second, operating as the bedside assistant helps the learner understand how the robotic arms interact with the patient to allow

effective surgical performance, and how to troubleshoot any issues that may interfere with the surgery. Cimen and colleagues[8] demonstrated improved console performance with trainees who had robotic bedside experience compared to those that did not. These findings were attributed to an increase in self-confidence and an ability to troubleshoot. Surgeons with bedside experience had the potential to handle challenging portions of a case at an earlier time than those with no experience. No learning curve for effective bedside experience has been established, and therefore a minimum number of cases to gain the necessary bedside assistant skills is unknown and likely varies based on the case. It is recommended that all robotic surgery trainees spend some time as a bedside assistant for all common robotic surgeries.

Laparoscopic Training

Robotic surgery is a form of minimally invasive surgery using a specialized tool that builds on the principles of standard laparoscopic surgery. Therefore, understanding the fundamentals of laparoscopic surgery is critical.

Appropriate patient positioning is an important step in successful robotic surgery. Proper positioning allows for optimization of patient safety and avoidance of complications, such as neurologic, musculoskeletal, and hemodynamic issues. Trainees should also understand how proper positioning and port placement allow for optimal spatial configuration and access to target organs while avoiding instrument clashes. Ergonomics for the bedside team (bedside assistant, scrub nurse, and anesthesia team) are also an important consideration when positioning the patient and robotic surgical arms. Trainees should develop comfort with the variations in patient positioning and port placement for transperitoneal and retroperitoneal cases.

Learners should become proficient in laparoscopic access, port placement, and creation of pneumoperitoneum. Insufflation leads to well-studied physiologic changes, and trainees should feel comfortable with both expected and unexpected hemodynamic changes during laparoscopic surgery. Although major complications occur in a small percentage of laparoscopic cases, trainees should understand the identification and management of both common and uncommon complications.[9] An excellent resource for laparoscopic fundamentals is the American Urologic Association (AUA) BLUS Handbook of Laparoscopic and Robotic Fundamentals[10] and its associated validated curriculum.[11,12]

CONSOLE-SIDE TRAINING

Most robotic surgery training focuses on developing the technical and cognitive skills required to operate at the surgical console. Once the basics of robotic and laparoscopic surgery are understood, this training should proceed concurrently with bedside training to help the learner develop a holistic understanding of the interactions between the patient, console surgeon, bedside assistant, robot instrumentation, and supporting team members. In our experience, most urologic training programs begin bedside assisting in the first 1 to 2 urology-focused years, transitioning to console training in the latter 1 to 2 years of residency.

Lee and colleagues[13] provided a 2-tiered framework for training of residents and fellows, divided into preclinical and clinical phases. In the preclinical phase, the learner is introduced to robotic surgery via didactics and hands-on familiarization with the platform, and then proceeds to develop his or her skills through a combination of virtual reality (VR), dry laboratory, and wet laboratory exercises. Once he or she passes a basic aptitude test, the learner is then allowed to proceed to the clinical phase of training. The trainee begins this phase by familiarizing themselves with specific procedures through reading and case observation, followed by bedsiding experience, and finally console operating time. For the surgery trainee who is beginning their robotic training, the authors recommend a graduated, stepwise progression of tasks under direct supervision of an expert surgeon. The goal is to learn the individual steps of an operation before putting them together to complete a case independently.

Simulation-Based Training

In preclinical robotic surgery training, surgical simulation can be achieved via dry laboratory, wet laboratory, and VR exercises. Each have unique advantages and disadvantages and are frequently combined in existing robotic surgery curricula. The term "dry laboratory" refers to skills practice using inanimate models such as transferring rings between pegs or suturing onto a sponge. In general, dry laboratories are a relatively inexpensive way to teach basic psychomotor skills, and therefore are often the preferred starting point in surgical skills curricula. However, dry laboratory tasks are also the most abstracted from real surgery, and continued practice is of limited utility once these basic skills have been acquired. Dry laboratories are typically succeeded by "wet laboratories," which replace the inanimate tasks with procedural practice using animal tissue, cadavers, or live animal subjects. With this increase in realism comes an increase in cost as well as the additional regulatory burdens involving cadaver and live animal use. In recent years, VR simulation has gained popularity in robotic surgery education as a complement and even a substitute for dry and wet laboratories. Compared with VR training in open and laparoscopic surgery, the loss of tactile feedback in VR robotics training is less of a factor. Current robotic surgery does not feature haptics, and future developments that allow for haptic feedback within the surgical platform can be adapted to simulators as well. Institutions hoping to include dry and wet laboratories in their curricula must consider either purchasing a dedicated platform reserved just for simulation, or using a clinically active robot that requires coordinating use with scheduled surgery. In comparison, VR trainers typically cost between $80,000 to $125,000 plus software and maintenance, depending on the platform. Hung and colleagues[14] compared the performances of novices and experts in structured (dry laboratory) inanimate tasks, simulated VR tasks, and a standardized live porcine model task. They found that performance on one type of tasks correlated significantly with performance on the other two, proposing the concept of "cross-method" validity in evaluation of surgical training modalities.

Virtual Reality Simulators

Purchasing a simulator as part of a robotics curriculum can be a large financial investment, and the curriculum developer should take into account cost, unique features, and validation status. Currently, there are 4 commercially available VR simulator platforms that have undergone validation studies: the dV-Trainer and da Vinci Skills Simulator (DVSS) (Mimic Technologies Inc., Seattle, WA), the Robotic Surgery Simulator (RoSS) (Simulated Surgical Systems LLC., San Jose, CA), and the RobotiX Mentor (3D Systems, Rock Hill, SC). A fifth simulator, the SEP robot (SimSurgery, Oslo, Norway), has been previously validated but is no longer available for purchase.[15,16] Common to all of these platforms are stereoscopic viewpieces, surgeon control handles, armrests, and foot pedals configured to mimic the da Vinci robot console, as well as software packages that include task-based (ie, knot-tying, suture-passing) and procedure-based (ie, radical prostatectomy) modules with built-in tracking of performance metrics.[17–19] The DVSS is unique in that it runs the same software as the dV-Trainer, but uses an existing da Vinci robot console as the physical interface, adding an extra layer of verisimilitude to the platform.[20] **Table 1** provides an at-a-glance summary of these platforms, their cost, and current validation status.

To understand the comparison of different simulators, a definition of relevant terminology is warranted. *Validity* refers to how well an instrument measures what it is intended to measure; subtypes of validity include *face* (does it look like what it is supposed to look like?), *content* (does it teach what it is supposed to teach?), *construct* (can it differentiate between experts and novices?), *concurrent* (does sim performance match real performance?), and *predictive* (does sim performance predict future real performance?).[21]

Of the 4, the dV-Trainer is the most well-established simulator, and supports the Mimic Technologies software suite which includes MSim psychomotor skills software, MaestroAR augmented reality procedure modules, and MScore proficiency tracking. The platform has multiple studies showing strong face and content validity even early on in development, with good data for construct and concurrent validity as well.[22–25] The estimated cost was approximately $110,000 in 2018.[26] In 2010, Mimic collaborated with Intuitive Surgical (Sunnyvale, CA) (developers of the da Vinci surgical robot) to adapt its software suite to the da Vinci console, creating the DVSS. The most obvious advantage of the DVSS is that the simulator and console are one and the same, but it is also the most well-validated: By virtue of using the same software, the validation studies for the dV-Trainer can be extrapolated to the DVSS, and additional studies have further supported the face, content, construct, concurrent, and predictive validity of the DVSS specifically.[27–31] The DVSS is officially supported by Intuitive in its *Da Vinci Residency and Fellowship Training Program Implementation Guide*.[32] Finally, it is the least expensive available option at $80,000 in 2018, though it becomes the most expensive by a large margin if factoring in the cost of the surgical console ($500,000) or the opportunity costs of not using said console for surgery.[26]

Similar to the dV-Trainer, the RoSS also contains independently-developed modules teaching basic psychomotor skills, as well as a procedure-based curriculum called Hands-on Surgical Training (HoST).[17] One unique feature of HoST is that it reverses the relationship between the surgeon control arms and the (simulated) robotic instruments to move the user's arms to match a recording of an actual surgery being performed on the console. Of note, the RoSS has only been validated for face and content, not construct, and these studies require external validation.[33,34] The platform's estimated cost was approximately $125,000 in 2011.[35]

Newest to the market is the RobotiX Mentor, which runs task-based and procedure-based modules developed in collaboration with Intuitive Surgical. So far, there has been one study validating to face, content, and construct.[36] The RobotiX Mentor was estimated to cost $137,000 in 2018.[26]

Two recent papers have been published comparing these platforms to one-another. Tanaka and colleagues (2015)[37] had participants complete one task each on the dV-Trainer, DVSS, and RoSS, and then complete questionnaires rating the validity and usability of each platform. In general, both the dV-Trainer and DVSS had favorable responses for face and content validity, whereas the RoSS did not. The RoSS also did not demonstrate construct validity in this limited study. In terms of usability, the DVSS was the most highly preferred. Hertz and colleagues[26] performed a similar study comparing the dV-Trainer, DVSS, and RobotiX Mentor. They found that all platforms had favorable ratings for face and content validity, but the scores for the DVSS were significantly higher.

Dual Console

Once a trainee advances to operating at the console, his or her learning experience becomes nearly completely determined by the teaching

Table 1
Commercially available robotic surgery simulators, cost, and validation status

Platform	Estimated Cost	Validation Status
dV-Trainer	$110,000	Face, content, construct, and concurrent
da Vinci Skills Simulator (DVSS)	$80,000 (console not included)	Face, content, construct, concurrent, and predictive
Robotic Surgery Simulator (RoSS)	$125,000	Face and content
RobotiX Mentor	$137,000	Face, content, construct

style of the supervising faculty surgeon. Nonetheless, there is one innovation in this space worth mentioning - the addition of a second surgical console in the operating room. In a dual-console setup, the trainee can sit down and see exactly what the surgeon is seeing as they operate, and control of instruments can be freely swapped between either console for effortless hand-off of the case between teacher and student. Morgan and colleagues (2015)[38] demonstrated the benefits of this system by examining 381 consecutive robot-assisted laparoscopic prostatectomies performed before (n = 185) and after (n = 196) introduction of a dual-console system at their teaching institution. On multivariable analysis, the cases performed with the dual-console setup had significantly lower average operative times (51 minutes) and intraoperative complication rates (1.5% vs 8.6%), without any statistically significant differences in blood loss, postoperative complication rates, surgical margin status, erectile function, continence rates, or biochemical recurrence rates.

Existing Curricula

Unlike the Fundamentals of Laparoscopic Surgery (FLS), which has become the preferred laparoscopic skills curriculum in most institutions and has been mandated by the American Board of Surgery for board eligibility,[39] no single curriculum has yet emerged as the gold standard in the field of robotic surgery. Many institutions and professional societies have published their own robotics curricula, with varying combinations of the educational tools described above. Given the numerous published robotic curricula, a few notable professionally supported and/or well-validated curricula worth elaborating on here. These can be adopted in their entirety, or can serve as useful templates in creating a curriculum that best suits the needs of a specific institution or learner population.

Of the existing published curricula, the Fundamentals of Robotic Surgery (FRS) curriculum published in 2013 by Smith and colleagues[40] is the most well-poised for widespread adoption. This comprehensive curriculum was developed over the course of 3 consensus conferences with multidisciplinary participation from surgeons, scientists, psychologists, educators, and representatives from 14 professional societies including the AUA and Society of American Gastrointestinal and Endoscopic Surgeons. After identifying consensus outcome measures for safe, effective robotic surgery, the development team split into 3 working groups to outline cognitive, psychomotor, and team-based curricula to target these core outcome measures. Additional

design goals included keeping the curriculum robotic-system agnostic (not limited to one robotic platform) and independent from industry influence. The final curriculum has been published online and is free-to-access at http://frsurgery.org/.[41] The 4 modules cover a basic introduction to laparoscopic and robotic surgery, didactics on the operation and troubleshooting of the surgical robot, a psychomotor skills curriculum, and nontechnical skills including team coordination, effective communication, and situational awareness. Progression through modules is proficiency-based. A 3D-printed physical trainer model (the "FRS dome") was created to test psychomotor skills in a dry laboratory setting, and a VR equivalent has also been developed. To date, one multi-institution multi-specialty study has been published evaluating the FRS and found that the curriculum led to comparable improvements in performance on an avian tissue model task when compared to preexisting robotics curricula.[42]

Other notable curricula include the Fundamental Skills of Robotic Surgery (FSRS), developed by the team behind the RoSS using their simulator, which is a fully VR curriculum with 4 modules covering basic console orientation, psychomotor skills training, basic surgical skills, and intermediate surgical skills. The group has published studies validating their curriculum to face, content, and construct validity.[43,44] For postgraduate urologists, McDougall and colleagues[45] described the creation of an intensive 5-day "mini-residency" for robot-assisted laparoscopic prostatectomy (RALP), combining didactic sessions, wet and dry laboratories, and operating room (OR) observation with the option for a proctored experience for attendee's first RALP at their home institution. In short term follow-up (median 7.2 months), the proportion of attendees performing RALP increased from 25% to 95%, and 25% also started doing robotic pyeloplasty. A follow-up study by Gamboa and colleagues[46] found that at 3 years, 81% of these original participants continued to include RALP as part of their practice, and several had expanded into robotic pyeloplasty, nephrectomy, and even cystectomy as well.

In 2018, Intuitive Surgical Inc. released its Da Vinci Residency and Fellowship Training Program Implementation Guide.[32] This guide presents a list of milestones to be met on the path to robotic surgery certification. Phase 1 covers online and in-service training to familiarize learners with the da Vinci platform. Phase 2 moves on to case observation and drills training through VR simulation and dry laboratory practicum. Phase 3 describes advanced skills practice and testing and initial operative experience as the bedside assistant. Finally, Phase 4 makes minimum case recommendations as bedside and console surgeon for completion of certification. Of note, the guide recommends the DVSS as the simulator to use for psychomotor skills exercises, and the FRS online curriculum as an alternative resource for robotic surgery training videos.

In terms of professional society participation, the European Association of Urology (EUA) section on robotic urologic surgery (ERUS) has developed an officially-endorsed robotics curriculum of its own.[47] Focus group interviews from EUA/ERUS meetings from 2012 to 2013 were analyzed and condensed into a proposed curriculum format that follows a familiar progression of online E-training modules, followed by simulation training in dry laboratory/wet laboratory/VR settings, then progressing to mentored OR training with progressive increase in responsibility. Unlike the other curricula described above, however, this format is then applied on a per-surgery basis. So far, versions of the ERUS curriculum have been developed and validated for robotic assisted radical prostatectomy and robotic assisted partial nephrectomy.[48,49] The AUA does not endorse one specific curriculum, but has made available a variety of resources including its BLUS handbook of laparoscopic and robotic fundamentals, a core curriculum module on the basics of laparoscopy and robotics, and guidelines regarding robotic urologic surgery standard operating procedure (SOP) covering minimum requirements for granting and maintaining urologic robotic privileges, and miscellaneous online and in-person courses.[10,50,51] Though resources are abundant, rates of utilization are unknown. Our own training program focuses heavily on patient-side training (both bedside and console-side), with most structured simulation training completed during a resident's preliminary year with the general surgery department.

ASSESSMENT TOOLS

Several validated tools have been developed to help standardize assessments of surgeon skill during robotic surgery. Chen and colleagues (2019) recently published a systematic review on this topic, providing a comprehensive overview of available robotic surgical skill assessment tools. Of these, the most widely-used and well-supported has been the Global Evaluative Assessment of Robotic Skills (GEARS).[52] Modeled after the Global Assessment for Open and Laparoscopic Surgery, with additions to reflect the unique challenges of robotic surgery, GEARS asks raters to rate surgeon performance on a scale from 1 to 5 in six domains: depth perception, bimanual

dexterity, efficiency, force sensitivity, autonomy, and robotic control. GEARS has demonstrated face, content, and construct validity in multiple studies.[52–54] It is quickly completed and procedure-agnostic, allowing for use in a wide range of applications, including the development of the ERUS and FRS robotic surgery curricula described above.[42,48] More recently, the use of crowdsourcing has come under investigation as a way to quickly and accurately complete surgeon performance assessments using large numbers of surgically-naive layperson raters.[55] Initial investigations of both simulated and real surgeries have demonstrated surprising levels of agreement between crowdsourced ratings obtained via the Crowd-Sourced Assessment of Technical Skill (C-SATS) and ratings by expert peer surgeons.[56–59]

NONTECHNICAL SKILLS

It is worth touching on the role of nontechnical skills in the successful performance of robotic surgery. Situational awareness, leadership, team coordination, and effective communication are all critical in maintaining a safe OR. Gawande and colleagues[60] examined a series of 146 surgical adverse events and the underlying contributing factors. Although inexperience/lack of competence was the most commonly cited contributing factor (53%), the next 5 most-common were all related to nontechnical skills: communication breakdown (43%), excessive workload/lack of staffing (22%), lack of supervision (21%), fatigue (16%), and interruptions/distractions (16%). These challenges are not unique to robotic surgery, but they can be exacerbated by the alterations to room dynamics that occur when the surgeon operates from a console that is physically separate from the OR table. This distance from the patient, monitoring hardware, and other members of OR team can negatively impact the surgeon's situational awareness. To address other team members, the surgeon speaks into a built-in microphone which transmits his or her voice through in-room speakers. The degradation of audio quality and the lack of nonverbal cues opens the door for communication breakdowns that may not occur in laparoscopic or open surgery. A growing recognition of the importance of nontechnical skills in these contexts led Raison and colleagues[61] to develop and validate an assessment tool specifically for robotic surgery, dubbed the Interpersonal and Cognitive Assessment for Robotic Surgery (ICARS). Nonetheless, formal instruction in developing these skills is lacking; of the notable published curricula described above, so far only the ERUS and FRS include modules on nontechnical skills.[40,47]

LEARNING CURVE

After completion of structured training, ongoing practice in robotic surgery is critical in improving surgeon efficiency and optimizing outcomes for patients. A 2017 review article by Mazzon and colleagues[62] on learning curves for robotic urologic surgeries paints a picture in which patient outcomes and surgeon comfort continue to improve well past the current minimum of 50 robotic surgery cases required by the Accreditation Council for Graduate Medical Education (ACGME) for graduation from residency.

For example, in RALP, the learning curve with respect to most measured outcomes (operative time, blood loss, early continence, potency, positive surgical margin rate) generally plateaued between 50 to 250 cases. However, there was significant heterogeneity in the referenced studies, and in one large study of 3794 patients the plateaus for operative time and positive surgical margins were reached at 750 and 1600 cases, respectively.

For robot-assisted radical cystectomy and robot-assisted partial nephrectomy, the learning curve plateaus appeared to be shorter, somewhere in the range of 20 to 100 cases depending on the study and the outcomes measured. Part of this may be explained in that surgeons attempting these procedures are likely already well-experienced in robotic surgery. Furthermore, there was once again significant variation in the data, and in some studies surgeons demonstrated continued improvement well beyond their initial 100 cases.

This need for additional experience has been recognized by the ACGME Review Committee for Urology, which is raising said minimum requirements from 50 cases to 80 cases for 2021 graduates.[63]

SUMMARY

Now is a critical period for robotic surgery education. Resources and references are in abundance, and the need for structured training has never been greater as the ability to perform robotic surgery has become a core competency for urology trainees. Advances in computing power and hardware development have pushed VR to the forefront of preclinical training, although wet and dry laboratories continue to help learners develop an intuition for the relationship between physical and virtual. In the clinical phase, there is broad agreement on a supervised, proficiency-based progression starting with case observation, then bedside assisting, followed by increasingly complex tasks at the console. Tools such as GEARS and ICARS have been developed as measures of proficiency, and crowd-sourcing is under investigation to facilitate this process. In the end, however, advancement is determined by the judgment of those supervising the trainees. Though a general consensus exists regarding the key components of training in robotic surgery, no single standard has emerged as a reference on which programs may build their curriculum. Programs such as the FRS and ERUS curricula are promising but have yet to achieve widespread adoption. As we prepare to enter the third decade of robotic surgery, the foundations have been laid for a standardized robotics curriculum, but much work remains to be done.

CLINICS CARE POINTS

1. The role of robotics in urology is increasing but training has lagged behind, with most graduating trainees reporting lack of comfort independently performing many robotic surgeries.

2. A complete robotic surgery curriculum should include formal didactics on the robotic platform, followed by a combination of patient-side and console-side training.

3. Patient-side training focuses on familiarization with the robotic setup, port placement, docking and undocking, using laparoscopic instruments, and troubleshooting common issues.

4. Console-side training starts with a combination of dry laboratory, wet laboratory, and VR simulation. Once proficiency has been demonstrated, trainees may advance to the clinical phase of training.

5. Currently, 4 VR simulator platforms are available for purchase to facilitate preclinical training. Selection should be guided by cost, availability, and validation status.

6. In the clinical phase, trainees should follow a graduated, stepwise progression of tasks under direct supervision of an expert surgeon, with the eventual goal of being able to perform the operation independently.

7. Numerous robotic surgery curricula have been published, but none have yet been adopted as the standard.

8. Nontechnical skills are a key component of robotic surgery and should be included in any comprehensive curriculum.

9. GEARS is an easy-to-use, well-validated assessment tool for technical performance during robotic surgery.

DISCLOSURE

No disclosures or Conflicts of Interest.

REFERENCES

1. Hu JC, O'Malley P, Chughtai B, et al. Comparative effectiveness of cancer control and survival after robot-assisted versus open radical prostatectomy. J Urol 2017;197(1):115–21.
2. Ghani KR, Sukumar S, Sammon JD, et al. Practice patterns and outcomes of open and minimally invasive partial nephrectomy since the introduction of robotic partial nephrectomy: results from the nationwide inpatient sample. J Urol 2014;191(4): 907–13.
3. Sukumar S, Sun M, Karakiewicz PI, et al. National trends and disparities in the use of minimally invasive adult pyeloplasty. J Urol 2012;188(3):913–8.
4. Duchene DA, Moinzadeh A, Gill IS, et al. Survey of residency training in laparoscopic and robotic surgery. J Urol 2006;176(5):2158–67.
5. Preston MA, Blew BDM, Breau RH, et al. Survey of senior resident training in urologic laparoscopy, robotics and endourology surgery in Canada. Can Urol Assoc J 2010;4(1):5.
6. Okhunov Z, Safiullah S, Patel R, et al. Evaluation of urology residency training and perceived resident abilities in the United States. J Surg Educ 2019; 76(4):936–48.
7. Sridhar AN, Briggs TP, Kelly JD, et al. Training in robotic surgery—an overview. Curr Urol Rep 2017; 18(8):58.
8. Cimen HI, Atik YT, Gul D, et al. Serving as a bedside surgeon before performing robotic radical prostatectomy improves surgical outcomes. Int Braz J Urol 2019;45(6):1122–8.
9. Soulié M, Salomon L, Seguin P, et al. Multi-institutional study of complications in 1085 laparoscopic urologic procedures. Urology 2001;58(6): 899–903.
10. Collins S, Lehman DS, McDougall EM, et al. AUA BLUS handbook of laparoscopic and robotic fundamentals. Linthicum Am Urol Assoc 2015;100: 200–300.
11. Kowalewski Timothy M, Sweet R, Lendvay TS, et al. Validation of the AUA BLUS Tasks. J Urol 2016;195(4 Part 1):998–1005.
12. Sweet RM, Beach R, Sainfort F, et al. Introduction and validation of the American Urological Association Basic Laparoscopic Urologic Surgery Skills Curriculum. J Endourol 2011;26(2):190–6.
13. Lee JY, Mucksavage P, Sundaram CP, et al. Best practices for robotic surgery training and credentialing. J Urol 2011;185(4):1191–7.
14. Hung AJ, Jayaratna IS, Teruya K, et al. Comparative assessment of three standardized robotic surgery training methods: Comparative assessment of standardized robotic surgery training methods. BJU Int 2013;112(6):864–71.
15. Gavazzi A, Bahsoun AN, Van Haute W, et al. Face, content and construct validity of a virtual reality simulator for robotic surgery (SEP Robot). Ann R Coll Surg Engl 2011;93(2):152–6.
16. van der Meijden OA, Broeders IA, Schijven MP. The SEP "robot": a valid virtual reality robotic simulator for the Da Vinci Surgical System? Surg Technol Int 2010;19:51–8.
17. RoSS II – Simulated Surgicals, LLC. Available at: http://simulatedsurgicals.com/projects/ross/. Accessed February 26, 2020.
18. RobotiX Mentor | Simbionix. Available at: https:// simbionix.com/simulators/robotix-mentor/. Accessed February 26, 2020.
19. dV-Trainer®. Mimic Simulation. Available at: https:// mimicsimulation.com/dv-trainer/. Accessed February 24, 2020.
20. Inside dV-Trainer®Partnership. Mimic Simulation. Available at: https://mimicsimulation.com/inside-dv-trainerpartnership/. Accessed February 26, 2020.
21. McDougall EM. Validation of surgical simulators. J Endourol 2007;21(3):244–7.
22. Lendvay TS, Casale P, Sweet R, et al. Initial validation of a virtual-reality robotic simulator. J Robot Surg 2008;2(3):145–9.
23. Kenney PA, Wszolek MF, Gould JJ, et al. Face, content, and construct validity of dV-Trainer, a novel virtual reality simulator for robotic surgery. Urology 2009;73(6):1288–92.
24. Sethi AS, Peine WJ, Mohammadi Y, et al. Validation of a novel virtual reality robotic simulator. J Endourol 2009;23(3):503–8.
25. Lee JY, Mucksavage P, Kerbl DC, et al. Validation study of a virtual reality robotic simulator—role as an assessment tool? J Urol 2012;187(3):998–1002.
26. Hertz AM, George EI, Vaccaro CM, et al. Head-to-head comparison of three virtual-reality robotic surgery simulators. JSLS 2018;22(1). https://doi.org/10.4293/JSLS.2017.00081.
27. Hung AJ, Zehnder P, Patil MB, et al. Face, content and construct validity of a novel robotic surgery simulator. J Urol 2011;186(3):1019–25.
28. Hung AJ, Patil MB, Zehnder P, et al. Concurrent and predictive validation of a novel robotic surgery simulator: a prospective, randomized study. J Urol 2012; 187(2):630–7.
29. Liss MA, Abdelshehid C, Quach S, et al. Validation, correlation, and comparison of the da Vinci Trainer TM and the da Vinci Surgical Skills Simulator TM Using the Mimic TM software for urologic robotic surgical education. J Endourol 2012;26(12):1629–34.
30. Kelly DC, Margules AC, Kundavaram CR, et al. Face, content, and construct validation of the da Vinci Skills Simulator. Urology 2012;79(5):1068–72.

31. Finnegan KT, Meraney AM, Staff I, et al. da Vinci Skills Simulator construct validation study: correlation of prior robotic experience with overall score and time score simulator performance. Urology 2012;80(2):330–6.

32. Da Vinci residency and fellowship training program implementation guide. 2018. Available at: https://www.intuitive.com/en-us/-/media/Project/Intuitive-surgical/files/pdf/davinci-resident-fellows-training-guide-1024650.pdf?la=en&hash=A755B62C01C010BA6C1A4F00EF7F2734. Accessed February 26, 2020.

33. Seixas-Mikelus SA, Kesavadas T, Srimathveeravalli G, et al. Face validation of a novel robotic surgical simulator. Urology 2010;76(2):357–60.

34. Seixas-Mikelus SA, Stegemann AP, Kesavadas T, et al. Content validation of a novel robotic surgical simulator. BJU Int 2011;107(7):1130–5.

35. Lallas CD, Davis JW, Members of the Society of Urologic Robotic Surgeons. Robotic surgery training with commercially available simulation systems in 2011: a current review and practice pattern survey from the Society of Urologic Robotic Surgeons. J Endourol 2012;26(3):283–93.

36. Whittaker G, Aydin A, Raison N, et al. Validation of the RobotiX Mentor Robotic Surgery Simulator. J Endourol 2015;30(3):338–46.

37. Tanaka A, Graddy C, Simpson K, et al. Robotic surgery simulation validity and usability comparative analysis. Surg Endosc 2016;30(9):3720–9.

38. Morgan MSC, Shakir NA, Garcia-Gil M, et al. Single- versus dual-console robot-assisted radical prostatectomy: impact on intraoperative and postoperative outcomes in a teaching institution. World J Urol 2015;33(6):781–6.

39. Okrainec A, Soper NJ, Swanstrom LL, et al. Trends and results of the first 5 years of Fundamentals of Laparoscopic Surgery (FLS) certification testing. Surg Endosc 2011;25(4):1192–8.

40. Smith R, Patel V, Satava R. Fundamentals of robotic surgery: a course of basic robotic surgery skills based upon a 14-society consensus template of outcomes measures and curriculum development: fundamentals of robotic surgery. Int J Med Robot 2014;10(3):379–84.

41. Fundamentals of robotic surgery. Available at: http://frsurgery.org/. Accessed March 3, 2020.

42. Satava RM, Stefanidis D, Levy JS, et al. Proving the effectiveness of the fundamentals of robotic surgery (FRS) skills curriculum: a single-blinded, multispecialty, multi-institutional randomized control trial. Ann Surg 2019. https://doi.org/10.1097/SLA.0000000000003220.

43. Stegemann AP, Ahmed K, Syed JR, et al. Fundamental skills of robotic surgery: a multi-institutional randomized controlled trial for validation of a simulation-based curriculum. Urology 2013;81(4):767–74.

44. Raza SJ, Froghi S, Chowriappa A, et al. Construct validation of the key components of Fundamental Skills of Robotic Surgery (FSRS) curriculum—a multi-institution prospective study. J Surg Educ 2014;71(3):316–24.

45. McDougall EM, Corica FA, Chou DS, et al. Short-term impact of a robot-assisted laparoscopic prostatectomy 'mini-residency' experience on postgraduate urologists' practice patterns. Int J Med Robot 2006;2(1):70–4.

46. Gamboa AJR, Santos RT, Sargent ER, et al. Long-term impact of a robot assisted laparoscopic prostatectomy mini fellowship training program on postgraduate urological practice patterns. J Urol 2009;181(2):778–82.

47. Ahmed K, Khan R, Mottrie A, et al. Development of a standardised training curriculum for robotic surgery: a consensus statement from an international multidisciplinary group of experts. BJU Int 2015;116(1):93–101.

48. Volpe A, Ahmed K, Dasgupta P, et al. Pilot validation study of the European Association of Urology Robotic Training Curriculum. Eur Urol 2015;68(2):292–9.

49. Larcher A, De Naeyer G, Turri F, et al. The ERUS Curriculum for Robot-assisted Partial Nephrectomy: structure definition and pilot clinical validation. Eur Urol 2019;75(6):1023–31.

50. AUA Core Curriculum - Laparoscopy and Robotics. Available at: https://university.auanet.org/modules/webapps/core/index.cfm#/corecontent/129. Accessed January 19, 2020.

51. AUA guidelines - Robotic Surgery (Urologic) Standard Operating Procedure (SOP). Available at: https://www.auanet.org/guidelines/robotic-surgery-(urologic)-sop. Accessed January 19, 2020.

52. Goh AC, Goldfarb DW, Sander JC, et al. Global evaluative assessment of robotic skills: validation of a clinical assessment tool to measure robotic surgical skills. J Urol 2012;187(1):247–52.

53. Sánchez R, Rodríguez O, Rosciano J, et al. Robotic surgery training: construct validity of Global Evaluative Assessment of Robotic Skills (GEARS). J Robot Surg 2016;10(3):227–31.

54. Aghazadeh MA, Jayaratna IS, Hung AJ, et al. External validation of Global Evaluative Assessment of Robotic Skills (GEARS). Surg Endosc 2015;29(11):3261–6.

55. Chen C, White L, Kowalewski T, et al. Crowd-sourced assessment of technical skills: a novel method to evaluate surgical performance. J Surg Res 2014;187(1):65–71.

56. Ghani KR, Miller DC, Linsell S, et al. Measuring to improve: peer and crowd-sourced assessments of

technical skill with robot-assisted radical prostatectomy. Eur Urol 2016;69(4):547–50.

57. Vernez SL, Huynh V, Osann K, et al. Assessing surgical skills among urology residency applicants. J Endourol 2016;31(S1):S–95.

58. Holst D, Kowalewski TM, White LW, et al. Crowdsourced assessment of technical skills: an adjunct to urology resident surgical simulation training. J Endourol 2014;29(5):604–9.

59. Powers MK, Boonjindasup A, Pinsky M, et al. Crowdsourcing assessment of surgeon dissection of renal artery and vein during robotic partial nephrectomy: a novel approach for quantitative assessment of surgical performance. J Endourol 2015;30(4):447–52.

60. Gawande AA, Zinner MJ, Studdert DM, et al. Analysis of errors reported by surgeons at three teaching hospitals. Surgery 2003;133(6):614–21.

61. Raison N, Wood T, Brunckhorst O, et al. Development and validation of a tool for non-technical skills evaluation in robotic surgery—the ICARS system. Surg Endosc 2017;31(12):5403–10.

62. Mazzon G, Sridhar A, Busuttil G, et al. Learning curves for robotic surgery: a review of the recent literature. Curr Urol Rep 2017;18(11):89.

63. ACGME Review Committee for Urology. New urology case log minimums: effective 2021 graduates. 2020. Available at: https://www.acgme.org/Portals/0/PFAssets/ProgramResources/480-Uro-Case-Log-Mins2021.pdf?ver=2020-02-24-161557-147. Accessed March 16, 2020.

Competing Robotic Systems: A Preview

Michael Wilson, DO[a],*, Ketan Badani, MD[b]

KEYWORDS

• Verb • Medtronic • DaVinci • Zeus • MEERE • TransEnterix • Titan • Robotic frontier

KEY POINTS

- Competing robotic systems are being developed with the goal to make smaller, cheaper, and more accessible robots worldwide.
- Each company is improving artificial intelligence to provide the best care for patients.
- The future of surgery is ultimately still undefined.

INTRODUCTION

The new frontier of robotic surgery is well under way and has begun to foster an industrial revolution in the medical community. Current research and development is rapidly progressing, allowing for the creation of many new companies. Each company has its own identity and platform for what their vision for the future entails. A driving force behind this revolution is a current surgical industry that accounts for $500 billion of health care spending with 5% to 10% of the market being allocated to robotics. This is estimated to grow to $20 billion by 2020.[1] Therefore, as history has taught us, competition will shortly be forcing newer, cheaper, more accessible robotic systems worldwide.

Since the early 2000s, robotics in urology has long been synonymous with DaVinci, with more than 1700 systems worldwide.[2] As competition increases, it is important to understand what each new robotic system offers and how it can benefit the medical community over what is offered today. There is one true fact for the new robotic frontier, "It's here and there are exciting things to come."

To discuss the future of robotics, we first need to understand how we arrived to the current robotic platform. The first Food and Drug Administration (FDA) approved surgical system on the market was the Automated Endoscopic System for Optimal Positioning (AESOP), which was created by Computed Motion Inc. in 1994. This was used for the master slave system called ZEUS in 2001. In 2003, it was acquired by Intuitive Surgical. This led to the creation of the first FDA-approved robotic laparoscopic surgical system, DaVinci.[3] At that time, Zeus was less expensive that DaVinci, at a rate of 975,000 to 1M, however, because of the superior adoption of DaVinci and its ergonomics, the Zeus was discontinued.

Intuitive Surgical (Sunnyvale, CA) has been considered the leader in the current robot marketplace since the early 2000s. Its DaVinci robotic system has been synonymous with robotic surgery, with more than 1700 systems worldwide. It was the first robotic platform commercially available for general laparoscopic surgery.[2]

Currently there are 4 DaVinci robotic systems in use, the Si, X, Xi, and SP.[1] The SP[1] is a single port system first approved for urologic procedures, followed by lateral oropharyngectomy and tongue-based resections.[4] The Xi is the most recent generation robotic system, with some major technological advancements over Si, notably the rotational boom. Approximately 86% of urology residencies have a DaVinci robotic system and more than 75% of all prostate surgeries are performed with a DaVinci robot.[2]

[a] Department of Urology, Icahn School of Medicine at Mount Sinai, 1425 Madison Avenue, 6th Floor, New York City, NY 10029, USA; [b] Department of Urology, Mount Sinai Hospital, Icahn School of Medicine at Mount Sinai Hospital, 5 East 98th Street, New York, NY 10029, USA
* Corresponding author.
E-mail address: Michael.Wilson@mountsinai.org

Urol Clin N Am 48 (2021) 147–150
https://doi.org/10.1016/j.ucl.2020.09.007
0094-0143/21/© 2020 Elsevier Inc. All rights reserved.

VERB

Verb Surgical (Santa Clara, CA) was created as a joint venture between Google and Johnson & Johnson, 9 months after their partnership began in 2015 with the goal to generate Surgery 4.0.[5] Since that time, the company has created its first digital prototype in January of 2017.[6] Much detailed information is still behind the veil of secrecy due to ongoing research and development. However, over the years since its conception, the company has acquired several other robotic-based companies such as Auris Health (Redwood City, CA), with the Monarch robotic system (bronchoscopy robotic platform) and Orthotaxy (orthopedic-based robotic company) to aid to its divisions.[7] The mission of the company is democratize surgery with goal of connecting surgeons to an end-to-end platform.[8]

One may wonder what exactly is Surgery 4.0. Well, Surgery 4.0 considered by VERB CEO Scott Huennekens as "If you think of open surgery as Surgery 1.0, minimally invasive surgery and laparoscopic surgery as Surgery 2.0, robotics surgery as 3.0, we really think that the next era is 4.0."[5] The clear understanding of what that new frontier of surgery 4.0 is yet to be defined. The goal, however, is clear: make robots smaller, more accessible, and cheaper. The company's goal is to make the robots 20% the size they currently are and allow the surgeon to be closer to the patient.[9] This new system would be able to incorporate preoperative, intraoperative, and postoperative imaging all while at bedside and performing procedures.

The VERB surgical system is based on 5 pillars that consist of Robotics, Advance instrumentation, Enhanced Visualization, Connectivity, and Machine Learning with data analytics.[10] The robot system itself is meant to provide machine learning in order to be an active bedside assistant. Again, allowing more surgeons to become facile with a goal to democratize surgery.

MEDTRONIC

Medtronic has joined the robotic revolution with its new system, HUGO. They have already been in the spine robotic surgery sector after acquiring Mazor Robotics in 2018. Medtronic partnered with Karl Storz SE & Co, in 2019 and unveiled HUGO in September of 2019 with its modularity and 3-dimensional (3-D) console being hallmarked. It has the standard tower, console, robotic arms cart, and surgical end effectors; however, the uniqueness of this new system is its robotic arms, which are individualized, on wheels, and modular. Therefore, arms can be maneuvered easily and help increase operative efficiency. The tower is multipurpose, as well. The main differences in the console compared with current standards, are its open nature with 3-D high-definition glass. Medtronic has even made the computer system easily compatible with upgrades. Some reports indicate that the system will be trialed outside of the United States, with aspirations of US approval in 2 years.[11]

MEERE

A new to the market Korean-based system is the Revo-I. It is currently based strictly out of Korea and produced by the Meere company. It is a 3-part system, similar to current models used elsewhere with a control console, operative cart, and vision cart. Recently it was approved by the Ministry of Food and Drug Safety in Korea. Revo-I was launched in 2018 in Seoul, South Korea. The hallmark for this new system is cost. The Revo-I is 42% less than the DaVinci system. It's unique software tailors to surgeon skill set, circumstances, and knowledge base. Currently it is approved for gynecology, cholecystectomy, and prostatectomy cases.[12]

AVATERA

Avatera (Jena, Germany) is a German-based company with a robotic system consisting of a 4-arm robot control unit and a flexible surgeon console seat with haptic manual input devices and footswitches. There are no external fans, allowing for low noise level. Instruments are 5 mm in size with $7°$ of freedom.[13] Each instrument is single-use only with the goal to improve function, reliability, and sterility. The company's goal was to eliminate contamination associated with the use of multiuse instruments.

Avatera's initial goal is to increase growth of robotic systems in Europe. This was based on the statistics that there are 8.5 robotic systems per 1 million people in the United States compared with 1 robot system to 1 million people in Europe. To increase robotic use in Europe, they have even developed a training center. Current cost is $1.1 million with plans to roll out production in 2020.[14,15]

MEDICAROID

Medicaroid (San Jose, CA) is a company that was established in 2013 in a joint venture between Kaawasaki Heavy Industries and SYSMEX, a Japan-based research and development Kobe Biomedical Innovation cluster. It currently has ongoing research and a robotic system under development.[16]

TransEnterix

TransEnterix (Morrisville, NC) is a surgical company that was founded in 2006. Its robotic system, SurgiBot, is a multiport robotic system with haptic feel and eye-sensing camera controls. Also tauted is the SPIDER system, which allows for more strength, ergonomics, and 360-degree control. A unique aspect of the system is there is no direct docking to the patient. The instruments are reusable and have a specific "pause" control, which allows instruments to stay in place when moved. There is a digital fulcrum on the instruments that help to minimize incision trauma. The learning curve is reportedly shorter than most systems. In the United States, the system is approved for hernias, cholecystectomy, gynecology, and colorectal surgery. In Europe, it currently is only approved for abdominal/pelvic surgery.[17,18]

The SurgiBot also takes aim at lowering the cost of a robotic system. Reportedly DaVinci costs approximately $1.5 million, plus $150,000 per year in system maintenance, with an average cost per procedure of $1600. In comparison, the Surgibot will cost approximately $800,000, with procedure costs of approximately $1600.[19]

TransEnterix has observed and made efforts to address performance-related injuries as well. There is an 87% performance-related injury associated with current robot use. The most common injuries reported are neck pain, rotator cuff injury, and carpal tunnel. In extreme cases, 12% of surgeons require a leave of absence due to their injuries. In response to these new data, TransEnterix developed the Senhance surgical system, which has already obtained numerous awards and is approved in the Japanese market (second largest robotic market) for general surgery, gynecology, urology, and thoracic surgery.[20]

TITAN MEDICAL

Titan Medical is a Toronto-based company with the goal of operating at a lower cost with more efficiency. They have created the Sport Surgical System. It consists of an open surgeon work station and a single arm mobile patient cart. It has multiarticulated instruments that are single use and specifically for small surgical spaces.[21] Outside of the Sport Surgical System, Titan has developed the single-incision laparoscopic surgery system that has two 8-mm arms that work via a 2.5-cm incision supraumbilically. The system also has a self-retaining retractor.[22]

Every one of the aforementioned robotic companies has their own unique style and vision of what the future of robotics will be. The goals of making more compact, cheaper, more accessible robotic systems seems to be a clear theme among all of them. Most of these companies use DaVinci as the gold standard for comparison due to their vast market presence and history. These companies will only continue to grow into established brands and continue to challenge current standards. As these robotics systems improve and become more automated, the days of the master slave control may be long gone.

Current improvements in surgery such as Firefly and the Micro Hand S (China-based aid for general surgery) are providing new ways to operate with the goal to not only improve overall care, but to decrease overall costs. One interesting area of which robotics has only scratched the surface is pediatrics. Given the small confined spaces, it would only seem plausible that robotics drastically would improve pediatric surgery. This could be why companies like Avatera and Titan Medical are focusing on smaller instruments and incisions.

In conclusion, the theme that has been present with every robotic company is to make surgery more cost-effective. Each company has tried to improve artificial intelligence in the interest of providing the best care for patients, whether it be decreasing infection risk by removing reusable instruments or to having more maneuverable arms to allow for more patients to be scheduled. The idea is clear, everyone has a different view of what is important in the new era of robotics.

DISCLOSURE

The author has nothing to disclose.

REFERENCES

1. Swanson C. Move over, Intuitive Surgical, here's How Johnson and Johnson and Google plan to build a better robot. The Motley Fool. 2016. Available at: https://www.fool.com/investing/2016/09/21/move-over-intuitive-surgical-heres-how-johnson-joh.aspx. Accessed February 3, 2020.
2. About the Davinci surgical system. UC Health. 2020. Available at: https://www.uchealth.com/services/robotic-surgery/patient-information/davinci-surgical-system/. Accessed February 20, 2020.
3. Schaaf T. MedTech Strategist History-Surigcal Robotics: Part 1. MedTech Strategist. 2018. Available at: https://www.mystrategist.com/blog/article/medtech-history-robotics-1. Accessed February 2, 2020.

4. About DaVinci systems. Davinci surgery. Available at: https://www.davincisurgery.com/da-vinci-systems/about-da-vinci-systems. Accessed February 20, 2020.

5. Al Idrus A. Verb Surgical. Fierce biotech. 2017. Available at: https://www.fiercebiotech.com/special-report/fiercemedicaldevices-2016-fierce-15-verb-surgical. Accessed February 2, 2020.

6. Verb Surgical delivers digital surgery prototype demonstration to collaborate partners. Verb Surgical. 2017. Available at: https://www.verbsurgical.com/media-article/verb-surgical-delivers-digital-surgery-prototype-demonstration-to-collaboration-partners/. Accessed February 2, 2020.

7. Pedersen A. J&J talks up Surgical Robotic plans. Medical Device and Diagnostic Industry. 2019. Available at: https://www.mddionline.com/jj-talks-surgical-robotics-plans. Accessed February 2, 2020.

8. About. Verb Surgical. 2020. Available at: https://www.verbsurgical.com/about/. Accessed January 31, 2020.

9. Pierson R. J&J, Alphabet aim for smarter, smaller, cheaper, surgical robot. Reuters. 2015. Available at: https://www.reuters.com/article/us-alphabet-johnson-johnson-robots-idUSKBN0TT1SB20151210. Accessed February 11, 2020.

10. Physicians. Verb Surgical. 2020. Available at: https://www.verbsurgical.com/physicians/. Accessed January 31, 2020.

11. Newmarker C. Medtronic finally unveils its new robot-assisted surgery system. Mass Device. 2019. Available at: https://www.massdevice.com/medtronic-finally-unveils-its-new-robot-assisted-surgery-system/. Accessed February 4, 2020.

12. Hye-seon L. Locally developed surgical robot unveiled, developer expects to reduce cost for patients, hospitals. Korean Biomedical Review. 2018. Available at: http://www.koreabiomed.com/news/articleView.html?idxno=2800. Accessed February 4, 2020.

13. Avatera system. Avatera. 2020. Available at: https://www.avatera.eu/en/avatera-system. Accessed February 14, 2020.

14. Cairns E. Avatera Medical becomes the newest robotic surgery group in Europe. Evaluate. 2019. Available at: https://www.evaluate.com/vantage/articles/interviews/avatera-medical-becomes-newest-robotic-surgery-group-europe. Accessed February 15, 2020.

15. CE mark for Avatera, the first German system for robot-assisted, minimally invasive surgery, setting the foundation for strategic growth plans. Avatera. 2019. Available at: https://www.avatera.eu/en/home/news-detail?tx_news_pi1%5Bnews%5D=19&cHash=0b499a1adf30ef40b4d441aa562e0a7b. Accessed February 16, 2020.

16. Medicaroid Corporation commences full-fledged development of medical robots. Medicaroid. 2015. Available at: http://www.medicaroid.com/en/pdf/20150402_01.pdf. Accessed February 2, 2020.

17. The first in digital laparoscopy: Senhance Surgical. Senhance. 2020. Available at: https://www.senhance.com/us/digital-laparoscopy. Accessed February 5, 2020.

18. Indications. Senhance. 2020. Available at: https://www.senhance.com/indications. Accessed February 5, 2020.

19. Parmar A. The robots have arrived. Medical device and diagnostic industry. 2016. Available at: https://www.mddionline.com/robots-have-arrived/page/4/0. Accessed January 28, 2020.

20. Perriello B. TransEnterix wins Japanese OK for Senhance in robot-assisted surgery. Mass Device. 2019. Available at: https://www.massdevice.com/transenterix-wins-japanese-ok-for-senhance-in-robot-assisted-surgery/. Accessed February 4, 2020.

21. Technology. Titian Medical. 2020. Available at: https://titanmedicalinc.com/technology/. Accessed February 6, 2020.

22. Estape R. Early acute in-vivo experience in gynecology oncology applications with the SPORT Surgical System Technology. Titan Medical. 2018. Available at: https://titanmedicalinc.com/wp-content/uploads/2018/01/Estape-TWP-GYO-Applications-Final-December-2017-1.pdf. Accessed February 6, 2020.

Current Trends in Artificial Intelligence Application for Endourology and Robotic Surgery

Timothy C. Chang, MD[a,b,*], Caleb Seufert, MD[a], Okyaz Eminaga, MD, PhD[a], Eugene Shkolyar, MD[a], Jim C. Hu, MD, MPH[c], Joseph C. Liao, MD[a,b]

KEYWORDS

• Artificial intelligence • Urology • Deep learning • Endourology

KEY POINTS

• Artificial intelligence algorithms are being used to process complex medical datasets to develop diagnostic, prognostic and therapeutic tools in urology.
• Endourology and robotic surgery are particular areas suitable for applications in artificial intelligence due to the optical imaging and robotic control systems data that is generated.
• Development of these tools are promising and still underway, but additional research to establish robust results is needed in order to achieve the goal of improving patient outcomes.

INTRODUCTION

First introduced 6 decades ago, artificial intelligence (AI) is a computational tool that reproduces or simulates human intellectual processes such as problem solving, reasoning, and learning. Although no universally accepted definition for AI exists,[1] Nil J. Nilsson, a pioneer in the field, described AI as machines that displayed the ability to function "appropriately" and with "foresight."[2] The development and application of AI technology has been historically confined by computational power and availability of high-quality big data. In the past decade, technological advances in AI, particularly in deep learning, and large-scale data digitalization have led to breakthroughs in the field. The biomedical research community has taken notice, and there has been a rapid increase in interest that is reflected by the exponential increase in health care–related AI publications in recent years.[3]

ARTIFICIAL INTELLIGENCE OVERVIEW

AI is rooted in cognitive science, statistical learning, optimization, and probability theories.[4] *Machine learning* is a form of AI where machines use algorithms to learn from data to refine the programmed outcomes. Alan Turing, an early pioneer in computer science and AI, wrote a seminal paper in 1950 entitled "Computing Machinery and Intelligence" that pondered whether a machine could demonstrate behavior or thinking similar to humans[5] and proposed the Turing Test to determine if a computer possessed AI with thought processes similar to humans. Over the following decades, the development of AI went through peaks and lulls until a renaissance in the 2010s following a breakthrough of a deep learning system in detecting and classifying objects for the 2012 ImageNet competition.[6] AI has been harnessed to produce self-driving motor vehicles, devices that execute voice commands, real-time

[a] Department of Urology, Stanford University School of Medicine, 300 Pasteur Drive, S-287, Stanford, CA 94305, USA; [b] Veterans Affairs Palo Alto Health Care System, 3801 Miranda Ave, Mail Code 112, Palo Alto, CA 94304, USA; [c] Department of Urology, Weill Cornell Medicine-New York Presbyterian Hospital, 525 E 68th Street, Starr Pavilion, Ninth Floor, New York, NY 10065, USA
* Corresponding author.
E-mail address: tcchang@stanford.edu

Urol Clin N Am 48 (2021) 151–160
https://doi.org/10.1016/j.ucl.2020.09.004

geographic directions, and ride-sharing apps. These advancements have been made possible through the convergence of 3 critical components: (1) sophisticated algorithms such as deep learning systems capable of deciphering significant signal from noise; (2) increasingly efficient microprocessors capable of quickly performing complex calculations; and (3) the acquisition, availability, and storage of large quantities of digital data.

AI aims to replicate human intellectual abilities by using computational algorithms and data analytics. This includes machine learning algorithms that help to solve classification, prediction, or anomaly problems. *Deep learning* is one of the advanced machine learning approaches used to solve various computer vision problems and modeling using artificial neural networks.[7] There have been different types of neural networks proposed, but a main driver in using neural networks to solve computer vision tasks has been the development of *convolutional neural networks* (CNNs). CNNs have recently come to the forefront of AI due to their efficacy in navigating different problems related to image classification, object detection, or segmentations based on representation or feature learning.[8,9] This breakthrough essentially allows machines to "see" objects that has revolutionized the field of computer vision.

ARTIFICIAL INTELLIGENCE IN HEALTH CARE

The use of AI is gaining prominence in the fields of biomedical science and clinical health care. Over the past decade, there has been an unprecedented growth in the volume of clinical data available in digital form through the wide-spread adoption of electronic medical health records and the emergence of data storage and sharing platforms. Currently, clinicians and researchers are faced with the challenge of attempting to synthesize and understand an overwhelming volume of health care data. As a result, AI has gained traction, as it harnesses the ever-increasing computational processing power available for data mining to extract meaningful signal from noisy background.

As noted, one of the major breakthroughs of AI is the ability for machines to essentially "see" objects through the development of CNNs. In radiology, AI has been used to recognize complex patterns in imaging data and provide quantitative assessments of imaging characteristics.[10] Examples include detection of suspicious nodules on chest radiographs[11] and liver masses on computed tomographic scans.[12] Pathology, with development of whole-slide imaging platforms and digital pathology, is another specialty ripe for

AI disruption. Digital image processing allows AI algorithms to detect complex patterns critical to pathologic diagnosis.[13] Examples include the detection of breast cancer metastases in digital pathology slides[14] and lymph node metastases of breast cancer in whole-slide images.[15] Examples of other medical fields well suited for AI applications include dermatology,[16] ophthalmology,[17] and gastroenterology,[18] as the increasing availability of big data curated across health care are driving the development of generalizable AI applications.

ARTIFICIAL INTELLIGENCE IN UROLOGY

Urology was an early adopter of AI going back over 2 decades in applications for prostate cancer diagnosis[19] and prognosis.[20,21] Given the scale of disease burden and unmet clinical needs, prostate cancer has fueled significant interest for the development of new diagnostic (eg, digital pathology, high throughput sequencing), imaging (eg, multimodal, multiparametric MRI), and surgical (image-guided and minimally invasive surgery) technologies, all of which have potential for integration with AI.

Increasingly, multiparametric MRI (mpMRI) is playing an important role in the detection and surveillance of prostate cancer.[22] The Prostate Imaging Reporting and Data System score is now the recognized standard to assess the significance of observed prostatic lesions on mpMRI, but there has been considerable variation in the reproducibility of the imaging findings.[23] Therefore, AI techniques are being explored to analyze these mpMRI images in order to optimize the accuracy of findings and overall diagnosis of prostate cancer.[24–27]

Beyond prostate cancer, recent AI-related studies in urology include detection of clinically significant hydronephrosis on renograms,[28] automated classification of sperm,[29] and predicting postoperative outcomes after percutaneous nephrolithotomy.[30] The AI applications described thus far, along with many others in all different areas of urology,[31–33] are being developed for the diagnostic and prognostic aspects of patient care. However, AI is proving to be a powerful tool in the active treatment of patients, as it is being used as an adjunctive tool in the operative setting (**Fig. 1**). The rest of this article focises on applications in endourology and robotic urologic surgery.

ARTIFICIAL INTELLIGENCE IN ENDOUROLOGY
Lower Urinary Tract

Lower and upper urinary tract endoscopy has long been integral in the diagnosis and treatment of

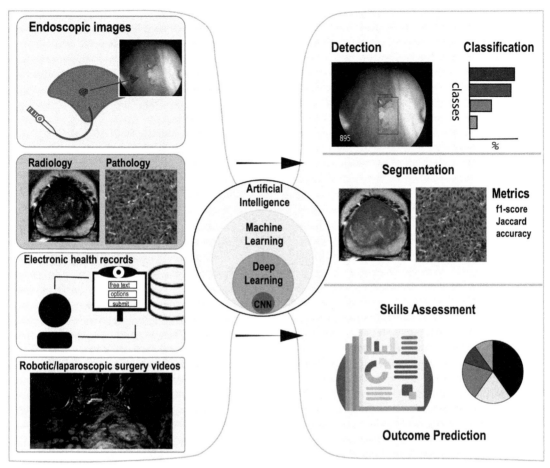

Fig. 1. Emerging applications of artificial intelligence (AI) in urology. AI has emerged as an enabling tool to manage and extract clinically meaningful signal from large, complex datasets curated from a variety of sources. Object detection, image classification, segmentation, skills assessment, and outcome prediction are examples of tasks that AI can apply to health care data. AI has been applied to endourology and robotic surgery, showing strong potential for improved bladder cancer detection and the development of surgical skill assessments and outcome prediction for complex urologic procedures.

urologic malignancies, urinary stones, and anatomic abnormalities within the genitourinary system. As such, significant efforts have been undertaken by multiple teams to develop AI applications for cystoscopic evaluation of the bladder, including deep learning for object detection, image classification, and image segmentation,[7] which allows machines to see and identify objects in cystoscopy images. Cystoscopies are one of the most common urologic procedures. The volume of cases, combined with an existing repository of data, makes this procedure an appropriate target for AI applications.

Bladder cancer is the 10th most common malignancy, with nearly 550,000 new cases globally in 2018.[34] Currently, bladder cancer diagnosis and tumor staging are completed by visual inspection of the bladder with cystoscopy and histopathological examination of tissue samples obtained by transurethral resection. Because of a wide spectrum of morphologic appearances and user experience, cystoscopy at times can be limited in differentiating between malignant and benign bladder lesions.

In 2018, Gosnell and colleagues investigated 3 different machine learning classifiers (linear regression, quadratic regression, and naïve Bayes) for bladder cancer detection.[35] They annotated 233 cystoscopy images (110 malignant and 123 benign) using pathologic examination as the standard. When machine learning algorithms were compared with the pathology assessments of specimens, linear regression demonstrated a higher overall accuracy and also a higher false-negative rate compared with the quadratic and naive Bayes classifiers. Quadratic and naive Bayes classifiers, in contrast, detected 100% of malignant images but had 50% to 60% false-positive rate, primarily of inflammation or scars. With the goal of developing a triaging system for cystoscopy that would favor detection of all malignancies, the investigators favored the quadratic or the naive Bayes classifiers over the linear classifier. Although this study approach was limited by accuracy and low sample size, it demonstrated the potential capability of machine learning for identifying bladder cancer on cystoscopy images.

In a separate study, Eminaga and colleagues was the first to apply deep learning with convolutional neural networks to analyze cystoscopy images derived from a digital atlas.[36] A total of 479 images representing 44 different benign and malignant bladder lesions were used to train, validate, and test 7 deep learning systems. The results showed greater than 95% accuracy of classification for all 7 models tested. Of the inaccurately classified images, 7.86% were of bladder stone images and 1.43% were of indwelling catheters. Limitations of the study include the highly selective nature of the images, thereby optimizing the performance of the system compared with real-world settings where image quality can be degraded by varying differences in magnification, contrast, and illumination.

Ikeda and colleagues obtained cystoscopy images from 109 patients (97 men, 12 women), encompassing 1671 normal images and 431 malignant images, to train a convolutional neural network.[37] Approximately 20% of the images were used for testing of the diagnostic algorithm. Overall area under the receiving operator characteristic curve was 0.98, with a sensitivity of 89.7% and specificity of 94.0% reported for the image classification task. The areas under the curve (AUCs) were all greater than 0.90 for the different types of tumors as well (elevated tumors 0.98, flat 0.96, mixed 0.99). The study noted that tumors comprising less than 10% of the image had a lower AUC of 0.88, whereas images with larger tumors comprising 10% to 50% and greater than 50% of the images both had AUC of 0.99, suggesting that smaller tumors may be missed or incorrectly identified compared with larger tumors using this model.

These early studies highlight the capability of AI in classifying cystoscopy images with the presence or absence of cancer. **Fig. 2**A illustrates an example of a *classification* task, where the algorithm provides a diagnosis and a measurement of its probability for an image. Deep learning systems are also capable of outlining and tracking objects of interest during real-time cystoscopic evaluation. **Fig. 2**B demonstrates an example of

object detection of a bladder tumor with bounding boxes. Similar to classification tasks, a diagnosis and confidence measurement can be provided for each box within images. Furthermore, deep learning systems can perform *semantic segmentation* as demonstrated in **Fig. 2**C, where the borders of the objects it detects in the images can be highlighted.

Incorporating object detection and semantic segmentation capabilities of deep learning to cystoscopy, Shkolyar and colleagues developed CystoNet, a convolutional neural network capable of tumor detection and dynamic tracking in cystoscopy videos.[38] Derived from a total of 100 patients, images from 141 videos were first used for model training, followed by a separate validation dataset of 57 videos from 54 patients. A per-frame sensitivity of 90.9% and specificity of 98.6% in identifying bladder tumors was achieved. Of the visualized tumors, 39 of 41 papillary tumors and 3 out of 3 flat tumors were detected. The videos obtained represented cases seen in clinical practice, with a range of tumor sizes from a few millimeters to greater than 5 cm, both solitary and multifocal tumors, and low- and high-grade tumors. Cystoscopic visibility and quality varied due to differences in patient physiology, illumination, cystoscopes (flexible vs rigid), and location of procedure (clinic vs operating room). The accuracy demonstrated by CystoNet in detecting multiple tumors and tracking them using high-definition video streaming holds promise for improving overall detection of tumors and may allow for more complete tumor resection. Future directions for use include model training to include flat tumors particularly carcinoma in situ and algorithm optimization to enable real-time operating room integration during transurethral resection.

Cystoscopy remains an essential but imperfect modality for bladder cancer detection, often missing multifocal, smaller tumors, and having limited accuracy with flat lesion malignancies.[39] Work done in applying AI to cystoscopy over the past few years has begun to demonstrate the capability AI has in improving the detection and localization of bladder tumors and atypical mucosa during cystoscopy. **Table 1** summarizes the studies to date in AI applications in cystoscopy. Future goals would include increasing the overall accuracy of detection, more refined tumor boundary segmentations, and real-time integration of this promising technology.

Finally, another promising adjunctive technology for bladder cancer imaging is confocal laser endomicroscopy (CLE). In contrast to the macroscopic bladder view visualized under standard white light cystoscopy, CLE provides microscopic

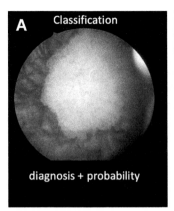
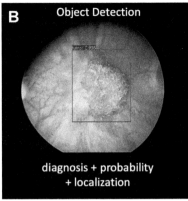
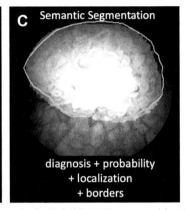

Fig. 2. Examples of image analysis capabilities of convolutional neural networks (CNNs). (*A*) CNNs are capable of classifying images to provide a diagnosis and a measurement of its probability. (*B*) Object detection provides localization of a diagnosed object within an image and also provides a measurement of its probability. (*C*) Semantic segmentation provides outlining of the borders of a given object in addition to the diagnosis, probability, and localization.

level imaging in real time similar in scale to the level of histopathology.[40] A probe is introduced into the working channel of the cystoscope, and objects of interest are imaged by direct contact of the probe on the object. Interpretation of the CLE images in real time depends on user experience level, as there is interobserver variation.[41] In a pilot study, AI was used with the goal of producing a reliable and automated interpretation of CLE images. Lucas and colleagues designed a recurrent neural network that was able to achieve accurate differentiation of benign versus malignant bladder urothelium in 79% of CLE images.[42] The system was also able to accurately differentiate high-grade and low-grade papillary tumors in 82% of CLE images. Although CLE is not widely adopted at this time, it suggests how AI can be applied as an enabling technology to facilitate introduction of new-generation enhanced imaging technologies with complex data output.

Table 1
Overview of studies using artificial intelligence for cystoscopy image analysis

Study	Data	AI Model	Accuracy
Gosnell et al,[35] 2018	233 still images from diagnostic and surveillance cystoscopy	Linear, quadratic, and naïve Bayes classifiers	100% detection of malignancy, 50%–60% false-positive rate for quadratic and naïve Bayes classifiers
Eminaga et al,[36] 2018	479 still images from digital atlas	7 deep learning models	>95% accuracy for all 7 models
Ikeda et al,[37] 2020	2102 still images from 124 cystoscopies. 431 images used for test set	Deep learning	Overall AUC 0.98, sensitivity 89.7%, specificity 94.0%
Shkolyar et al,[38] 2019	198 videos from cystoscopies. 2335 normal and 417 tumor annotated frames used for training set. 1002 normal and 211 tumor frames used for validation set	Deep learning	Perframe sensitivity 90.9% and specificity 98.6% Pertumor sensitivity 95.5%

Data from Refs.[35–38]

Upper Urinary Tract

Most of the AI applications in endourology to date have focused on lower urinary tract and bladder cancer, but AI concepts are also applicable to the upper urinary tract and noncancerous indications, particularly urinary stones. Identification of anatomic structures or stones during ureteroscopy could prove to be a valuable tool for surgical decision-making. Two studies looked at automated classification of stone composition based on ex vivo images taken after stone extraction. Serrat and colleagues used a traditional machine learning approach with the random forest classifier to achieve an accuracy of 63% for classifying 8 different kidney stone compositions from 454 stones.[43] Using a deep learning algorithm for image classification, Black and colleagues trained a convolutional neural network by presenting 127 digital images from 63 stones (17 uric acid, 21 calcium oxalate monohydrate, 7 struvite, 4 cystine, and 14 brushite stones). This model achieved an overall weighted recall of 85% for stone composition.[44] These studies were not performed with images obtained during ureteroscopy, and further work is needed for translation of the ex vivo work to clinical practice.

There are no known reports of AI applications to upper tract urothelial carcinoma, where the need for image classification is arguably greater than the bladder, given the challenges of obtaining high-quality biopsy samples. As AI application in the upper urinary tract remains in the earliest stage, there are opportunities for research through groundwork laid out in work with imaging in the lower urinary tract.

ARTIFICIAL INTELLIGENCE IN ROBOTIC SURGERY
Artificial Intelligence in Surgical Skills

Surgical skill and performance assessment have traditionally been completed through peer assessment, which requires an expert surgeon to evaluate a less-experienced surgeon's performance. This process is often considered laborious, time intensive, introduces significant interobserver variability, and is overall nonscalable. The importance of surgical skill could also be a key determinant of patient outcomes,[45] and as a result there has been growing interest to improve the assessment of surgical skill.

Over the past 25 years, many traditional open urologic surgeries have been replaced by minimally invasive approaches, first laparoscopic then robotic. The instruments for traditional laparoscopic and robotic-assisted surgery are capable of capturing kinematic data and high-quality surgical footage through a laparoscopic camera. Specifically, robotic surgery platforms are capable of outputting metrics such as instrument position, total distance traveled, speed, curvature, time to task completion, camera movement, and grip force.[46,47] These metrics can be recorded from the robot and analyzed to give objective data related to a particular surgical operator. The availability of kinematic data and high-quality endoscopic camera footage provides the potential to evaluate surgical performance more effectively and objectively through the use of AI applications.

There are several studies that have paved the way for integration of AI into improving the assessment of surgical skills. Ghani and colleagues assessed whether peer surgeons and crowd-sourced evaluation of robotic-assisted radical prostatectomy could distinguish technical skill among the recorded surgeon. The study revealed a strong correlation in the assessment of surgical skills between a group of peer surgeons and crowd-sourced review,[48] which suggests that the 2 groups agreed on the rank order of lower scoring surgeons. However, the study lacked information tied to patient outcomes, which would quantify the clinical significance of these findings. Later, a validated surgical skills evaluation tool called the Global Evaluative Assessment of Robotic Skills (GEARS) noted a correlation with surgeon skill and clinical outcomes for radical prostatectomies. GEARS score, which indicates increased surgical competency, were independently predictive of 3-month continence status following robotic-assisted surgery.[49] However, similar to peer review, the use of GEARS to assess surgical performance is limited by the time consuming nature of video reviews and relatively subjective assessments of viewers.

To develop a more objective approach to assessing surgical skill level, Law and colleagues developed an instrument-associated tracking system using video data and computational deep learning to create a model to assess technical skill.[50] With the tracking data obtained from a limited set of 12 videos, a separate support vector machine (SVM) classifier was trained to categorize high or low surgeon skill based on the tracking data. The performance of this system was greater than 83.3%, meaning the SVM classifier system accurately predicted skill level, albeit on a limited data set. Although this study used video files from robotic surgeries, this approach has possible applications in the assessment of surgical skills during laparoscopic procedures, because only video data are needed.

Hung and colleagues (Jan. 2018) successfully conducted a pilot study that explored and validated surgeon performance metrics while completing a robotic-assisted radical prostatectomy. A novel recorder, "dVLogger," was used to directly capture several objective metrics, which were then compared between novice and expert robotic surgeons. Parameters that were assessed included the differences between the 2 groups in task completion time, instrument travel distance, and camera movement.[46] The assessed metrics demonstrated experts to be more efficient and directed during surgery and provided a foundation for developing standardized metrics for surgical training and assessment.

In a follow-up study by Hung and colleagues (May 2018) using the same data sets, machine learning algorithms were used to process automated performance metrics (APMs) data to predict clinic outcomes in the form of length of hospital stay.[51] APMs are data describing instrument motion tracking, and the goal of the study was to process the APMs to determine what metrics led to the best short-term clinical outcome, measured by the patient's length of hospital stay (≤ 2 days and >2 days). Of the 3 traditional machine learning algorithms used, the random forest–50 model resulted in an accuracy of 87.2% for predicting hospital length of stay. APMs such as camera manipulation were associated with surgeon performance, but this skill may be one that is passively developed and demonstrated in highly skilled surgeons but not actively developed.[52]

Using APMs from robotic-assisted radical prostatectomy procedures, Hung and colleagues (2019)[53] developed a deep learning algorithm to predict postoperative urinary continence. The APMs from 8 surgeons were analyzed with a conventional Cox regression model, a machine learning model with random survival forests, and a deep learning algorithm named "DeepSurv." The top 5 APM features predicting continence were used to separate the surgeons into 2 groups (group 1 vs group 2). The higher scoring group had superior rates of urinary continence at 3 months (47.5% vs 36.7%, $P = .034$) and 6 months (68.3% vs 59.2%, $P = .047$) postoperatively. The investigators note limitations of the study including the small sample set of 8 surgeons and the unbalanced number of cases per surgeon, which may have contributed to a C-index score of 0.599. Further evaluations will be necessary to understand the relevance and predictive values of APM scores and clinical outcomes. Both machine learning algorithms ("DeepSurv" and random survival forests) were overall superior to the Cox regression model in predicting postoperative urinary continence.

To further build on the previously cited studies, Zia and colleagues (2018)[54] described a methodology using both video and APM data to develop a system capable of recognizing 12 key steps during RARP surgery. This was in contrast to the previous studies that analyzed data from the entire surgery to assess surgical skill using either video data alone or APM data alone. Collected data in the study by Zia and colleagues (2018) was presented to several deep learning systems for testing, including a CNN called "RP-Net" based on InceptionV3. A dataset of 100 RARPs surgeries were used to develop this system. The highest performance metrics recognizing the key steps was achieved by the "RP-Net" based algorithm. Subsequent work by the Zia and colleagues (2019) led to the development of a new deep learning system called "RP-Net-V2" that recognizes the 12 steps of RARP that outperformed its predecessor.[55]

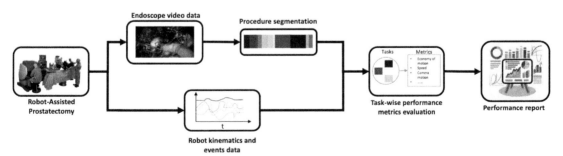

Fig. 3. Automated performance report generation from analysis of video, kinematic and events data from robotic surgery. Robotic systems generate digital data such as video, robot kinematic and events data, which can be segmented into different parts of surgical procedures. AI algorithms process these data to generate performance reports based on clinically relevant endpoints. (*From* Zia A, Guo L, Zhou L, Essa I, Jarc A. Novel evaluation of surgical activity recognition models using task-based efficiency metrics. *International journal of computer assisted radiology and surgery.* 2019;14(12):2155-2163.)

Surgeon performance metrics computed for the automatically identified tasks overall showed correlation with tasks labeled by clinicians, although there were some tasks that performed worse than others.

This series of studies in robotic surgery demonstrates the feasibility of obtaining objective metrics that can be analyzed with machine learning and deep learning algorithms to evaluate surgeon performance (**Fig. 3**). The overall results are limited at this time due to the relatively small data sets and size of the studies, but the studies suggest the potential capability of AI in processing larger datasets to elucidate relationships and correlations within a sea of APM data. With this capability, more objective assessments of surgical skill can be developed. Surgical performance on robotic procedures and clinical outcomes using objective data are beginning to be evaluated in surgical training programs.[56,57] However, further development of robust models will be needed to promulgate widespread use of AI in training programs and ultimately improve patient outcomes.

SUMMARY

Recent advances in AI and its initial applications in endourology and robotic surgery have provided a glimpse of the strong potential AI holds to improve diagnosis and treatment of urologic diseases, as well as the potential to assist in the development of skill acquisition required for complex urologic surgeries. Although deep learning enables the investigation of large data sets, the implementation of AI still faces considerable obstacles such as heterogenous data infrastructure between different health care organizations and the need for collaboration between computer scientists and surgeons. Modalities such as cystoscopy and robotic video/image-based data have shown promise, with initial studies however requiring additional research to establish more robust results and better ways to incorporate AI in an effort to improve patient outcomes.

REFERENCES

1. Stone P, Brooks R, Brynjolfsson E, et al. Artificial intelligence and life in 2030. One hundred year study on artificial intelligence: report of the 2015-2016 study panel, vol. 6. Stanford (CA): Stanford University; 2016. Available at: http://ai100.stanford.edu/2016-report. Accessed September, 2016.
2. Nilsson NJ. The quest for artificial intelligence : a history of ideas and achievements. Cambridge (United Kingdom): Cambridge University Press; 2010.
3. Tran BX, Vu GT, Ha GH, et al. Global evolution of research in artificial intelligence in health and medicine: a bibliometric study. J Clin Med 2019;8(3):360.
4. Vapnik VN. An overview of statistical learning theory. IEEE Trans Neural Netw 1999;10(5):988–99.
5. Turing AM. I.—Computing machinery and intelligence. Mind 1950;LIX(236):433–60.
6. Krizhevsky, Alex, Ilya Sutskever, and Geoffrey E. Hinton. "Imagenet classification with deep convolutional neural networks." In Advances in neural information processing systems, pp. 1097-1105. 2012.
7. Schmidhuber J. Deep learning in neural networks: An overview. Neural Networks 2015;61:85–117.
8. Nanni L, Ghidoni S, Brahnam S. Handcrafted vs. non-handcrafted features for computer vision classification. Pattern Recognition 2017;71:158–72.
9. LeCun Y, Bengio Y, Hinton G. Deep learning. Nature 2015;521(7553):436–44.
10. Giger ML. Machine learning in medical imaging. J Am Coll Radiol 2018;15(3):512–20.
11. Nam JG, Park S, Hwang EJ, et al. Development and validation of deep learning–based automatic detection algorithm for malignant pulmonary nodules on chest radiographs. Radiology 2019;290(1):218–28.
12. Yasaka K, Akai H, Abe O, et al. Deep learning with convolutional neural network for differentiation of liver masses at dynamic contrast-enhanced CT: a preliminary study. Radiology 2018;286(3):887–96.
13. Serag A, Ion-Margineanu A, Qureshi H, et al. Translational AI and deep learning in diagnostic pathology. Front Med 2019;6:185.
14. Liu Y, Kohlberger T, Norouzi M, et al. Artificial intelligence–based breast cancer nodal metastasis detection: Insights into the black box for pathologists. Arch Pathol Lab Med 2019;143(7):859–68.
15. Bejnordi BE, Veta M, Van Diest PJ, et al. Diagnostic assessment of deep learning algorithms for detection of lymph node metastases in women with breast cancer. JAMA 2017;318(22):2199–210.
16. Esteva A, Kuprel B, Novoa RA, et al. Dermatologist-level classification of skin cancer with deep neural networks. Nature 2017;542(7639):115–8.
17. Wong TY, Bressler NM. Artificial intelligence with deep learning technology looks into diabetic retinopathy screening. Jama 2016;316(22):2366–7.
18. Wang P, Xiao X, Brown JRG, et al. Development and validation of a deep-learning algorithm for the detection of polyps during colonoscopy. Nat Biomed Eng 2018;2(10):741–8.
19. Snow PB, Smith DS, Catalona WJ. Artificial neural networks in the diagnosis and prognosis of prostate cancer: a pilot study. J Urol 1994;152(5):1923–6.
20. Partin AW, Kattan MW, Subong EN, et al. Combination of prostate-specific antigen, clinical stage, and Gleason score to predict pathological stage of

localized prostate cancer: a multi-institutional update. Jama 1997;277(18):1445–51.
21. Anagnostou T, Remzi M, Lykourinas M, et al. Artificial neural networks for decision-making in urologic oncology. Eur Urol 2003;43(6):596–603.
22. Ahmed HU, Bosaily AE-S, Brown LC, et al. Diagnostic accuracy of multi-parametric MRI and TRUS biopsy in prostate cancer (PROMIS): a paired validating confirmatory study. Lancet 2017;389(10071):815–22.
23. Sonn GA, Fan RE, Ghanouni P, et al. Prostate magnetic resonance imaging interpretation varies substantially across radiologists. Eur Urol Focus 2019;5(4):592–9.
24. Ishioka J, Matsuoka Y, Uehara S, et al. Computer-aided diagnosis of prostate cancer on magnetic resonance imaging using a convolutional neural network algorithm. BJU Int 2018;122(3):411–7.
25. Algohary A, Viswanath S, Shiradkar R, et al. Radiomic features on MRI enable risk categorization of prostate cancer patients on active surveillance: Preliminary findings. J Magn Reson Imaging 2018;48(3):818–28.
26. Ginsburg SB, Algohary A, Pahwa S, et al. Radiomic features for prostate cancer detection on MRI differ between the transition and peripheral zones: preliminary findings from a multi-institutional study. J Magn Reson Imaging 2017;46(1):184–93.
27. Toivonen J, Montoya Perez I, Movahedi P, et al. Radiomics and machine learning of multisequence multiparametric prostate MRI: Towards improved non-invasive prostate cancer characterization. PLoS One 2019;14(7):e0217702.
28. Blum ES, Porras AR, Biggs E, et al. Early detection of ureteropelvic junction obstruction using signal analysis and machine learning: a dynamic Solution to a dynamic Problem. J Urol 2018;199(3):847–52.
29. Riordon J, McCallum C, Sinton D. Deep learning for the classification of human sperm. Comput Biol Med 2019;111:103342.
30. Aminsharifi A, Irani D, Pooyesh S, et al. Artificial neural network system to predict the postoperative outcome of percutaneous nephrolithotomy. J Endourol 2017;31(5):461–7.
31. Suarez-Ibarrola R, Hein S, Reis G, et al. Current and future applications of machine and deep learning in urology: a review of the literature on urolithiasis, renal cell carcinoma, and bladder and prostate cancer. World J Urol 2020;38(10):2329–47.
32. Checcucci E, Autorino R, Cacciamani GE, et al. Artificial intelligence and neural networks in urology: current clinical applications. Minerva Urol Nefrol 2019;72(1):49–57.
33. Chen J, Remulla D, Nguyen JH, et al. Current status of artificial intelligence applications in urology and their potential to influence clinical practice. BJU Int 2019;124(4):567–77.
34. Bray F, Ferlay J, Soerjomataram I, et al. Global cancer statistics 2018: GLOBOCAN estimates of incidence and mortality worldwide for 36 cancers in 185 countries. CA Cancer J Clin 2018;68(6):394–424.
35. Gosnell ME, Polikarpov DM, Goldys EM, et al. Computer-assisted cystoscopy diagnosis of bladder cancer. Urol Oncol 2018;36(1):8.e9-15.
36. Eminaga O, Eminaga N, Semjonow A, et al. Diagnostic Classification of Cystoscopic Images Using Deep Convolutional Neural Networks. JCO Clin Cancer Inform 2018;2:1–8.
37. Ikeda A, Nosato H, Kochi Y, et al. Support System of Cystoscopic Diagnosis for Bladder Cancer Based on Artificial Intelligence. J Endourol 2020;34(3):352–8.
38. Shkolyar E, Jia X, Chang TC, et al. Augmented Bladder Tumor Detection Using Deep Learning. Eur Urol 2019;76(6):714–8.
39. Grossman HB, Soloway M, Messing E, et al. Surveillance for recurrent bladder cancer using a point-of-care proteomic assay. JAMA 2006;295(3):299–305.
40. Wu K, Liu J-J, Adams W, et al. Dynamic real-time microscopy of the urinary tract using confocal laser endomicroscopy. Urology 2011;78(1):225–31.
41. Chang TC, Liu J-J, Hsiao ST, et al. Interobserver agreement of confocal laser endomicroscopy for bladder cancer. J Endourol 2013;27(5):598–603.
42. Lucas M, Liem EI, Savci-Heijink CD, et al. Toward Automated In Vivo Bladder Tumor Stratification Using Confocal Laser Endomicroscopy. J Endourol 2019;33(11):930–7.
43. Serrat J, Lumbreras F, Blanco F, et al. myStone: A system for automatic kidney stone classification. Expert Syst Appl 2017;89:41–51.
44. Black KM, Law H, Aldoukhi A, et al. Deep learning computer vision algorithm for detecting kidney stone composition. BJU Int 2020;125(6):920–4.
45. Birkmeyer JD, Finks JF, O'Reilly A, et al. Surgical skill and complication rates after bariatric surgery. N Engl J Med 2013;369(15):1434–42.
46. Hung AJ, Chen J, Jarc A, et al. Development and Validation of Objective Performance Metrics for Robot-Assisted Radical Prostatectomy: A Pilot Study. J Urol 2018;199(1):296–304.
47. Judkins TN, Oleynikov D, Stergiou N. Objective evaluation of expert and novice performance during robotic surgical training tasks. Surg Endosc 2009;23(3):590–7.
48. Ghani KR, Miller DC, Linsell S, et al. Measuring to Improve: Peer and Crowd-sourced Assessments of Technical Skill with Robot-assisted Radical Prostatectomy. Eur Urol 2016;69(4):547–50.
49. Goldenberg MG, Goldenberg L, Grantcharov TP. Surgeon Performance Predicts Early Continence After Robot-Assisted Radical Prostatectomy. J Endourol 2017;31(9):858–63.

50. Law, H., Ghani, K. & Deng, J.. (2017). Surgeon Technical Skill Assessment using Computer Vision based Analysis. Proceedings of the 2nd Machine Learning for Healthcare Conference, in PMLR68:88-99.

51. Hung AJ, Chen J, Che Z, et al. Utilizing Machine Learning and Automated Performance Metrics to Evaluate Robot-Assisted Radical Prostatectomy Performance and Predict Outcomes. J endourology 2018;32(5):438–44.

52. Hung AJ, Chen J, Gill IS. Automated Performance Metrics and Machine Learning Algorithms to Measure Surgeon Performance and Anticipate Clinical Outcomes in Robotic Surgery. JAMA Surg 2018; 153(8):770–1.

53. Hung AJ, Chen J, Ghodoussipour S, et al. A deep-learning model using automated performance metrics and clinical features to predict urinary continence recovery after robot-assisted radical prostatectomy. BJU Int 2019;124(3):487–95.

54. Zia A, Hung A, Essa I, Jarc A. Surgical activity recognition in robot-assisted radical prostatectomy using deep learning. InInternational Conference on Medical Image Computing and Computer-Assisted Intervention 2018 Sep 16 (pp. 273-280). Springer, Cham.

55. Zia A, Guo L, Zhou L, et al. Novel evaluation of surgical activity recognition models using task-based efficiency metrics. Int J Comput Assist Radiol Surg 2019;14(12):2155–63.

56. Chen J, Oh PJ, Cheng N, et al. Use of Automated Performance Metrics to Measure Surgeon Performance during Robotic Vesicourethral Anastomosis and Methodical Development of a Training Tutorial. J Urol 2018;200(4):895–902.

57. Chen A, Ghodoussipour S, Titus MB, et al. Comparison of clinical outcomes and automated performance metrics in robot-assisted radical prostatectomy with and without trainee involvement. World J Urol 2019;38(7):1615–21.